This book is due for return on or before the last date shown below.

SEPSIS: NEW INSIGHTS, NEW THERAPIES

Novartis Foundation Symposium 280

SEPSIS: NEW INSIGHTS, NEW THERAPIES

John Wiley & Sons, Ltd

Published in 2007 by John Wiley & Sons Ltd,
The Atrium, Southern Gate,
Chichester PO19 8SQ, UK

National   01243 779777
International (+44) 1243 779777
e-mail (for orders and customer service enquiries): cs-books©wiley.co.uk
Visit our Home Page on http://www.wileyeurope.com
or http://www.wiley.com

This publication is designed to provide accurate and authoritative information in regard to
the subject matter covered. It is sold on the understanding that the Publisher is not engaged
in rendering professional services. If professional advice or other expert assistance is
required, the services of a competent professional should be sought.

Other Wiley Editorial Offices

John Wiley & Sons Inc., 111 River Street, Hoboken, NJ 07030, USA

Jossey-Bass, 989 Market Street, San Francisco, CA 94103-1741, USA

Wiley-VCH Verlag GmbH, Boschstr. 12, D-69469 Weinheim, Germany

John Wiley & Sons Australia Ltd, 33 Park Road, Milton, Queensland 4064, Australia

John Wiley & Sons (Asia) Pte Ltd, 2 Clementi Loop #02-01, Jin Xing Distripark, Singapore
129809

John Wiley & Sons Canada Ltd, 6045 Freemont Blvd, Mississauga, Ontario, Canada L5R 4J3

Wiley also publishes its books in a variety of electronic formats. Some content that appears
in print may not be available in electronic books.

Novartis Foundation Symposium 280
x + 280 pages, 34 figures, 6 tables

Anniversary Logo Design: Richard J. Pacifico

British Library Cataloguing in Publication Data

A catalogue record for this book is available from the British Library

ISBN 978-0-470-02798-1

Typeset in 10½ on 12½ pt Garamond by SNP Best-set Typesetter Ltd., Hong Kong
Printed and bound in Great Britain by T. J. International Ltd, Padstow, Cornwall.
This book is printed on acid-free paper responsibly manufactured from sustainable forestry,
in which at least two trees are planted for each one used for paper production.

Contents

Participants

Djillali Annane Address Service de Reanimation, Hôpital Raymond Poincaré (AP-HP), Faculté de Médecine Paris Ile de France Ouest (UVSQ), 104 Boulevard Raymond Poincaré, 92380 Garches, France

Alfred Ayala Aldrich 227, Division of Surgical Research/Shock-Trauma Research Laboratories, Rhode Island Hospital / Brown University School of Medicine, 593 Eddy Street, Providence, RI 02903, USA

Jean-Marc Cavaillon UP Cytokines and Inflammation, Institut Pasteur, 28 rue Dr Roux, 75015 Paris, France

Augustine M. K. Choi Division of Pulmonary, Allergy and Critical Care Medicine, University of Pittsburgh School of Medicine, MUH628, 3459 5th Avenue, Pittsburgh, PA 15213, USA

Jon Cohen Brighton and Sussex Medical School, University of Sussex, Falmer, Brighton BN1 9PX, UK

Tom J. Evans Level 4, Glasgow, Biomedical Research Centre, University of Glasgow, 120 University Place, Glasgow G12 8TA, UK

Mitchell P. Fink *(Chair)* Department of Critical Care Medicine, University of Pittsburgh, 616 Scaife Hall, 3550 Terrace Street, Pittsburgh, PA 15261, USA

Derek Gilroy Division of Medicine, BHF Laboratories, University College London, 5 University Street, London WC1E 6JJ, UK

Richard D. Griffiths Intensive Care Research Group, Division of Metabolic & Cellular Medicine, School of Clinical Science, Faculty of Medicine, University of Liverpool, Liverpool L69 3GA, UK

Paul G. Hellewell Division of Clinical Sciences North, Northern General Hospital, University of Sheffield, Sheffield S5 7AU, UK

David N. Herndon Chief of Staff, Shriners Hospitals for Children, Director of the Blocker Burn Unit, University of Texas Medical Branch, Galveston, TX 77550, USA

Xavier Leverve LBFA-INSERM 221, Nutrition Humaine et Sécurité des Aliments, Université Joseph Fourier, Institut National de la Recherche Agronomique (INRA), 147, Rue de l'Université, Paris 75007, France

John C. Marshall Department of Surgery and the Interdepartmental Division of Critical Care Medicine, St Michael's Hospital, University of Toronto and Room 4–007, 30 Bond Wing, Toronto, Ontario M5B 1W8, Canada

Claude A. Piantadosi Division of Pulmonary and Critical Care Medicine, Duke University Medical Center, Durham, NC 27710, USA

Jérôme Pugin Division of Medical Intensive Care, University Hospital, 24, r. Micheli-du-Crest, Geneva 14, CH-1211, Switzerland

Peter Radermacher Sektion Anästhesiologische Pathophysiologie und Verfahrensentwicklung, Universitätsklinik für Anästhesiologie, Universität Ulm, Parkstrasse 11, 89073 Ulm, Germany

Anne Marie Schmidt Division of Surgical Science, Columbia University Department of Surgery, New York, NY 10032, USA

Mervyn Singer Department of Medicine and Wolfson Institute of Biomedical Research, University College London, Cruciform Building, Gower Street, London WC1E 6BT, UK

Csaba Szabó Department of Surgery, University of Medicine and Dentistry of New Jersey, 185 South Orange Avenue, University Heights, Newark, NJ 07103-2714, USA

Chris Thiemermann The Department of Experimental Medicine, Nephrology and Critical Care, William Harvey Research Institute, St Bartholomew's and The Royal London School of Medicine and Dentistry, London EC1M 6BQ, UK

Jack Tinker Royal Society of Medicine, 1 Wimpole Street, London W1G 0AE, UK

Pierre Tissières *(Novartis Foundation Bursar)* Laboratory of Intensive Care, Department of Microbiology and Molecular Medicine, University of Geneva Medical Center, CMU-1, Rue Michel Servet, 1211 Geneva 4, Switzerland

Luis Ulloa North Shore University Hospital, 350 Community Drive, Manhasset, NY 11030, USA

Greet Van den Berghe Department of Intensive Care Medicine, Catholic University of Leuven, B-3000 Leuven, Belgium

Haichao Wang Laboratory of Emergency Medicine, Feinstein Institute for Medical Research, North Shore-Long Island Jewish Health System, 350 Community Drive, New York, NY 11030, USA

Chair's introduction

Mitchell P. Fink

Department of Critical Care Medicine, University of Pittsburgh, 616 Scaife Hall, 3550 Terrace Street, Pittsburgh, PA 15261, USA

Let me try to set the stage for this symposium. We will be discussing new treatments for sepsis. In 1992 a landmark publication appeared, which attempted to create some definitions that would bring order to the field of sepsis research (American College of Chest Physicians/Society of Critical Care Medicine 1992). At this time the concept of a tiered approach to diagnosing systemic inflammation, sepsis and severe sepsis was developed. The notion was that the combination of the cardinal signs of inflammation and infection constituted sepsis. If organ dysfunction is layered on this mix, the condition is now severe sepsis, and if arterial hypotension is included in the mix, this condition is septic shock.

In 2001 another consensus conference was held that slightly modified this concept (Levy et al 2003). This meeting recognized that there are many findings that tip clinicians off to the possibility that a patient has a deleterious response to infection. The list is long and complete. To keep peace, the notion was adopted that everything should be listed and the new definition does not specify how many features are needed for a diagnosis of sepsis. This is one of the current weaknesses in our field: unlike our brethren in oncology and cardiology, we don't have a tissue diagnosis for the disease we are interested in, and we don't have a biochemical marker. So we are not all studying the same thing, and when we enrol patients in clinical trials we tend to enrol a very heterogeneous group of people, poorly characterized with respect to genotype and phenotype.

This being said, no matter how you diagnose sepsis, it is an important public health problem. Angus et al (2001) published a paper that has been cited more than 900 times. The findings in the paper were the result of a thorough epidemiological analysis of the incidence of sepsis in the USA, using data from seven states and then generalizing it to the rest of the population. This study showed that sepsis is a disease of the very young and very old, and there are about three cases per 1000 in the population. This incidence translates to about 750000 cases annually, with a mortality rate of about 30%. To put this into context, colon cancer (a common form of cancer in the USA) has an incidence of about 50 cases per 100000 people, and breast cancer has an incidence of about 110 cases per 100000 women. AIDS gets an enormous amount of research funding, and has an incidence of

1

17 cases per 100 000 people, and the incidence of congestive heart failure is about 130 cases per 100 000. Sepsis is truly a major public health problem.

In the developed world, the most costly health problems are the neurodegenerative diseases of ageing, such as Alzheimer's disease. Congestive heart failure and type 2 diabetes mellitus are also epidemics. In this same category of huge public health problems is sepsis. In the developing world the list looks very different; malnutrition heads the list. Malaria remains a huge public health problem internationally, and cerebral malaria is a cytokine-driven illness that is very reminiscent of sepsis. Diarrhoeal diseases, AIDS and schistosomiasis are also enormous worldwide public health problems. Even in the developing world, because of the importance of cerebral malaria, I think sepsis is an important public health problem.

About six years ago a number of us in the Department of Critical Care Medicine at the University of Pittsburgh wrote a proposal to the NIH. Professor Derek Angus was the principal investigator on this project. The goal was to do the largest and best large-scale observational study of human sepsis, focusing in particular on the genetic and biochemical markers associated with development and progression of the syndrome. We chose to study patients with community-acquired pneumonia, because of the diagnostic problems mentioned at the outset. Accordingly, we wanted to study as homogeneous a population as possible. We enrolled patients from 38 hospitals from four states, and the enrolment was concluded in November 2003.

We enrolled 2300 patients, and of these about 2100 were shown to have community-acquired pneumonia. Of these, the vast majority were admitted to the hospital. About 70% of these admitted patients did not have a diagnosis of severe sepsis (no evidence of organ dysfunction). Of these, only 4% died over a 60 day observation period. On the other hand, about 30% did have a diagnosis of severe sepsis, and in this group about 30% died. The difference in the shape of the mortality curves was not just apparent during the acute period, when the patients were in the hospital, but it persisted for months afterwards.

The cytokine profiles for different groups of patients are interesting. At admission, almost all the patients had high circulating concentrations of interleukin (IL)6. In general, the patients who were discharged alive normalized their circulating IL6 level. In contrast, the patients who succumbed to their illness tended to have biochemical evidence of persistent systemic inflammation. This can be shown by plotting the log circulating concentrations for IL6, IL10 and tumour necrosis factor (TNF). There are a couple of messages here: first of all, everyone with sepsis is admitted to the hospital with biochemical evidence of systemic inflammation. The peak inflammatory and counter-inflammatory response is at the time of admission. The notion that there is a delayed anti-inflammatory response that comes up 3, 5 or 7 days after admission is probably wrong. Circulating cytokine levels tend to normalize relatively quickly in patients who are destined to survive. In contrast, both pro-inflammatory and anti-inflammatory cytokine levels tend to remain elevated in patients who are destined for a bad outcome. Additionally, it is worth noting that circulating levels of TNF are not very valuable as a prognostic marker, and it is not too surprising that TNF has not proven to be a useful drug target for the development of therapeutic agents for sepsis.

The history of research in our field can be defined in three epochs. The first is the period prior to the publication of the Beutler et al (1985) paper in *Science*, which identified for the first time that TNF is a mediator of lipopolysaccharide (LPS)-induced lethality in rodents. The premodern era of sepsis research is the period before this paper. The modern era comes after this publication. Another landmark was the report of the results of the PROWESS study in 2001 (Bernard et al 2001). This report led to the approval in many countries of Xigris® as an adjuvant therapy for the management of severe sepsis. The approval of Xigris® doesn't mean that research in our field is over (Carlet 2006).

In the era before the PROWESS study was published, several clinical trials were carried out using drugs directed at a number of targets. TNF was the favourite target for a long time. Another alarm-phase cytokine, IL1β, was a target of several studies. There were numerous studies of drugs that targeted platelet activating factor (PAF), thromboxane A_2, cyclooxygenase isoforms, bradykinin, endotoxin, nitric oxide (NO) and reactive oxygen species. The results of all of these studies were negative. In February 2006, the current list of drug targets includes TLR4 (including components of a proximal TLR4 signalosome), GSK3β, Fas/FasL, caspases, histone deacetylase, HMGB1, RAGE, the α7 nicotinic receptor and reactive oxygen species. There are also some therapeutics under development that seem to work in sepsis models but no one knows why. These include ethyl pyruvate, carbon monoxide and inosine. Then there is Xigris®, which also has demonstrable efficacy in humans without a clearly delineated mechanism of action.

I think this will have teed up the subject. Sepsis is an enormous public health problem. There has been much progress over the last 20 years, but I think the real progress will be made in the next few years because our understanding of the biology has improved so much.

References

American College of Chest Physicians/Society of Critical Care Medicine Consensus Conference 1992 Definitions for sepsis and organ failure and guidelines for the use of innovative therapies in sepsis. Crit Care Med 20:864–874
Angus DC, Linde-Zwirble WT, Lidicker J, Clermont G, Carcillo J, Pinsky MR 2001 Epidemiology of severe sepsis in the United States: analysis of incidence, outcome, and associated costs of care. Crit Care Med 29:1303–1310

Bernard GR, Vincent JL, Laterre PF et al 2001 Recombinant human protein C Worldwide
    Evaluation in Severe Sepsis (PROWESS) study group. Efficacy and safety of recombinant
    human activated protein C for severe sepsis. N Engl J Med 344:699–709
Beutler B, Milsark IW, Cerami AC 1985 Passive immunization against cachectin/tumor necro-
    sis factor protects mice from lethal effect of endotoxin. Science 229:869–871
Carlet J 2006 Prescribing indications based on successful clinical trials in sepsis: a difficult
    exercise. Crit Care Med 34:525–529
Levy MM, Fink MP, Marshall JC et al 2003 2001 SCCM/ESICM/ACCP/ATS/SIS Interna-
    tional Sepsis Definitions Conference. Crit Care Med 31:1250–1256

DISCUSSION

Marshall: As someone who has contributed to the 940 citations of Derek Angus'
paper, I want to challenge the notion that sepsis is a common disease. Sepsis in
the abstract is common in the same way that cancer is common. Cancer is very
common if you include diseases such as carcinoma of the prostate, basal cell cancer
and metastatic small cell cancer. The reality is that when we have actually studied
it, the disease we think we are modelling in our animals is in fact quite rare. One
of the challenges we have is deconstructing a lot of the assumptions we have made
in the past and refocusing them on the reality. High profile victims of sepsis have
included Jim Henson and that is the disease that we would like to treat. They have
also included Pope John Paul II who had a urinary tract infection that the doctors
decided not to treat. He died of sepsis as well. We need to recognize that this
complex polyglot of diseases is not a single common process that we want to treat
in every patient.

Fink: I beg to differ. In the context of doing the GeNIMS study, where our goal
was to study patients with community-acquired pneumonia, we had no difficulty
enrolling. Busy emergency rooms, such as the one at the University of Pittsburgh,
were enrolling at the rate of three or four cases a week. This makes it a common
disease. We admit patients to the hospital with community-acquired pneumonia
during the winter at the rate of at least one per day. We admit congestive heart
failure patients at about one per day. These are diseases of comparable epidemiological significance.

Marshall: Only a third of the patients you recruited had severe sepsis.

Fink: Among the patients who were admitted, about one third had severe sepsis.
This means that we admit two to three patients per week with severe sepsis. This
number is not a trivial number.

Marshall: Look at the people who come in with community-acquired pneumonia.
My father died of sepsis but he was 86 years old and had Alzheimer's disease;
it was the appropriate end for his life. I guess the point I am trying to make is
that we have to be a bit more critical at looking at the population of patients
we want to target with aggressive, expensive, biologically complex treatments.

Probably for the majority of people this is not such a bad way to leave this planet.

Fink: My dad died of sepsis as well; he was 91 years old. To a certain extent I agree with you; some of these deaths are appropriate. How many of these in the fifth decade and beyond are inappropriate?

Cohen: One of the points John Marshall was making is this question of definition. We probably don't want to spend the whole meeting rehearsing the definition of sepsis, but we should flag this up because it is a real issue. Because what we are talking about is so vague and nebulous, we will inevitably be dealing with a heterogeneous population and the polar examples you give are bound to occur. We are coming to the end of another era, that of thinking of sepsis as a disease or diagnosis. I don't think it will be helpful to continue to do this. Should we not perhaps be reverting to a situation where we talk about severe infection complicated by organ failure. This might be pneumonia or it might be peritonitis. This is different from the syndromic approach to sepsis, which is that a slight fevered brow is suddenly sepsis.

Fink: I agree with you. As we improve our level of precision in diagnosis, the whole field will be able to move forward in leaps and bounds. Now we are setting up a disease instead of a loose collection of clinical features or a syndrome. The haematologists and oncologists used to define cancer on the basis of histology. Now they do it on the basis of genetics. They are way ahead of us. Cardiologists have a blood test that establishes the diagnosis of myocardial infarction in the emergency department. We need to move to that biochemical level, phenotyping patients on the basis of biochemistry rather than syndrome description.

Griffiths: One of the things that has always dogged me from a clinical perspective has been the timeline of severe sepsis. Mortality is still progressing, even a year after the event. This has troubled a lot of our understanding of sepsis. We need a pathological explanation for how and why people die at different time points. It may well be that we're not dealing with a single phenomenon but rather a cascade of events. This could explain why there has been disappointment with Xigris®.

Fink: This gets at John Marshall's point. Part of the reasons for those excess deaths out at three months, six months and a year is because the people who get sepsis are not healthy people to begin with. They are dying after their sepsis, but what they are really dying from is their pancreatic carcinoma, for example.

Griffiths: That is an assumption I'm not sure of. You can match people to different ages and illness and there outcomes can be quite different. We must not forget the legacy of the septic illness itself.

Fink: This is just some of it. For any of you who have followed your patients out months afterwards, there is clearly a nutritional hit that is associated with two or three weeks in an intensive care unit. It is non-trivial. Patients lose enormous amounts of lean body mass as a result of this acute illness, and they don't recover that for months. There is also a neurocognitive hit that is enormous. I don't think we understand the implications of this and its effect on survival at all: it is currently a black box.

Herndon: The prolonged response to sepsis may be one of the most poignant observations you have made. Individuals do have a cascade of events. There is a prolonged hypermetabolic response, and a prolonged catabolic response. It is not just the loss of weight that occurs during the intensive care unit stay. There is another aspect to this: people who develop sepsis may well be genetically different. There are two aspects of this shift in curve that you mentioned: first, the response or the genetic make-up of the individual as they come in, and second, the prolonged response, which we have studied little if at all. Perhaps we should focus on this prolonged response more to separate out those who may benefit from therapy.

Singer: It is interesting to hear this discussion develop. Certainly, my experience of community sepsis is that it is now relatively rare. These are ones we are waiting to recruit into studies, but we don't see many. The ones we do get are those who develop sepsis as a complication of another problem. This could be a different population, or there could be syndromes within a syndrome. Could we therefore argue that sepsis is a human-induced disease? We are admitting fewer and fewer people from the community into our intensive care units with sepsis. The sepsis patients we do see come predominantly from the ward, or they are on the unit already recovering from surgery or trauma. Perhaps we have created the monster?

Fink: This may be one difference between the way that healthcare is done in the USA and the UK. At the University of Pittsburgh Medical Center we have more than 150 ICU beds. This is roughly one-quarter of the beds in the adult Medical Surgical hospital. In the medical ICU, I suspect that the vast majority of patients with sepsis or severe sepsis have acquired this in the community.

Marshall: Mervyn Singer's point is an important one. This is one of the ways that we need to parse this entity. The reality is, if we look at severe sepsis as a construct, it is entirely iatrogenic. We are dealing with organ dysfunction that is lethal if we don't intervene. We know that many of the interventions we use can become a second hit, or something that modifies the response, such as mechanical ventilation and the cytokine response. This is one of the groups that we systematically exclude from studies. It is probably the group that we should be most keen on studying, although it is also the most difficult to describe.

Strategies to modulate cellular energetic metabolism during sepsis

Alessandro Protti and Mervyn Singer[1]

Bloomsbury Institute of Intensive Care Medicine, University College London, Gower Street, London WC1E 6BT, UK

Abstract. Growing evidence suggests that mitochondrial inhibition plays a major role in the development of multiple organ failure during sepsis. Early correction of tissue hypoxia, strict control of glycaemia and modulation of oxidative and nitrosative stress may protect mitochondria during the acute inflammatory response. Once mitochondrial dysfunction has developed, the regulated induction of a hypometabolic state, analogous to hibernation, may protect the cells from severe bioenergetic failure and a critical fall in ATP. Though this is clinically manifest as organ dysfunction, it may actually represent an adaptive response to a prolonged, severe inflammatory stress. Repair of damaged organelles, stimulation of mitochondrial biogenesis and re-activation of cellular metabolism may accelerate the recovery phase and thus improve clinical outcomes. The aim of this review is to discuss putative interventions aimed at preventing or reversing mitochondrial dysfunction that may have possible clinical relevance, and to stress the importance of the correct timing of intervention.

2007 Sepsis—new insights, new therapies. Wiley, Chichester (Novartis Foundation Symposium 280) p 7–20

Sepsis is the systemic inflammatory response to infection and represents a major cause of morbidity and mortality in patients admitted to intensive care units (Padkin et al 2003). Despite recent advances, many aspects of the pathophysiology of sepsis remain to be elucidated. Findings of reduced oxygen consumption, elevated tissue oxygen tension and the absence of significant histological changes in most of the affected organs suggest that multiple organ failure (MOF) during sepsis may be due to an acquired inability of the cells to use oxygen (Fink 2002).

Mitochondria utilize >90% of total body oxygen consumption to produce energy as adenosine triphosphate (ATP). The electron transport chain consists of enzyme complexes and carrier molecules associated to the inner membrane. The reduced nicotinamide (NADH) and flavin ($FADH_2$) adenine dinucleotides produced by the oxidation of nutrients donate electrons to complex I and complex II, respectively. The electrons then flow through complex III and complex IV

---

[1]This paper was presented at the symposium by Mervyn Singer, to whom correspondence should be addressed.

(cytochrome oxidase) transported by coenzyme Q and cytochrome C, and finally reduce oxygen to water. Electron transfer through complexes I, III and IV generates a proton gradient across the inner mitochondrial membrane that is used by a specific ATP synthase to generate ATP from ADP.

Studies on the early phase of sepsis have produced conflicting results with increases, decreases or no change in mitochondrial function all being reported (Singer & Brealey 1999). Nonetheless, mitochondrial structure and activity were consistently shown to be damaged in studies lasting more than 12–16 hours, in both a time- and a severity-dependent manner. ATP levels were variably affected, depending on the balance between energy production and consumption. A reduction in the latter, eventually leading to MOF, may represent a cellular adaptive strategy to preserve ATP levels above a threshold compatible with survival (Singer et al 2004). Restoration of mitochondrial activity may drive the recovery of these 'failed' organs, a hallmark of survival from MOF. Accordingly, the need for long-term support (e.g. renal dialysis, mechanical ventilation) in septic survivors is very uncommon in those whose organs were healthy before the septic insult. This finding suggests that organ failure in sepsis differs from organ-specific diseases (e.g. glomerulonephritis) as it predominantly represents a potentially reversible, functional problem.

Early tissue hypoxia, excess production of inflammatory mediators, and hormonal changes are all implicated in the pathogenesis of mitochondrial abnormalities during sepsis. Nitric oxide (NO) production rises significantly, mainly as a consequence of increased expression of a specific inducible synthase (iNOS) and, possibly, of a mitochondrial isoform of the enzyme. Activation of phagocytic cells accounts for most of the increased production of reactive oxygen species. However, NO-mediated inhibition of cytochrome oxidase increases electron leak from the respiratory chain and subsequent generation of superoxide (O_2^-). NO and O_2^- accumulating within the mitochondria will react together to generate peroxynitrite and other nitrogen species. These are able to alter the structure and function of several mitochondrial proteins. Changes occurring at the electron transport chain are likely to impair cellular energy production (Liaudet et al 2000).

Only a few specific therapeutic approaches are currently available for treating sepsis. The aim of this chapter is to discuss some putative interventions that could prevent or reverse mitochondrial dysfunction, or that could modulate cellular metabolic activity both during the development of sepsis and in the recovery phase.

Prevention and early reversal of mitochondrial dysfunction

If the development of MOF following sepsis or any other major insult (e.g. major trauma) is related to a cellular energetic failure, then strategies aimed at preventing the impairment of mitochondrial energy production may be potentially beneficial.

Septic mitochondrial dysfunction can occur despite adequate tissue perfusion. Nonetheless, cellular hypoxia resulting from an unresuscitated shock state will limit aerobic ATP generation and will thus contribute to the development of progressive mitochondrial damage. We have recently demonstrated that activated macrophages experience an earlier impairment of mitochondrial oxygen consumption when incubated in 1% oxygen compared to room air (Frost et al 2005). The competitive NO-mediated inhibition of cytochrome oxidase is more likely to occur at low oxygen tension; this, in turn, may accelerate the production of highly reactive species that are able to persistently impair mitochondrial respiration.

At a cellular level, optimization of oxygen delivery can ameliorate energy failure as long as mitochondria retain their ability to produce energy. Patients with severe sepsis or septic shock clinically managed to achieve an adequate balance between global oxygen supply and demand (defined as a central venous oxygen saturation, SvO_2, $\geq 70\%$) early after admission to an Emergency Department experienced significantly better survival than control patients; the faster normalization of lactate levels, arterial base deficit and pH was consistent with an improvement in aerobic cellular metabolism (Rivers et al 2001). When critically ill patients with established MOF were treated in a similar way, often after several days in intensive care, there was either no benefit (Gattinoni et al 1995) or harm (Hayes et al 1994). Thus the same intervention, performed at different time points, had a different clinical impact: in the early phase, when the cellular energetic machinery is still likely to be functional and oxygen delivery may represent a limiting factor (as suggested by a baseline SvO_2 around 49% in the Rivers' study), it may correct the impending cellular energetic failure and reduce the incidence of organ dysfunction. In a late phase, when mitochondrial inhibition and damage have eventually occurred, and the cell has become 'intrinsically' unable to produce ATP, such an approach may not provide any benefit. Lack of improvement of oxygen consumption despite a re-established oxygen supply has been associated with unfavourable outcomes in septic patients (Hayes et al 1997).

Hyperglycaemia and insulin resistance are common among critically ill patients and represent an additional potential threat to mitochondrial integrity. Even though most of the evidence comes from studies on diabetes, recently published work suggests that acute hyperglycaemia can dramatically increase the mitochondrial production of reactive oxygen species in normal bovine aortic endothelial cells (Nishikawa et al 2000). Moreover, insulin may contribute to the regulation of mitochondrial protein synthesis and oxidative phosphorylation (Stump et al 2003). Maintenance of normoglycaemia with intensive insulin therapy has been demonstrated to improve outcomes in a surgical intensive care unit population

(Van den Berghe et al 2001). The greatest reduction in mortality was seen in deaths due to sepsis-related MOF in patients requiring intensive care for more than five days. A study performed on a subgroup of non-survivors found a protective effect of intensive insulin therapy on hepatocyte mitochondrial ultrastructure and respiratory enzyme activities (Vanhorebeek et al 2005).

Oxidative and nitrosative stress occur within the mitochondria during sepsis. Reactive oxygen and nitrogen species are overproduced whereas mitochondrial antioxidants (reduced glutathione [GSH] and manganese superoxide [MnSOD]) are depleted because of increased oxidation and altered metabolism. In the presence of persistently high levels of NO and other free radicals, mitochondrial proteins may undergo (semi-)permanent modifications. Damage to the iron-sulfur centres, nitros(yl)ation of thiol groups and nitration of tyrosine residues of complex I may occur in a stepwise process, leading to a prolonged inhibition of mitochondrial respiration (Brown & Borutaite 2004).

Studies performed on cells in culture demonstrated that the membrane permeable glutathione ethyl ester can protect the functioning of complex I in an early phase, by either preventing or reversing its oxidation and nitros(yl)ation (Clementi et al 1998). Reduced concentrations of GSH and increased levels of nitrite and nitrate (products of NO metabolism) were associated with greater inhibition of complex I in skeletal muscle biopsies taken within 24 hours of admission to intensive care from patients in septic shock (Brealey et al 2002). Incubation of the tissue samples with exogenous glutathione did not ameliorate the activity of the mitochondrial enzyme, suggesting that GSH-irreversible changes, such as nitration, may have occurred by this point. Provision of glutamine, N-acetylcysteine and other precursors may stimulate glutathione synthesis and potentially enhance the mitochondrial antioxidant state.

Manganese superoxide dismutase (MnSOD) scavenges superoxide anions, preventing them from further reacting with NO to generate peroxynitrite within the mitochondria. Nitration and inactivation of the enzyme may occur in the presence of high levels of reactive nitrogen species (MacMillan-Crow et al 1996). MnSOD mimetics may exert a protective effect towards oxidative and nitrosative damage, possibly reducing mitochondrial superoxide accumulation and peroxynitrite generation (Salvemini et al 2002).

Prevention of cellular energetic failure in the presence of mitochondrial dysfunction

Once permanent mitochondrial dysfunction has developed, optimization of the residual cellular ability to produce energy, and/or a reduction in metabolic requirements, may prevent the ATP level from dropping below the threshold that stimulates cell death pathways.

Electron donors able to 'bypass' defective components of the respiratory chain may help in attaining the former objective. Within the inner mitochondrial membrane, complex II works in parallel with complex I, transferring electrons from $FADH_2$ produced during oxidation of succinate to coenzyme Q. The contribution of this pathway to oxidative phosphorylation is normally minimal, since glucose metabolism mainly leads to the synthesis of the complex I-specific electron donor, NADH. However, unlike complex I, the activity of complex II is relatively preserved during sepsis (Brealey et al 2002, 2004). Thus, when complex I is inhibited, administration of succinate may potentially increase the electron flow through the respiratory chain and the generation of ATP, provided that any inhibition of the electron transport chain distal to complex II has not become rate-limiting (Protti et al 2006). In two animal models of sepsis, infusion of succinate dimethyl ester prevented a fall in liver ATP content (Malaisse et al 1997) and prolonged survival time (Ferreira et al 2000). Compared to glucose, lipids are a better source of $FADH_2$: as with succinate, they may improve mitochondrial respiration when electron flow through complex I is impaired.

Another possible strategy to adopt once mitochondrial dysfunction is established is a controlled reduction in cellular energetic expenditure. Multi-organ failure secondary to sepsis may actually represent an adaptive hypometabolic response to preserve ATP homeostasis in the face of a prolonged inflammatory insult (Singer et al 2004). This metabolic shutdown may be triggered by a progressive and sustained reduction in energy production. Hibernating and aestivating animals depress their metabolic rate when the climate changes and food and water provision become restricted; similarly, oxygen-conforming organisms such as deep sea diving turtles tolerate hypoxia by suppressing ATP turnover (Hochachka et al 1996). Humans do not hibernate or aestivate and have only a limited tolerance to inadequate oxygenation. Nonetheless, patients with chronic coronary artery disease frequently develop myocardial contractile dysfunction—termed myocardial hibernation—that may represent an adaptive response to ischaemia. Lack of necrosis and improvement of function upon reperfusion are commonplace findings in this condition. Similarly, the majority of failing organs during sepsis retain their normal morphology (Hotchkiss et al 1999) and an ability to recover function. Activated macrophages exposed to endotoxin undergo an initial increase followed by a progressive reduction in ATP consumption. Through a mechanism resembling hibernation, they transiently manage to maintain stable ATP levels despite an inhibition of cellular respiration (Frost & Singer 2005).

The mechanisms governing hibernation remain to be clarified. Efforts have been made to identify compounds able to induce a controlled hypometabolic state in animals that do not normally hibernate. The natural peptide 'hibernation induction trigger', its synthetic analogue [D-Ala[2], D-Leu[5]] enkephalin (DADLE) and other δ-opioids might act in such a way; in animal studies, these have been shown to prolong survival time of organs for transplantation and protect cardiac and neuronal tissue against ischaemia (Su 2000). Carbon monoxide (CO) and NO may mediate the active, hibernation-like, decrease in energy demand occurring in cells lacking oxygen. CO exposure prevented the hypoxia-induced drop in ATP levels and significantly reduced death in mouse primary hepatocytes (Zuckerbraun et al 2005). Administration of NO to *Drosophila* embryos reversibly arrested development, gene expression and protein turnover, and afforded protection against cyanide poisoning. Conversely, NO scavenging reduced embryonic survival during hypoxia (Teodoro & O'Farrell 2003). Mice exposed to the complex IV inhibitor, hydrogen sulfide (H_2S) experienced a dramatic decrease in their metabolic rate and became poikilothermic (Blackstone et al 2005); after 6 hours of exposure to H_2S, oxygen consumption and CO_2 production dropped by around 90% and core body temperature approached that of the environment. Such a suspended animation-like state fully reversed when the H_2S was discontinued, without any permanent behavioural or functional damage. Rapid induction of profound cerebral hypothermia may also preserve the organism during prolonged cardio-circulatory arrest; survival without brain damage was reported in an animal study when resuscitation attempts were commenced as late as 120 minutes after exsanguination (Behringer et al 2003). Perhaps even during sepsis, we can speculate that inducing hibernation (possibly through one of the above mentioned approaches) may protect the organism from prolonged energetic failure and enable faster recovery on resolution of the inflammatory insult.

Once mitochondrial dysfunction has occurred it may be equally important to avoid inappropriately stimulating cellular metabolism. Administration of thyroid or growth hormone to critically ill patients has been reported to cause harm (Acker et al 2000, Takala et al 1999). Following an acute insult, anabolic target organ hormones are usually inactivated: energy consumption is (beneficially) reduced and redirected. Any attempt to interfere with this (adaptive) initial neuroendocrine response may need to be discouraged (Van den Berghe et al 1998), at least until we better understand when and how to modultate it. Anabolic hormonal interventions during the acute phase of sepsis may be even more inappropriate, due to the concomitant impairment in cells' capacity to produce energy.

Resolution of mitochondrial dysfunction: arousal from 'hibernation'

Sepsis is a dynamic process. Recovery from mitochondrial dysfunction is likely to depend on both the resolution of the acute inflammatory response *and* the repair or replacement of damaged organelles. Preliminary results show an association between a progressive improvement in mitochondrial respiration and organ function in survivor septic patients (Brealey et al 2003).

Mitochondrial biogenesis relies on the growth and division of pre-existing mitochondria. The overall process seems to be regulated at a transcriptional level. Peroxisome proliferator-activated receptor γ coactivator 1α (PGC1α) can stimulate mitochondrial biogenesis. It increases the expression of nuclear respiratory factors (NRFs) and mitochondrial transcription factor A (mtTFA), initiating the transcription of both nuclear and mitochondrial genes encoding for mitochondrial proteins. Replication of the mitochondrial genome is also controlled by mtTFA (Wu et al 1999).

The proximal steps of the signalling pathway regulating mitochondrial proliferation still need to be elucidated. Nitric oxide has been recently suggested to have a major role. Long-term exposure to low concentration of the gas triggered the expression of PGC1α, NRFs and mtTFA and significantly increased mitochondrial mass in different cells in culture. Similar results were obtained when 8 Br-cGMP, a membrane permeable analogue of the cyclic guanosine $3',5'$-monophosphate (cGMP) was used (Nisoli et al 2003). Once again, NO seems to exert different actions depending on the rate, amount and site of production. The high quantity synthesized by iNOS during the initial inflammatory response to sepsis will block mitochondrial respiration and can be cytotoxic. On the other hand, the smaller amounts of NO produced by the specific constitutive endothelial synthase (eNOS) may trigger mitochondrial biogenesis in a late phase. Nitration also dramatically accelerates mitochondrial protein turnover, from days to hours (Elfering et al 2004). Taken together, these results suggest that recovery from mitochondrial dysfunction may depend on a NO/cGMP-dependent signalling pathway.

Hormones may also have an equally important role. Thyroid hormones stimulate mitochondrial activity; moreover, injection of triiodothyronine (T_3) to hypothyroid rats will up-regulate PGC1α and NRF1 (Weitzel et al 2001). In contrast to the acute response, persistently low circulating levels of T_3 during the prolonged phase of critical illness may be related to neuroendocrine dysfunction (Van den Berghe et al 1998). Directed hormonal therapy given at this time, when cells have regained the ability to increase their metabolic rate, might beneficially arouse cellular (and possibly organ) activity.

Leptin is a hormone/cytokine secreted by adipose tissue. It regulates food intake and energy balance to maintain constancy of total body fat mass. Ectopic hyperleptinaemia increased expression of PGC1α in diabetic fatty rats and transformed white adipocytes into mitochondria-rich, fat-oxidizing cells. Such a response apparently depended on leptin-induced phosphorylation and activation of AMP-activated protein kinase (AMPK) (Orci et al 2004). Similarly, chronic activation of AMPK through injection of 5-aminoimidazole-4-carboxamide 1-β-D-ribofuranoside (AICAR) increased PGC1α expression and mitochondrial enzyme activities in rat skeletal muscle (Suwa et al 2003).

Oestrogen and anti-androgen administration after trauma-haemorrhage also up-regulated PGC1α and NRF2 in rat heart tissue. Relative to sham operated animals, mitochondrial enzyme activities and protein synthesis, ATP levels and cardiac function all increased in similar fashion (Hsieh et al 2005).

A further biological equivalent to sepsis-induced hibernation is bacterial dormancy. This is a reversible, low-growth state well recognized in mycobacteria; it explains the ability of these microorganisms to survive for a long time without infecting their host, yet to withstand any antibiotic onslaught. *Micrococcus luteus* can enter a similar quiescent phase and can be then aroused by an endogenous protein named 'resuscitation promoting factor' (Mukamolova et al 1998). It is pertinent to remind the reader that mitochondria descend from a bacterial endosymbiont and many similarities exist between the mitochondrial and bacterial genome. Identification and application of a similar protein able to specifically stimulate mitochondrial activity may well yield beneficial results.

Conclusions

Prevention and correction of mitochondrial dysfunction and cellular energetic failure may represent novel strategies that can improve the clinical outcomes of septic patients. Timing of intervention appears to be critical and the adaptive role of some of the major acute changes needs to be considered. The regulated induction of a hypometabolic state resembling hibernation may help the cell to face a reduced capacity to generate energy. The stimulation of mitochondrial activity and biogenesis during the late phase of sepsis may accelerate the recovery process. This increasing insight into underlying mechanisms promises to be an exciting era of novel therapeutic developments.

References

Acker CG, Singh AR, Flick RP, Bernardini J, Greenberg A, Johnson JP 2000 A trial of thyroxine in acute renal failure. Kidney Int 57:293–298

Behringer W, Safar P, Wu X et al 2003 Survival without brain damage after clinical death of 60–120 mins in dogs using suspended animation by profound hypothermia. Crit Care Med 31:1523–1531

Blackstone E, Morrison M, Roth MB 2005 H$_2$S induces a suspended animation-like state in mice. Science 308:518

Brealey D, Brand M, Hargreaves I et al 2002 Association between mitochondrial dysfunction and severity and outcome of septic shock. Lancet 360:219–223

Brealey DA, Hargreaves I, Heales S, Land J, Smolenski R, Singer M 2003 Recovery from organ failure is associated with improved mitochondrial function in septic patients. Intensive Care Med 29 (Suppl 1): S134 (abstract)

Brealey D, Karyampudi S, Jacques TS et al 2004 Mitochondrial dysfunction in a long-term rodent model of sepsis and organ failure. Am J Physiol Regul Integr Comp Physiol 286: R491–497

Brown GC, Borutaite V 2004 Inhibition of mitochondrial respiratory complex I by nitric oxide, peroxynitrite and S-nitrosothiols. Biochim Biophys Acta 165:844–849

Clementi E, Brown GC, Feelisch M, Moncada S 1998 Persistent inhibition of cell respiration by nitric oxide: crucial role of S-nitrosylation of mitochondrial complex I and protective action of glutathione. Proc Natl Acad Sci USA 95:7631–7636

Elfering SL, Haynes VL, Traaseth NJ, Ettl A, Giulivi C 2004 Aspects, mechanism, and biological relevance of mitochondrial protein nitration sustained by mitochondrial nitric oxide synthase. Am J Physiol Heart Circ Physiol 286:H22–29

Ferreira FL, Ladriere L, Vincent JL, Malaisse WJ 2000 Prolongation of survival time by infusion of succinic acid dimethyl ester in a caecal ligation and perforation model of sepsis. Horm Metab Res 32:335–336

Fink MP 2002 Cytopathic hypoxia. Is oxygen use impaired in sepsis as a result of an acquired intrinsic derangement in cellular respiration? Crit Care Clin 18:165–175

Frost MT, Singer M 2005 ATP turnover rises then falls in J774 macrophages exposed to endotoxin. Intensive Care Med 31 (Suppl 1): S150 (abstract)

Frost MT, Wang Q, Moncada S, Singer M 2005 Hypoxia accelerates nitric oxide-dependent inhibition of mitochondrial complex I in activated macrophages. Am J Physiol Regul Integr Comp Physiol 288:R394–400

Gattinoni L, Brazzi L, Pelosi P et al 1995 A trial of goal-oriented hemodynamic therapy in critically ill patients. N Engl J Med 333:1025–1032

Hayes MA, Timmins AC, Yau EH, Palazzo M, Hinds CJ, Watson D 1994 Elevation of systemic oxygen delivery in the treatment of critically ill patients. N Engl J Med 330:1717–1722

Hayes MA, Timmins AC, Yau EH, Palazzo M, Watson D, Hinds CJ 1997 Oxygen transport patterns in patients with sepsis syndrome or septic shock: influence of treatment and relationship to outcome. Crit Care Med 25:926–936

Hochachka PW, Buck LT, Doll CJ, Land SC 1996 Unifying theory of hypoxia tolerance: molecular/metabolic defense and rescue mechanisms for surviving oxygen lack. Proc Natl Acad Sci USA 93:9493–9498

Hotchkiss RS, Swanson PE, Freeman BD et al 1999 Apoptotic cell death in patients with sepsis, shock, and multiple organ dysfunction. Crit Care Med 27:1230–1251

Hsieh YC, Yang S, Choudhry MA et al 2005 PGC-1 upregulation via estrogen receptors: a common mechanism of salutary effects of estrogen and flutamide on heart function after trauma-hemorrhage. Am J Physiol Heart Circ Physiol 289:H2665–2672

Liaudet L, Soriano FG, Szabo C 2000 Biology of nitric oxide signaling. Crit Care Med 28 (4 Suppl):N37–52

MacMillan-Crow LA, Crow JP, Kerby JD, Beckman JS, Thompson JA 1996 Nitration and inactivation of manganese superoxide dismutase in chronic rejection of human renal allografts. Proc Natl Acad Sci USA 93:11853–11858

Malaisse WJ, Nadi AB, Ladriere L, Zhang TM 1997 Protective effects of succinic acid dimethyl ester infusion in experimental endotoxemia. Nutrition 13:330–341

Mukamolova GV, Kaprelyants AS, Young DI, Young M, Kell DB 1998 A bacterial cytokine. Proc Natl Acad Sci USA 95:8916–8921

Nishikawa T, Edelstein D, Du XL et al 2000 Normalizing mitochondrial superoxide production blocks three pathways of hyperglycaemic damage. Nature 404:787–790

Nisoli E, Clementi E, Paolucci C et al 2003 Mitochondrial biogenesis in mammals: the role of endogenous nitric oxide. Science 299:896–899

Orci L, Cook WS, Ravazzola M et al 2004 Rapid transformation of white adipocytes into fat-oxidizing machines. Proc Natl Acad Sci USA 101:2058–2063

Padkin A, Goldfrad C, Brady AR, Young D, Black N, Rowan K 2003 Epidemiology of severe sepsis occurring in the first 24 hrs in intensive care units in England, Wales, and Northern Ireland. Crit Care Med 31:2332–2338

Protti A, Carrè J, Frost MT et al 2006 Succinate improves mitochondrial oxygen consumption in septic rat skeletal muscle. Intensive Care Med 32 (Supl 13): 0273 (abstract)

Rivers E, Nguyen B, Havstad S et al 2001 Early goal-directed therapy in the treatment of severe sepsis and septic shock. N Engl J Med 345:1368–1377

Salvemini D, Riley DP, Cuzzocrea S 2002 SOD mimetics are coming of age. Nat Rev Drug Discov. 1:367–374

Singer M, Brealey D 1999 Mitochondrial dysfunction in sepsis. Biochem Soc Symp 66: 149–166

Singer M, De Santis V, Vitale D, Jeffcoate W 2004 Multiorgan failure is an adaptive, endocrine-mediated, metabolic response to overwhelming systemic inflammation. Lancet 364:545–548

Stump CS, Short KR, Bigelow ML, Schimke JM, Nair KS 2003 Effect of insulin on human skeletal muscle mitochondrial ATP production, protein synthesis, and mRNA transcripts. Proc Natl Acad Sci USA 100:7996–8001

Su TP 2000 Delta opioid peptide[D- Ala(2),D-Leu(5)]enkephalin promotes cell survival. J Biomed Sci 7:195–199

Suwa M, Nakano H, Kumagai S 2003 Effects of chronic AICAR treatment on fiber composition, enzyme activity, UCP3, and PGC-1 in rat muscles. J Appl Physiol 95:960–968

Takala J, Ruokonen E, Webster NR et al 1999 Increased mortality associated with growth hormone treatment in critically ill adults. N Engl J Med 341:785–792

Teodoro RO, O'Farrell PH 2003 Nitric oxide-induced suspended animation promotes survival during hypoxia. EMBO J 22:580–587

Van den Berghe G, de Zegher F, Bouillon R 1998 Clinical review 95: Acute and prolonged critical illness as different neuroendocrine paradigms. J Clin Endocrinol Metab 83:1827–1834

Van den Berghe G, Wouters P, Weekers F et al 2001 Intensive insulin therapy in the critically ill patients. N Engl J Med 345:1359–1367

Vanhorebeek I, De Vos R, Mesotten D, Wouters PJ, De Wolf-Peeters C, Van den Berghe G 2005 Protection of hepatocyte mitochondrial ultrastructure and function by strict blood glucose control with insulin in critically ill patients. Lancet 365:53–59

Weitzel JM, Radtke C, Seitz HJ 2001 Two thyroid hormone-mediated gene expression patterns in vivo identified by cDNA expression arrays in rat. Nucleic Acids Res 29:5148–5155

Wu Z, Puigserver P, Andersson U et al 1999 Mechanisms controlling mitochondrial biogenesis and respiration through the thermogenic coactivator PGC-1. Cell 98:115–112

Zuckerbraun BS, McCloskey CA, Gallo D et al 2005 Carbon monoxide prevents multiple organ injury in a model of hemorrhagic shock and resuscitation. Shock 23:527–532

DISCUSSION

Radermacher: I am fascinated by the concept that multiple organ failure is a type of hibernation. When we have patients in the intensive care unit (ICU), probably most of us will have the idea to support whatever the failing organ function is. Could you comment on the reversal of this idea, which is suspended animation? You could take up your idea and add something to switch down the system to wait until the repair of the damage has been done. This has for example been shown as an effect of CO inhalation (Nystul & Roth 2004).

Singer: There was a great paper in Science where H_2S was given to mice (Blackstone et al 2005). The authors alleged that H_2S is a specific blocker of mitochondrial complex IV. These mice essentially went into hibernation mode. Four hours later they stopped giving H_2S and the mice bounced back, with normal psychometric testing. They repeated the insult on a number of occasions and the animals were not perturbed by this. I guess the issue is whether or not animals would be better protected against a septic insult in this state.

Griffiths: The word 'hibernation' is the challenge. If I was a hedgehog and I had adapted my genetic system to hibernate over winter, my intention is to survive at the end of the day without anyone else doing anything. I can understand that there will be highly interactive mechanisms that try to preserve cell systems to prevent damage and failure. But this isn't necessarily 'hibernation'.

Singer: I am simply using the analogy. Perhaps we could be more accurate in talking about aestivation. Animals, fish or trees aestivate when there's a severe heat or drought and go into a state of torpor. We are a product of nature. Perhaps our inability to recognize this leads to problems. Look at the use of inotropes. Early use before the patient has developed established organ failure is related to outcome benefit. But once it has shut down the last thing the body needs is inotropes to push things along.

Gilroy: Animals who have learned to hibernate can recover. As humans, when our organs shut down we don't seem to be able to recover.

Singer: The cardiologists recognize this in the heart.

Gilroy: From a true hibernation state, the trick is to understand how the biochemistry kicks in to reverse the hibernation state. From this perspective we want to understand the basic biochemistry of the hibernation state.

Fink: I have got to know Mark Roth who wrote this paper on H_2S and mice (Blackstone et al 2005). We have funding on a project to identify novel approaches for extending the ability of animals to survive being subjected to massive haemorrhage for extended periods. Mark Roth is part of this program, and I have heard his story. He begins his account by saying how he got interested in this field. He read about a teenage girl from Norway who was buried in an avalanche. She spent 16 h buried under a mountain of snow. When they recovered her, she wasn't breathing, she didn't have a detectable pulse and her core temperature was in single digits. They took her to a hospital in Norway, put her on cardiopulmonary bypass, slowly warmed her and she is now fine. He read this story and decided that humans really can hibernate.

Gilroy: Hibernation as a consequence of multiple organ failure brought about by severe inflammation will be very different from a biochemical point of view.

Fink: Our notion that if energetics are such that if you aren't making ATP at a certain rate, then cellular metabolism falls apart irrevocably is wrong. In Roth's work, he took this case report and then went to *Caenorhabditis elegans*. He showed that if he made the worms hypoxic, he killed them. But if he made them anoxic they did fine. Then he poisoned them with CO to induce a hibernation state and found that he could do almost anything to them as long as they were in a gas mixture of CO or HCN or H_2S (Nystul & Roth 2004). The more noxious the stuff, the better the *C. elegans* did. They couldn't tolerate hypoxaemia, though. They either wanted to be in air or in an atmosphere of pure nitrogen; something in between wasn't good for them. It is a fascinating story.

Piantadosi: This discussion raises a very interesting idea: how do we define these concepts of homeostasis, adaptation and injury response? We have to be careful about conflating the concepts because they are unique. It isn't fair to say that when you have an injury, the response to that injury also recruits an adaptive or homeostatic mechanism, because these are different mechanisms. This is not to say that the body can't use those mechanisms in the injury state, but we can't forget what the primary injury does. Even the homeostatic or adaptive mechanisms have a chance to become deranged. Whether they will then benefit the injury state is an open question.

Evans: I appreciate Mervyn Singer's point about some aspects of septic patient responses being a quasi-hibernation state. We have all seen patients whose marrow has shut down and who have stopped producing neutrophils, and with renal failure and so on. Uniquely different is the fact that everyone who is septic, almost without exception, is extremely catabolic. This is a big difference.

Singer: Are they catabolic because of what we do to them? We keep them warm and give them inotropes. We even give them food. You could make the teleological argument that the fat patients lose body weight, because in an evolutionary environment when you have been injured by a sabre-toothed tiger then you aren't well enough to go and hunt and forage, so you consume your own body reserves.

Evans: I don't think so. Most people become febrile.

Piantadosi: If you take a malnourished person and make them septic they will more likely die. I don't think the catabolic state is particularly unexpected. It fits with the higher mortality with severe sepsis in third world countries. We need nutrition to survive a severe stress like this. We are mixing concepts of normal homeostatic mechanisms with the host response to infection.

Singer: Certainly, I don't starve my patients—I feed them. Yet they still waste away.

Piantadosi: Some do, but not all.

Van den Berghe: I'd like to comment on the adaptive response. Adaptation only makes sense in a natural environment. We only talk about adaptation for a few days, because then the time comes that your body says 'let's die'. In clinical practice, if we don't intervene the patients die. If we continue to support them we are in a different pathophysiological situation which I can't see as adaptive any more. Evolution hasn't allowed us to adapt to this situation because it occurs when we have passed our reproductive age.

Fink: One thing that Mervyn Singer says rings very true: the vast majority of what we do for these patients in the ICU is untested. When we have subjected interventions to rigorous testing we have had some surprises. The best example is the result of the ARDSNet trial (ARDSNet 2000), which showed that ventilating patients at a lower tidal volume improved their outcome, at a cost of decreasing their arterial oxygen saturation. Without those data we all would have thought that having the ventilator set up in such a way to optimise PO_2 (making it higher) would have been best. The results of this trial suggest that setting up the ventilator badly is better for the patients. We all feed patients because the data from burn and trauma patients is that if you don't feed them in the early days after a burn or trauma injury, they do badly. It is not clear that 2 weeks into an ICU experience that feeding is still good at that point. It is a question that hasn't been asked. Also, how long should we be giving antibiotics to these patients? Should the patients be kept warm or cool?

Piantadosi: I have to address these comments about feeding. From my point of view, feeding is necessary to restore cell health. There is limited mileage from autophagic metabolism and recycling; new nutrients are needed.

Singer: That is compatible with the point that Greet Van den Berghe made earlier: we'd be dead without this prolonged care. Now we are pushing beyond the bounds. But we still don't know quite how to feed. We throw feed at the patients, with a one-feed-fits-all approach, but we might do better with different feeds at different stages of the disease process.

Piantadosi: I am sure that is true. This is one of the insights that I have got from Greet's work: the use of carbon sources is different than we had expected.

Van den Berghe: You compared reports of death rates in septic patients, but it is difficult to know what people we are talking about: is this 28 day, or 90 day mortality; is it hospital or ICU mortality? These things ought to be clarified each time we mention the death rate.

Singer: What would be your ideal?

Van den Berghe: It should be clarified, so that we know what we are talking about.

Fink: Some have suggested that the right way to do this is to analyse the shape of the survival curve. Oncologists do it this way.

Ulloa: One of the problems in this field is that we still don't really understand the pathogenesis of sepsis. We try to normalize the metabolism and the inflammatory response according to normal physiological conditions. But in some cases, this strategy may interfere with some of the metabolic or immunological mechanisms of defence. This is a characteristic example in the immunological response during sepsis, where different authors appear to suggest a contradictory strategy and argue whether to increase or decrease the production of pro-inflammatory cytokines.

References

ARDSNet 2000 Ventilation with lower tidal volumes as compared with traditional tidal volumes for acute lung injury and the acute respiratory distress syndrome. The Acute Respiratory Distress Syndrome Network. N Engl J Med 342:1301–1308

Blackstone E, Morrison M, Roth MB 2005 H$_2$S induces a suspended animation-like state in mice. Science 308:518

Nystul TG, Roth MB 2004 Carbon monoxide-induced suspended animation protects against hypoxic damage in *Caenorhabditis elegans*. Proc Natl Acad Sci USA 101:9133–9136

Immunostimulation is a rational therapeutic strategy in sepsis

Jérôme Pugin

Intensive Care, University Hospital of Geneva, 1211 Geneva 14, Switzerland

Abstract. It has recently been appreciated that patients with severe sepsis and septic shock suffer from altered innate and adaptive immune responses, leading to an impaired clearance of microorganisms. This explains their difficulty to fight their primary bacterial infection and their propensity to develop superinfections. A depressed immunological surveillance in some of these patients is also responsible for a reactivation of dormant viruses, such as cytomegalovirus. Leukocyte functions are profoundly affected during sepsis. Circulating phagocytes show a marked decrease in their capacity to mount a pro-inflammatory reaction in response to microorganisms. Monocytes express low levels of major histocompatibility class II molecules. These phenotypic changes are known as 'immune paralysis'. Massive lymphocyte and dendritic cell apoptosis has also been reported in patients dying of sepsis, responsible, at least in part, for the impairment of adaptive responses. This was highlighted by the defective skin tests to common antigens documented already three decades ago in patients with sepsis. Patients with severe sepsis and septic shock may therefore benefit from treatments aimed at stimulating innate and adaptive immune responses. The aims of immune stimulation are: (1) to help bacterial killing at the primary focus of infection; (2) to prevent the development of nosocomial infections; and (3) to prevent the reactivation of dormant viruses. Therapeutic strategies based on 'boosting' immune responses with interferon γ, G-CSF, and more recently with GM-CSF have been initiated. Although results of pilot studies are encouraging, these will need to be confirmed in larger clinical studies. As a word of caution, one should not induce deleterious overwhelming inflammatory reactions, and therefore close monitoring of immune and inflammatory responses during immune stimulation therapy is necessary.

2007 Sepsis—new insights, new therapies. Wiley, Chichester (Novartis Foundation Symposium 280) p 21–36

In the 1970s and 1980s, it was believed that septic shock and sepsis-related organ dysfunction were caused by overwhelming pro-inflammatory and hyperimmune responses induced by bacterial products, such as lipopolysaccharide (LPS, endotoxin), and were mediated by circulating pro-inflammatory cytokines, such as tumour necrosis factor (TNF)α and interleukin (IL)1β. Animal studies largely supported this theory. The parenteral administration of LPS to animals and healthy human volunteers was associated with a syndrome that closely resembled that of sepsis. Moreover, the blockade of pro-inflammatory cytokines was invariably associated with a better outcome in these models. These experiments served as a basis for the development of anti-cytokine therapeutic strategies in sepsis, such as inhibitors of TNFα, IL1β and platelet-activating factor. Several large-scale multicentre randomized controlled trials failed to show a benefit from the administration of cytokine blockers (Abraham 1999). It was even demonstrated that blocking TNFα was associated with a worse outcome in some patient populations.

This led to a complete reappraisal of the 'pro-inflammatory' pathophysiological concept of sepsis. A series of animal experiments were subsequently published showing that when live bacteria instead of LPS were injected into animals, anti-cytokines were not only non-protective, they even proved to be detrimental. This was particularly verified in the case of models with true bacterial infections, such as pneumonia and peritonitis (Schultz & van der Poll 2002). These experiments indicated that the initial inflammatory response elicited by the presence of live bacteria was essential to mount a beneficial immune reaction, necessary for the clearance of the infection.

Earlier, the notion of a compartmentalized immune response arose (Meakins 1975). It was recognized that the inflammatory response was very different in organs and usually the mirror image of that measured in the circulation. During sepsis-related acute respiratory distress syndrome (ARDS), for example, whereas a net pro-inflammatory response was observed within the airspace, the circulatory compartment was at the same time profoundly anti-inflammatory (Pugin et al 1996, 1999).

Furthermore, the circulating anti-inflammatory response observed during sepsis induces an immunosuppression that starts very early after the onset of sepsis (Munford & Pugin 2001a, 2001b). There are several lines of evidence supporting the fact that patients with severe sepsis and septic shock are immunocompromised, rather than 'hyperimmune', and that boosting their immunity might actually be beneficial.

Pro- vs. anti-inflammatory response

For a long period of time only the 'pro-inflammatory' reaction to bacteria or bacterial products was appreciated and studied (Dinarello 1991). This concept was essentially based on experiments showing that LPS and other bacterial products induced a 'pro-inflammatory' response, both *in vitro* and *in vivo*. The detection of pro-inflammatory cytokines was essentially performed using ELISA techniques, detecting the total cytokine antigen. This largely oversaw the simultaneous anti-inflammatory reaction that took place in patients with sepsis, particularly in the systemic compartment. A vast excess of natural inhibitors of TNFα and IL1β circulated and was measured in the plasma from patients with sepsis (soluble receptors, receptor antagonists, IL10) (Goldie et al 1995). Bioassays indicated that these inhibitors completely blocked the activity of circulating pro-inflammatory cytokines, and that the net activity of septic plasma was 'anti-inflammatory' (Pugin et al 1996, 1999). This contrasted with a net 'pro-inflammatory' reaction measured in organs from critically ill patients with sepsis, ARDS and pancreatitis (Pugin et al 1996, 1999, Dugernier et al 2003).

This, in part, explains why the parenteral administration of cytokine inhibitors failed in the treatment of patients with severe sepsis and septic shock (Abraham 1999). Adding high doses of recombinant soluble TNF receptors or the IL1 receptor antagonist to the plasma compartment of patients having already extremely high circulating levels of the natural antagonists was certainly not helpful. The potential beneficial effect of targeting these inhibitors directly to organs, such as the lung where an excess of bioactive pro-inflammatory cytokines could be demonstrated, was never tested in patients. The use of 'non-specific' anti-inflammatory agents (high doses of glucocorticoids, non-steroidal anti-inflammatory drugs) did not show any benefit in patients with sepsis either.

It is also important to realize that the initial pro-inflammatory response at the site of a bacterial infection is essential for the clearance of the infection. Cytokine inhibitors were protective in numerous animal studies when a sepsis syndrome was induced with purified bacterial products such as LPS. The opposite effect was observed in infectious models. Blocking TNFα or IL1β results in a worst outcome when the animal suffers from pneumonia or peritonitis. The same phenomenon has been reported in TNFα and IL1β knockout mice. It remains however to be determined whether cytokine inhibitors may be beneficial in infectious models of sepsis treated with antibiotics.

Immune suppression during sepsis

Nowadays, patients with severe sepsis and septic shock survive longer with improved support therapy, while they enter into a new phase of the disease evolution. They most frequently die from multiple organ dysfunction. Many patients fail to correctly clear the primary bacterial infection, or acquire secondary, nosocomial infections perpetrating the sepsis syndrome. Interestingly, the majority of secondary infections are due to commensals, which become pathogenic in a fragile, immunocompromised host. Accumulating evidence indicates that superinfection as well as the failure to clear the primary bacterial infection is related to an acquired immunosuppressed state. When looked at carefully, a significant number of septic patients reactivate dormant viral infections, such as cytomegalovirus (Kutza et al 1998). This also demonstrates an acquired failure of the immune system to keep those viruses in check.

The adaptive immunity is profoundly perturbed in patients with sepsis, as demonstrated as long as three decades ago by a decreased delayed-type hypersensitivity (DTH) and cutaneous anergy to common antigens. Lymphoid organs from patients dying of sepsis show a marked decrease in lymphocyte and dendritic cell concentrations, principally due to a sepsis-related programmed cell death (Hotchkiss et al 1999, Hotchkiss & Karl 2003). Circulating monocytes, the precursors of antigen-presenting cells, show a marked decrease in the surface expression of major histocompatibility complex (MHC) proteins, such as HLA-DR. This phenomenon is in part due to the effect of the anti-inflammatory molecule IL10 inducing the intracellular sequestration of MHC proteins (Fumeaux & Pugin 2002). A correlation has recently been identified between the level of the monocyte HLA-DR expression and the outcome (Monneret et al 2006).

As indicated above, the production of pro-inflammatory cytokines such as TNFα and IL1β seems to be essential to mount an initial and beneficial inflammatory and innate immune response. Phagocytes from patients with sepsis are also deficient in the production of TNFα and IL1β, when stimulated with bacteria or bacterial products. This phenomenon, together with a low expression of HLA-DR in monocytes is known as 'immune paralysis' (Volk et al 2000). It has been proposed that either low HLA-DR expression or TNF production in whole blood could serve as markers for the competence of the innate immunity in septic patients, and to use these tests for immunomonitoring to guide future immunotherapies (Payen et al 2000, Fumeaux et al 2004).

Recently, Cavaillon et al (2005) have revisited the concept of 'immune paralysis' in sepsis. They have proposed use of the term 'leukocyte reprogramming', instead. Indeed, although a low capacity of TNFα and IL1β production is evident in septic leukocytes, the secretion of other growth factors does not seem to be affected (G-CSF and GM-CSFs). The production of the anti-inflammatory cytokine IL10 has even been found to be elevated in leukocytes from patients with sepsis stimulated with LPS.

The physiological reasons for a systemic immunosuppressive response to severe infections are not entirely clear (Munford & Pugin 2001a, 2001b). One possible explanation is that this response avoids the circulation of potentially deleterious bioactive pro-inflammatory molecules in the vascular compartment. Active pro-inflammatory cytokines produced in this compartment would certainly induce leukocyte hyperactivity, non-specific adherence to the endothelium, capillary sludging and intravascular coagulation. The circulating anti-inflammatory milieu allows leukocyte adhesion to be concentrated at the site of an infection, where chemokine gradients exist and the transmigration of phagocytes is required. We believe that when this immune suppression is too important, or localized at sites where commensals or pathogens are present, it becomes deleterious, allowing the infection to develop (Munford & Pugin 2001a, 2001b).

Rationale for immune stimulation

Both arms of the immune system (innate and adaptive) are markedly altered in patients with sepsis. This is likely to participate in the propensity of our patients to develop superinfection and in their failure to adequately clear their primary infection. It seems therefore reasonable to develop therapeutic strategies aimed at boosting immunity, i.e. to restore a capacity to present antigens and a beneficial pro-inflammatory response.

In their seminal study, Döcke et al proposed the use of interferon (IFN)γ in patients with sepsis (Döcke et al 1997). They succeeded in reversing the immune paralysis both *in vitro* and *in vivo*, monitoring monocyte expression of HLA-DR and LPS-induced TNFα production in whole blood. The patients treated with IFNγ tended to have a better outcome, although the study was not powered to show an effect on mortality (Döcke et al 1997). Interestingly, IFNγ used as a prophylactic therapy failed to influence the outcome of trauma and burn patients.

Growth factors such as G-CSF and GM-CSF boost several anti-bacterial functions of phagocytes, and are of potential interest to reverse the immune dysfunction of patients with sepsis. While G-CSF has not been properly tested in sepsis clinical trials, GM-CSF has shown preliminary but encouraging results (Rosenbloom et al 2005, Nierhaus et al 2003). Like IFNγ, GM-CSF was capable of reversing the immune paralysis, and increasing phagocytic activity. In addition, GM-CSF accelerated the resolution of the clinical and microbiological resolution of the bacterial infection in patients with sepsis (Rosenbloom et al 2005). Currently, a large-scale NIH-sponsored trial is testing the hypothesis that GM-CSF may be beneficial in patients with severe sepsis.

IFNγ and, to a lesser extent, GM-CSF, induce a large number of genes and cause significant side effects, such as fever and a flu-like syndrome, which may limit their future use as therapeutic agents in this indication. The identification of a causative deactivating factor, such as IL10, opens new strategies with IL10 antagonists. The timing of the administration of immune-boosting therapies remains unclear. However, severe immune dysfunction has been measured very early after the onset of sepsis. It would be reasonable to propose initiating such therapies after the shock period has been controlled, i.e. 2–3 days after intensive care unit (ICU) admission, in most of the cases. Effects of the drugs would need to be monitored using appropriate immmunomonitoring tools (Payen et al 2000, Fumeaux et al 2004).

An efficient primary immune response is, at least in part, dependent on soluble mediators such as natural antibodies to bacterial molecules. High levels of natural anti-LPS IgM antibodies have for example shown to be protective in human sepsis (Goldie et al 1995). The potential benefit of passive immunotherapy in patients with severe infections might be revisited, particularly polyclonal immunoglobulin preparations containing high IgM titres (Lissner et al 1999, Rodriguez et al 2005). Along the same lines, and since septic patients survive longer in the ICU, vaccines with conserved surface bacterial antigens coupled with adequate adjuvants may also help innate immune responses and prove to be beneficial in the future.

In conclusion, patients with severe sepsis suffer from a profound dysfunction of both the innate and adaptive arms of immunity. This is a major reason why these patients develop superinfections with commensals, which will eventually lead to persistent organ dysfunction and death. In this context it is reasonable to test the hypothesis that boosting immunity using IFNγ, GM-CSF, anti-IL10, IgM-enriched immunoglobulins, or antibacterial vaccines might prove to be beneficial in patients with severe sepsis and septic shock.

References

Abraham E 1999 Why immunomodulatory therapies have not worked in sepsis. Intensive Care Med 25:556–566

Cavaillon JM, Adrie C, Fitting C Adib-Conquy M 2005 Reprogramming of circulatory cells in sepsis and SIRS. J Endotox Res 11:311–320

Dinarello CA 1991 The proinflammatory cytokines interleukin-1 and tumor necrosis factor and treatment of the septic shock syndrome. J Infect Dis 163:1177–1184

Docke WD, Randow F, Syrbe U et al 1997 Monocyte deactivation in septic patients: restoration by IFN-gamma treatment. Nat Med 3:678–681

Dugernier TL, Laterre PF, Wittebole X et al 2003 Compartmentalization of the inflammatory response during acute pancreatitis: correlation with local and systemic complications. Am J Respir Crit Care Med 168:148–157

Fumeaux T, Pugin J 2002 Role of interleukin-10 in the intracellular sequestration of human leukocyte antigen-DR in monocytes during septic shock. Am J Respir Crit Care Med 166: 1475–1482

Fumeaux T, Dufour J, Stern S, Pugin J 2004 Immune monitoring of patients with septic shock by measurement of intraleukocyte cytokines. Intensive Care Med 30:2028–2037

Goldie AS, Fearon KC, Ross JA et al 1995 Natural cytokine antagonists and endogenous antiendotoxin core antibodies in sepsis syndrome. The Sepsis Intervention Group. JAMA 274:172–177

Hotchkiss RS, Karl IE 2003 The pathophysiology and treatment of sepsis. N Engl J Med 348:138–150

Hotchkiss RS, Swanson PE, Freeman BD et al 1999 Apoptotic cell death in patients with sepsis, shock, and multiple organ dysfunction. Crit Care Med 27:1230–1251

Kutza AS, Muhl E, Hackstein H, Kirchner H, Bein G 1998 High incidence of active cytomegalovirus infection among septic patients. Clin Infect Dis 26:1076–1082

Lissner R, Struff WG, Autenrieth IB, Woodcock BG, Karch H 1999 Efficacy and potential clinical applications of Pentaglobin, an IgM-enriched immunoglobulin concentrate suitable for intravenous infusion. Eur J Surg Suppl 17–25

Meakins JL 1975 Host defence mechanisms: evaluation and roles of acquired defects and immunotherapy. Can J Surg 18:259–268

Monneret G, Lepape A, Voirin N et al 2006 Persisting low monocyte human leukocyte antigen-DR expression predicts mortality in septic shock. Intensive Care Med 32:1175–1183

Munford RS, Pugin J 2001a Normal responses to injury prevent systemic inflammation and can be immunosuppressive. Am J Respir Crit Care Med 163:316–321

Munford RS, Pugin J 2001b The crucial role of systemic responses in the innate (non-adaptive) host defense. J Endotox Res 7:327–332

Nierhaus A, Montag B, Timmler N et al 2003 Reversal of immunoparalysis by recombinant human granulocyte-macrophage colony-stimulating factor in patients with severe sepsis. Intensive care Med 29:646–651

Payen D, Faivre V, Lukaszewicz AC, Losser MR 2000 Assessment of immunological status in the critically ill. Minerva Anesthesiol 66:351–357

Pugin J, Ricou B, Steinberg KP, Suter PM, Martin TR 1996 Proinflammatory activity in bronchoalveolar lavage fluids from patients with ARDS, a prominent role for interleukin-1. Am J Respir Crit Care Med 153:1850–1856

Pugin J, Verghese G, Widmer MC, Matthay MA 1999 The alveolar space is the site of intense inflammatory and profibrotic reactions in the early phase of acute respiratory distress syndrome. Crit Care Med 27:304–312

Rodriguez A, Rello J, Neira J et al 2005 Effects of high-dose of intravenous immunoglobulin and antibiotics on survival for severe sepsis undergoing surgery. Shock 23:298–304

Rosenbloom AJ, Linden PK, Dorrance A, Penkosky N, Cohen-Melamed MH, Pinsky MR 2005 Effect of granulocyte-monocyte colony-stimulating factor therapy on leukocyte function and clearance of serious infection in nonneutropenic patients. Chest 127:2139–2150

Schultz MJ, van der Poll T 2002 Animal and human models for sepsis. Ann Med 34:573–581

Volk HD, Reinke P, Docke WD 2000 Clinical aspects: from systemic inflammation to 'immunoparalysis'. Chem Immunol 74:162–177

DISCUSSION

Ayala: I want to ask you the question that everyone asks me. What would you see as the ideal way of monitoring immune status? If systemic circulation doesn't always carry the best markers and you want a local perspective, how would you get that?

Pugin: I don't think we are well equipped with a good marker. I would like a marker so I can make sure I am doing something that is good for treating the infection. We have some data showing that the way daily procalcitonin measurements decrease tell us a lot about how the patient is doing in terms of clearing the primary infection. The immunity question is more difficult. The two assays that have been used in the immunomodulatory studies are HLA-DR expression and the capacity of whole blood to respond to a lipopolysaccharide (LPS) challenge (TNFα). Michael Pinsky and his colleagues have proposed another marker: the expression of CD11b on neutrophils. CD11b still needs to be tested as a useful immunomonitoring tool.

Fink: Let me take a sceptic's stance, even though in reality I'm not. A famous US surgeon, Dr Hiram Polk, organized a series of trials with IFNγ in trauma and burn patients. These were big multicentric studies and the results were negative;

if anything there was a trend towards a deleterious effect. Dr Steve Nelson organized a series of trials with G-CSF and there was no evidence at all of a signal in favour of efficacy. Two potent immunostimulating agents, evaluated in the crucible of multicentre trials, didn't work. The only things that have seemed to work are hydrocortisone, insulin and APC. These are all anti-inflammatory agents. So the sceptical view is that pro-inflammatory factors don't work, but anti-inflammatory things do, so what are you trying to sell us here?

Pugin: If we think of IFNγ and GM-CSF, they are doing a lot of things apart from restoring immunity. This is one of the problems: they are basically bombs that are being given to the patients. Perhaps we need to find a drug that is doing only the work that we want it to do, which is restoring immunity. Blocking deleterious molecules, such as IL10, might be another way to go. We could be more 'surgical' in terms of the way we attack the problem.

Cavaillon: I would like to challenge the concept of compartmentalization. I strongly support this concept, but I admit that there are some examples suggesting that it is not that simple. One is the work of Standiford and colleagues (Reddy et al 2001), studying the macrophages from alveolar lavages of mice that had peritonitis: they showed that those cells were deactivated, explaining the sensitivity of the mice to lung infection. This is an example for the lung compartment. The other examples are from the blood compartment. Your own work showing high levels of soluble MD2 in plasma of septic patients (Pugin et al 2004) demonstrates that the blood is carrying a molecule that can not only down-regulate the inflammatory process (Munford & Pugin 2001), but also allow cell activation within tissues in response to LPS. There is also our observation in sepsis: the immune depression for leukocytes has been mainly addressed with endotoxin, but when we studied cellular reactivity with whole heat-killed bacteria, the cells responded normally and produced a normal amount of TNF (Adib-Conquy et al 2006). I like the concept, because it is a dichotomy, but the reality is more complex: the blood compartment is not always associated with a dampened reactivity of circulating cells, and tissue compartments are not always associated with an on-going inflammatory process and the presence of activated cells.

Pugin: I agree. In the lung (which is an easy compartment to study and sample from) there are probably two things going on. There is depressed immunity, but there is also excess inflammation. This could be deleterious for the lung tissue. I think this is what is going on. Clearly, the alveolar macrophages are less responsive and do not express many molecules that would eventually present antigens. The MD2 story is very interesting. Here you have a molecule that is a soluble protein circulating in the body which will increase during sepsis, just like an acute phase reactant. When it is in the circulation it behaves as a sink for LPS. When it goes out of the circulation together with soluble CD14, then it can reconstruct, together with TLR4, a potent LPS receptor and fire up the epithelial compartment. There are other examples of proteins which have dual functions as an anti-inflammatory within one compartment and a proinflammatory in another compartment.

Marshall: The concept you raised of time dependence (which is really the stage dependence) of the process is an important one. It certainly works in cancer, where treatments depend on the stage. One of the lessons here is that treatments depend on the stage of the septic process. But I want to challenge two pieces of nihilism that I have heard so far this morning. First, the idea that we don't have a 'troponin' for sepsis. I think we do have some quite promising candidates to be useful bio-markers. The reality is that we just don't use them. The other thing I want to challenge is Mitch's comment about the fact that we know that some things work and some things don't. This is dangerous ground. It is a crude categorization to say, for example, that insulin doesn't work in medical patients in the ICU for less than 3 days. The other side is that TNF does work very well: the literature for TNF in rheumatoid arthritis shows that if you have the −308 polymorphism you do better. We haven't stratified patients this way. It is tempting to see it all as a big homogeneous process, but we do have to parse it out to understand where there is activity and where there is a lack of activity.

Ayala: I find it hard to view sepsis solely as a response to a pro-inflammatory aspect. Insulin or any of the drugs (e.g. steroids or activated protein C) that were described (to have shown clinical efficacy) have multiple effects. The mechanism that underpins them does not necessarily relate to an ability to alter the proinflam-matory response. If it was just proinflammation that's affected, then it is a drug that fights rheumatoid arthritis like anti-TNF (Enebrel© or Remicade©) and fits with why we can mirror it with LPS challenge: those are clear aspects of pro-inflammation. Those drugs work in those scenarios. However, this is why I think these same drugs don't work in sepsis and multiple organ failure.

Radermacher: While I like the nice up and down time-course concept that you outlined, I would like to pick up Mervyn Singer's idea and play the devil's advocate: how much of the anti-inflammatory state of the immune paralysis is physician-made? We administer sedatives, catecholamines, insulin and other drugs, which are supposed to have anti-inflammatory effects. I'd like to challenge your concept in the sense that it is not the natural time-course, but what we add upon this time course.

Pugin: I agree with you. I didn't say that IL10, for example, is doing all the work. We have also published that β agonists will decrease cell responsiveness. We discussed the signalling behind this. But at some point, when you are a patient you also want to have pressure perfusion for the organs. I don't know what to do about this.

Radermacher: It's not that I ignore the concept—of course, I would also like to have some perfusion pressure—it is a question of whether we do the right things when we manipulate the perfusion pressure using a compound X or Y, or we sedate the patient and suppress the neuroendocrine coupling. I can't answer this. But what I am getting at is whether we are talking about a natural disease, or a mix of something which is a disease plus our intervention on top of this.

Evans: I think we are in danger of being too negative about anti-inflammatory therapies. Certainly, there is the risk of reactivation of infection. This is seen in the animal models where anti-infective antibiotics aren't used. But most patients are pretty effectively sterilized by antibiotics and their blood is cleared of micro-organisms. In animal models which have been treated with anti-infectives, anti-inflammatory approaches work well in live models of sepsis. If we look at the slope of survival curves, most of the excess mortality of sepsis is in this first period. Sure, there is a tail that goes out, but the hit is the inflammatory response in that first period.

Pugin: I agree. That is probably why there is still a window of opportunity for molecules that block interactions between bacterial molecules and receptors, or are just downstream of these receptors.

Cavaillon: It is not only the doctors who are causing the immune depression. We have investigated patients who have been resuscitated after cardiac arrest (RCA) (Adrie et al 2002). We studied them at admission in the ICU, three hours after the cardiac arrest; the reactivity of their circulating leukocytes to LPS was already very low. It is clearly a natural response to a stressful event. I would like to challenge one other point: you presented a two-way curve. This is a very popular one. However, the up part and down part of the curve are more or less concomitant. In RCA patients we measured IL10 at admission. IL10 was already a marker of severity and of outcome. Thus, the anti-inflammatory response is occurring very rapidly, and almost concomitantly with the pro-inflammatory part. I have another point to make about the balance between the pro- and anti-inflammatory mediators in the bloodstream. You showed the bioactivity of TNF. We should not forget that the very first demonstration of TNF by Waage et al (1987) in patients with meningococcal infection was obtained measuring bioactivity; thus, TNF was discovered as present in the bloodstream because it was a bioactive molecule. In a lethal endotoxin model in rabbits, we studied the effect of endotoxin absorption (Tetta et al 2000). The rabbits were protected by the treatment but TNF bioactivity in their plasma was unchanged as compared to animals that died in the absence of treatment. Thus, there is no clear relationship between the level of TNF, its bioactivity and survival.

Gilroy: When you dissect experimental models of defined innate immune responses, or something far more complex like sepsis which is an experimental nightmare, there are pro and anti-inflammatory signals which coexist at the very early phase. But the progression and resolution phase has predominantly pro-resolution/immunosuppression factors. IL10, for example, is up within an hour or two in most experimental models, but it is never present during resolution until you introduce a bacterial infection. The system has some sort of innate ability to respond even during resolution. I am not at all surprised when you say that there are pro and anti inflammatory factors occurring at the same time. It is almost a regression to normal physiological processes rather than active anti-inflammation that we want to be aiming towards in sepsis.

Fink: I completely agree with John; I was being deliberately argumentative, setting up a dichotomy that doesn't exist. My own experience with some of these therapeutics is exactly that way. I know we have to be distrustful of experiments with $n = 1$, yet that is how penicillin was discovered. Penicillin has never been subjected to a randomized clinical trial, nor will it be, because this would be unethical. When we do these randomized trials of sepsis patients, we are observing population phenomena, and there are subsets of patients who are getting benefit, and there are those who we are hurting. When we aggregate the data over a large number of patients, we see perhaps a little trend towards benefit or a little trend towards harm. I agree with you: the problem is that we haven't figured out how to identify the right patients in prospective studies. This dichotomy of inflammation/anti-inflammation is a dichotomy that humans are imposing on nature. I don't think the immune system thinks of things in this way at all. It's a lot more complicated than that.

Choi: Picking up on what you have just said, the problem with a therapy targeting sepsis is that the same molecule could have opposing functions. We know that NF-κB is a pro-inflammatory mediator, but there is now evidence showing that depending on the kinetics it can be anti-inflammatory. If you target this with a drug, the chance of it working is probably zero. Another classic story is iNOS: it is not about kinetics, but compartmentalization. In the lung it is pro-inflammatory, in the liver it is cytoprotective. If you target iNOS with a drug, because of its differential function the drug might not work. You can pick your molecular targets, but they can have opposing functions.

Wang: Which is worse? The over-activation of immune cells in the tissue, versus immunosuppression in the circulation? In other words, is the cytokine activity differentially regulated in the tissue versus the circulation?

Pugin: I think the two coexist. There are cells that are circulating which will eventually be recruited in the tissues which might have an immunosuppression phenotype. At the same time within the organs there might be a pro-inflammatory reaction that might be deleterious.

Griffiths: Many of these signals have a U-shaped relationship. When we don't have them we have a worse outcome than when we have them, but if we have too much of them we do badly, too. We live in a system where we need to have these signals, so we are always being exposed to stimuli to keep them. The trouble with our therapies is that we don't know where on this curve we are shifting: are we shifting it into the beneficial area, or too far one way or another?

Fink: It is even more complicated than that: it is not just a signal, it's a signal transduction chain. There may be up-regulation of a ligand and down-regulation of a receptor, and up-regulation of the signal transduction stuff that is downstream of the receptor. The final read out of all this will be multivariate algebra at a level we are not capable of doing right now. The cells aren't just responding to TNF at a moment in time; they are responding to TNF and a host of other cytokines, some of which have synergistic effects and some of which have counter-regulatory effects.

Choi: You mention the complex signalling transduction pathways. But the bottom line is that if it goes back to homeostasis the cell survives, and if it doesn't the cell doesn't. Although it is complex, the homeostatic drive is there, whether it is through cytoprotective factors such as heat shock protein or something else.

Ayala: I like this idea, but tissues are like signals, and there is complexity of the different characters involved. There are cases in regeneration where you will ask a cell to die because it is a better choice. You use the same system that in an injury situation might be triggered as pathology. This is like the question with systemic cytokines: even the cytokines we see systemically are often a reflection of some tissue that is more injury. The liver is an example of a source of a lot of cytokines, but not all of them. Then we look at blood monocytes which really aren't very good producers of cytokines as models for what happened in the liver.

Cavaillon: There is an interesting literature on eye inflammation after the injection of LPS. When researchers look at the eye and ocular inflammation, all that has been described for pro- and anti-inflammatory agents is reversed. TNF is an anti-inflammatory cytokine for inflammation in the eye, and IL10 is pro-inflammatory. The concept depends on the compartments, and probably many other parameters. Let me give an example: we have incubated whole blood samples with IL10, and then we prepared the monocytes and triggered them with LPS (Petit-Bertron et al 2005). The monocytes derived from the blood incubated with IL10 were producing more TNF than the cells derived from the blood samples without IL10. Indeed, it appeared that adherence is a parameter that completely modifies the behaviour of the cells. If we worked with monocytes adhering to plastic or with monocytes maintained on teflon (preventing adhesion), IL10 did not behave the same way.

Fink: You don't need to go to the eye literature to find this. In our own literature, Peter Ward treated septic mice with antibody to IL6 (Riedemann et al 2005). If he gave a lot he killed them, but if he gave just the right amount they survived better, and if he didn't give enough it didn't work. It's like Goldilocks and the three bears. There was a very small range of therapeutic benefit for this one antibody against one target. If this is the case in the clinic, but the dose–response curve is different for every patient in the ICU, this is a pessimistic situation to be working in.

Pugin: To add to this complexity, hydrocortisone has been shown to restore immune function when given at low doses, so it cannot be considered only as an anti-inflammatory agent. I am not sure about IL6: it is always labelled as pro-inflammatory, but it isn't. It increases antibody production and the acute phase response.

Fink: If you want to become hopelessly confused read the IL6 literature!

Marshall: If you don't treat diabetic ketoacidosis with insulin, the patient will die, but if you give too much, he or she might also die. This is simply the kinetics of an endocrine response.

Gilroy: I have a question about the HLA-DR expression and general adaptive immune status of patients that you described getting sepsis. You said that they are suppressed for a long time after they become septic. Is that a consequence of receiving a high dose of LPS, or is this a subpopulation with substandard adaptive immune capabilities?

Pugin: Our first thought when we did that study and looked at survivors was that it would come back up very quickly, suggesting that it was an acquired deficiency. Infection would lower the HLA-DR expression. Perhaps septic patients are selected for low expressors. No one knows this because we can't study people before sepsis.

Cohen: We all agree it is very complicated. I can understand why you might want to treat someone who has an excessive pro-inflammatory response, because inflammation is bad and it injures tissues. And I can understand why you would want to reverse an inappropriate immunosuppression, because of the problems of secondary infection. But that aside, in what way would reversing an inappropriate immunosuppression actually cure sepsis? Immune status should be normal, but even taking into account the apoptosis, I am not sure why it makes sense to reverse immunosuppression in terms of curing the sepsis episode.

Pugin: We don't have clear evidence that these patients who don't do well, don't clear their primary infection well. But this is the general feeling. Perhaps by boosting the immunity in that time frame would help these patients clear their primary infection.

Cohen: If you have empyema, the best way to treat it is insert a chest drain and get the pus out.

Pugin: If it is pneumonia you can't put a chest tube in.

Cohen: Antibiotics kill germs. I am not sure that these subtle modifications of immune status are beneficial. If they are, it is because of the failure to resolve the primary infection.

Singer: The timing issue is important. Many people die because of the secondary hit, and perhaps due to therapeutic fatigue. It also strikes me that perhaps we are lumping sepsis into a one-size-fits-all condition. We see the meningococcal or toxic shock patient who can be dead within a few hours, and they are very different from your 'average' sepsis patient who has developed the problem over a couple of days. Perhaps we should decompartmentalize the problem as well as the immunity.

Marshall: The other question is, are we missing another diagnosis? Suppose there is a problem with clearing infection: are we missing viral infections occurring in a compromised host? Is it possible that there is prolonged survival of an intracellular pathogen?

Fink: I'll introduce an additional complexity that we haven't raised. This is the concept that John Alverdy at the University of Chicago has been pushing for the last three or four years (Wu et al 2005). The bacteria and host are not living on two islands, but talk to each other. In response to you being sick, the bacteria in your GI tract and lungs change their phenotype, becoming nastier. It is as if they sense that you are weak, then this is the time to pounce. In your gut at least, in response to catecholamines or other factors, *Pseudomonas aeruginosa* increases its expression of virulence proteins.

Pugin: There is also the concept that molecules from the host can impact on the way that bacteria grow.

Fink: G-CSF is one of those molecules (Held et al 1998).

Hellewell: I have a comment about low-grade infection and the role of endogenous cells. We did some studies in mice, where we gave them a low-grade infection with streptococcal pneumonia. This didn't induce a neutrophilic response into the airways as soon as the bacteria instilled into the lungs. If we depleted alveolar macrophages, then that low dose of bacteria induced a florid neutrophil influx and the animals got very sick. The implication is that these endogenous macrophages are providing some sort of protective mechanism to the low-grade infection.

Griffiths: With the PCR diagnostic methods coming on stream, aren't we starting to recognize a lot more fungal infection in the bloodstream?

Cohen: The PCR diagnostics for fungi aren't terribly good, and aren't being used systematically in a way that would allow us to answer that question.

Griffiths: I raise this because the studies of prophylactic use of antifungal therapy are highlighting that perhaps we underestimate the impact of fungal infections and is one area where there may be some chance of improved clinical outcome.

Cohen: Rather than fungal infections, I think herpes virus infections is quite an interesting area here. There are published data about unappreciated reactivation of herpes virus infections in ICU patients (e.g. Razonable et al 2002, Bruynseels et al 2003). Indeed, we can demonstrate that there are some clinical outcomes associated with those reactivations.

Evans: It is important to make a distinction between classic infections of yesteryear and infections that evolve as patients are on ICUs. We are now confronted by organisms that thrive on plastic devices and which are multi-antibiotic resistant. Fungi are very much emerging pathogens in this group.

Griffiths: The argument can be turned round. How much are the immune features that we are seeing causal or a consequence of this process?

Fink: Do you think the FDA in the USA is ready to register a drug with the indication being PCT-aemia?

Marshall: I couldn't speak for the FDA, but it is an interesting idea. We use insulin based on a glucose level, not on the basis of polyuria and weight loss, which is how diabetes was originally defined clinically. It's an important next step in the progression to change sepsis from a physiological diagnosis to a biochemical one.

Cohen: Right at the beginning, you made a comment about how it didn't seem logical for there to be an inflammatory response in the circulation. The acute phase response, which we all recognize as being absolutely fundamental, is there for a reason. If you induce an acute phase response and challenge with bacteria, then all survive.

Pugin: We don't know what those proteins are doing in terms of helping infection. But it is certainly protective.

References

Adib-Conquy M, Adrie C, Fitting C, Gattolliat O, Beyaert R, Cavaillon JM 2006 Up-regulation of MyD88s and SIGIRR, molecules inhibiting Toll-like receptor signaling, in monocytes from septic patients. Crit Care Med 34:2377–2385

Adrie C, Adib-Conquy M, Laurent I et al 2002 Successful cardiopulmonary resuscitation after cardiac arrest as a 'sepsis-like' syndrome. Circulation 106:562–568

Bruynseels P, Jorens PG, Demey HE et al 2003 Herpes simplex virus in the respiratory tract of critical care patients: a prospective study. Lancet 362:1536–1541

Held TK, Mielke ME, Chedid M, Unger M, Trautmann M, Huhn D, Cross AS 1998 Granulocyte colony-stimulating factor worsens the outcome of experimental Klebsiella pneumoniae pneumonia through direct interaction with the bacteria Blood 91:2525–2535

Munford RS, Pugin J 2001 Normal responses to injury prevent systemic inflammation and can be immunosuppressive. Am J Respir Crit Care Med 163:316–321

Petit-Bertron AF, Pedron T, Gross U, Coppee JY, Sansonetti PJ, Cavaillon JM, Adib-Conquy M 2005 Adherence modifies the regulation of gene expression induced by interleukin-10. Cytokine 29:1–12

Pugin J, Stern-Voeffray S, Daubeuf B, Matthay MA, Elson G, Dunn-Siegrist I 2004 Soluble MD-2 activity in plasma from patients with severe sepsis and septic shock. Blood 104: 4071–4079

Razonable RR, Fanning C, Brown RA et al 2002 Selective reactivation of human herpesvirus 6 variant a occurs in critically ill immunocompetent hosts. J Infect Dis 185:110–113

Reddy RC, Chen GH, Newstead MW, Moore T, Zeng X, Tateda K, Standiford TJ 2001 Alveolar macrophage deactivation in murine septic peritonitis: role of interleukin 10. Infect Immun 69:1394–1401

Riedemann NC, Neff TA, Guo RF et al 2003 Protective effects of IL-6 blockade in sepsis are linked to reduced C5a receptor expression. J Immunol 170:503–507

Tetta C, Gianotti L, Cavaillon JM et al 2000 Coupled plasma filtration-adsorption in a rabbit model of endotoxic shock. Crit Care Med 28:1526–1533

Waage A, Halstensen A, Espevik T 1987 Association between tumour necrosis factor in serum and fatal outcome in patients with meningococcal disease. Lancet 8529:355–357

Wu L, Estrada O, Zaborina O et al 2005 Recognition of host immune activation by Pseudomonas aeruginosa. Science 309:774–777

Blockade of apoptosis as a rational therapeutic strategy for the treatment of sepsis

Alfred Ayala, Doreen E. Wesche-Soldato, Mario Perl, Joanne L. Lomas-Neira, Ryan Swan and Chun-Shiang Chung

Shock-Trauma Research Laboratory, Division of Surgical Research, Department of Surgery, Rhode Island Hospital / Brown University School of Medicine, Providence, RI 02903, USA

Abstract. Over time it has become clear that, much like other organ systems, the function and responsiveness of the immune system is impaired during the course of sepsis and that this is a precipitous event in the decline of the critically ill patient/animal. One hypothesis put forward to explain the development of septic immune dysfunction is that it is a pathological result of increased immune cell apoptosis. Alternatively, it has been proposed that the clearance of increased numbers of apoptotic cells may actively drive immune suppression through the cells that handle them. Here we review the data from studies involving septic animals and patients, which indicate that loss of immune cells, as well as non-immune cells, in some cases, is a result of dysregulated apoptosis. Subsequently, we will consider the cell death pathways, i.e. 'extrinsic' and/or 'intrinsic', which are activated and what cell populations may orchestrate this dysfunctional apoptotic process, immune and/or non-immune. Finally, we will discuss potentially novel therapeutic targets, such as caspases, death receptor family members (e.g. tumour necrosis factor, Fas) and pro-/anti-apoptotic Bcl-family members, and approaches such as caspase inhibitors, the use of fusion proteins, peptidomimetics and siRNA, which might be considered for the treatment of the septic patient.

2007 Sepsis—new insights, new therapies. Wiley, Chichester (Novartis Foundation Symposium 280) p 37–52

The incidence of sepsis in the USA as of the year 2000 was ~700 000 cases per year, with an overall mortality rate reported to be nearly 30% (Angus et al 2001). And as the American population ages, it is expected that the occurrence of sepsis will only increase (Angus et al 2001). Unfortunately, with respect to the development of new drug therapies that might substantially impact morbidity and mortality of sepsis, with the exception of recombinant human activated protein C, this has proven to be a difficult task (Rice & Bernard 2005). Even appreciating the important advancements made in the treatment of the critically ill patient through the application of low-dose corticosteroids (Annane et al 2002) and the improved control of blood glucose (van den Berghe et al 2001), these still provide a relatively modest survival benefit. Another important difference between these therapies, where some benefit has been seen, is that they have divergent modes of action. With the possible exception of low-dose steroids, they do not directly act on inflammation, in a fashion comparable to that of the failed anti-inflammatory drugs, such as anti-tumour necrosis factor (TNF) and anti-interleukin (IL)1 receptor antagonist, trialed in septic patients over the last 10 years. Taken another way, this suggests that the pathology behind the septic condition in the patient/animal is not simply about inflammation. Thus much more needs to be understood about sepsis and processes underpinning its development if we are either to optimize these present clinical therapies or develop novel approaches.

In this respect, it is now understood that essentially all cells in the body have within them the capacity to undergo cell suicide. This process is referred to as apoptosis or programmed cell death and is described as an energy-requiring process (unlike necrotic cell injury) that can be initiated by intra- as well as extracellular events. This is also largely a non-inflammatory event in which cells are actively eliminated via this pathway during processes as diverse as morphogenesis, tissue remodelling, and the regulation/resolution of the immune response. However, it is also now evident that overt activation or suppression of the apoptotic pathway can contribute to a variety of pathological conditions, such as HIV immune depression, cancer, autoimmune disorders, neurodegenerative diseases, inflammatory bowel disease and ischaemic injury (Li et al 1995, Liles 1997, Barinaga 1998, Barr & Tomei 1994). Therefore, the objective of this review is to discuss the evidence that has accumulated over the last 10 years that supports not only the concepts that change in the septic animal/patient's apoptotic process and/or the interaction of the immune system/body with these apoptotic materials contribute to septic morbidity and mortality, but also that components of the apoptotic process represent potential novel therapeutic targets.

Apoptotic pathways

Apoptotic cell death occurs primarily through three general pathways: the extrinsic or death receptor pathway (type I cells), the intrinsic or mitochondrial pathway (type II cells) and the endoplasmic reticulum (ER) or stress-induced pathway (Fig. 1) (Hotchkiss et al 2003, Wesche et al 2005). In brief, with respect to the extrinsic pathway it is thought that ligation of the death receptors (i.e. Fas, TNF receptor [TNFR], Trail, etc.), leads to activation of apoptosis (type I cells) through the recruitment of Fas-associated death domain protein (FADD), procaspase 8 (an initiator caspase), etc. via formation of a death-inducing signalling complex (DISC) and activation of caspase 3. Several counter-regulatory proteins, such as FADD-like interleukin-1-converting enzyme (FLICE)-inhibitory protein (FLIP)

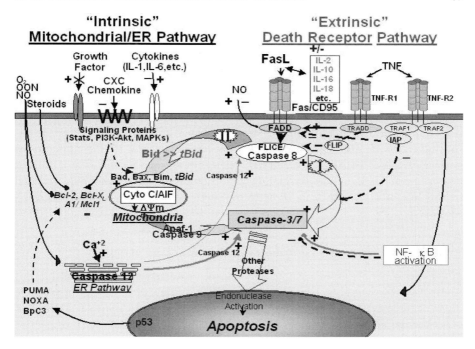

FIG. 1. Apoptotic signalling pathways as seen through death receptor ligation of TNFR or Fas (extrinsic signalling, type I cells) or through activation of the mitochondrial pathway through Bcl-2 family members (intrinsic signalling, type II cells).

and inhibitor of apoptosis protein (IAP), are also present at the level of the DISC and caspase 8 activation.

Alternatively, activation of the intrinsic pathway (type II cells) is regulated by the interaction of various anti- (B-cell CLL/lymphoma 2 [Bcl-2], myeloid cell leukaemia sequence 1 [Mcl-1], etc.) and/or pro-apoptotic members (Bcl-2/Bcl-XL-associated death promoter [Bad], Bcl-2-associated X protein [Bax], Bcl-2 interacting mediator of cell death [Bim], BH3 interacting death domain agonist [Bid], etc.) of the Bcl-2 family of proteins, which control mitochondrial ion permeability/flux (ΔΨm) and function. If this process is dysfunctional it culminates in the release of various proteins that contribute to apoptosome formation (cytochrome C, Smac/Diablo, apaf-1 and caspase 9) and the eventual activation of caspase 3/7 (an executioner caspase). Intrinsic pathway regulation appears to be a general product of cytokine/chemokine/growth factor regulation via signalling or the lack thereof (due to growth factor removal); through phosphatidylinositol-3-kinase (PI3K)/Akt, the mitogen-activated protein kinases (MAPK), steroid receptors, nuclear factor κB (NF-κB), signal transducers and activators of transcription (STAT), etc. These in turn act either on the various Bcl-2 family members or effect initiator/regulatory caspases (i.e. caspases 1, 8, 10) or IAP activity. The intrinsic pathway is also affected by changes in p53 status mediated through NOXA, PUMA, BbC3, etc., which also act on Bcl-2 family members' function/ expression, that link to processes affecting the cell cycle. Activation of caspase 12 in the endoplasmic reticulum (ER) potentially represents a third possible pathway that is activated by oxidant/calcium stress; however, this appears to be a species-specific apoptotic effector. That said, these pathways are not wholly autonomous as the cleavage of BID to truncated BID (tBID) by caspase 8 exhibits a significant aspect of cell death pathway cross-talk and a number of the regulators mentioned in the intrinsic pathway can directly/indirectly affect the extrinsic pathway's activity.

Evidence that apoptosis contributes to the pathology of sepsis

Studies in recent years have suggested that dysregulated apoptotic immune cell death may play a role in contributing to the immune dysfunction and multiple organ failure observed during sepsis and that blocking it can improve survival of experimental animals (Chung et al 2003, Hotchkiss et al 2003). With respect to the immune system, those cells most commonly reported to exhibit evidence of dysregulated apoptotic cell death appear to be lymphocytes (Fig. 2). That the loss of lymphocytes is detrimental to the survival of septic mice is documented by the observation that RAG$^{-/-}$ mice are markedly more susceptible to lethal effects of polymicrobial septic challenge, caecal ligation and puncture (CLP), than their background controls (Hotchkiss et al 2003). Typically, lymphocyte apoptosis has been seen following the onset of experimental sepsis in the thymus, spleen and gut-associated lymphoid tissues (GALT). The most basic hypothesis arising from these observations is that the overt apoptotic loss of these lymphocytes in the septic animal/patient reduces the number of functional immune cells available to ward off the lethal effects of septic challenge (Fig. 3A). Probably the most potent support for this hypothesis comes from the data indicating that if the development of lymphocyte apoptosis is blocked via the restricted overexpression of Bcl-2, this ameliorates much of the mortality seen in the CLP model of sepsis in mice (Hotchkiss et al 2003).

Other immune cell types, that have been reported to exhibit an increased incidence of apoptosis in sepsis, are CD8$^+$ lymphoid-derived dendritic cells of the spleen after CD3$^+$CD4$^+$ T cell activation (Hotchkiss et al 2003) (Fig. 2). Interestingly, the potential impact of the loss of dendritic cells, via apoptosis or some other process, on the septic animal's ability to survive experimental sepsis, is illustrated by the increased mortality seen in conditionally-induced dendritic cell deficient

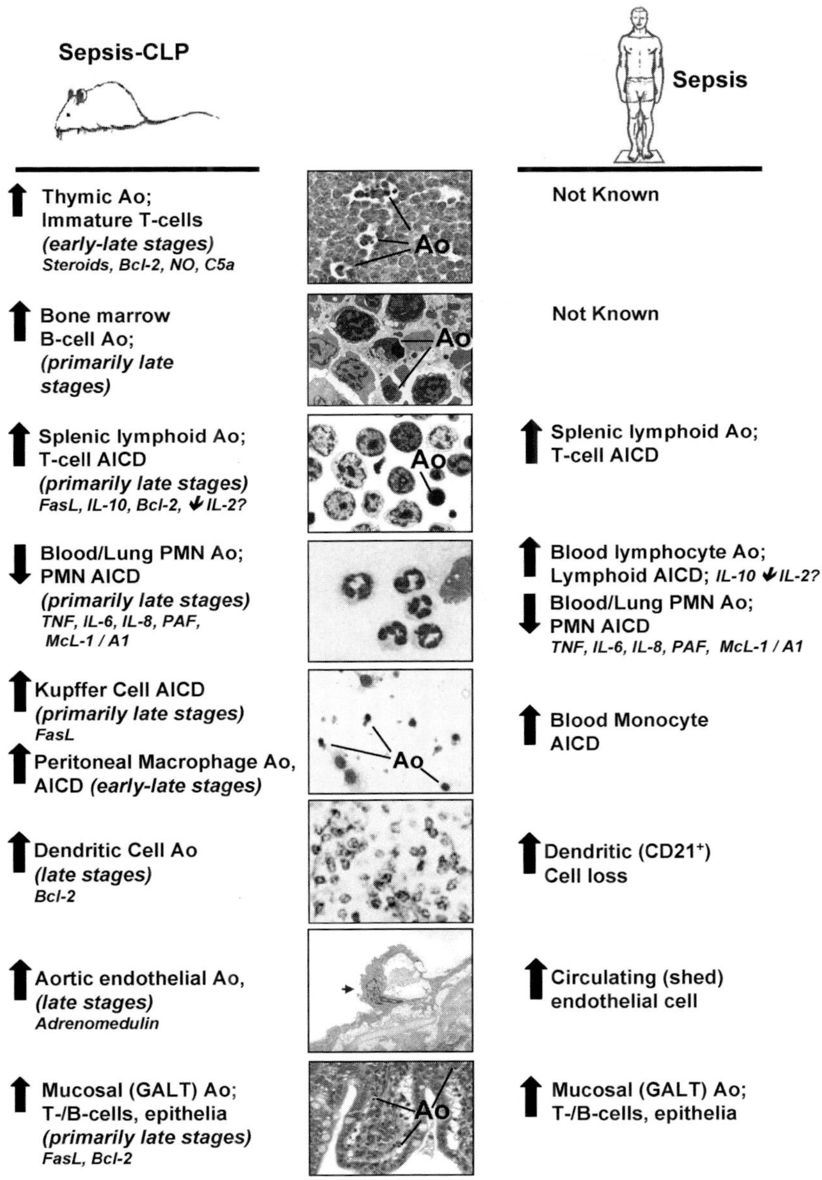

Sepsis-CLP

Sepsis

↑ Thymic Ao;
Immature T-cells
(early-late stages)
Steroids, Bcl-2, NO, C5a

Not Known

↑ Bone marrow
B-cell Ao;
*(primarily late
stages)*

Not Known

↑ Splenic lymphoid Ao;
T-cell AICD
(primarily late stages)
FasL, IL-10, Bcl-2, ↓IL-2?

↑ Splenic lymphoid Ao;
T-cell AICD

↓ Blood/Lung PMN Ao;
PMN AICD
(primarily late stages)
*TNF, IL-6, IL-8, PAF,
McL-1 / A1*

↑ Blood lymphocyte Ao;
Lymphoid AICD; *IL-10 ↓IL-2?*
↓ Blood/Lung PMN Ao;
PMN AICD
TNF, IL-6, IL-8, PAF, McL-1 / A1

↑ Kupffer Cell AICD
(primarily late stages)
FasL
↑ Peritoneal Macrophage Ao,
AICD *(early-late stages)*

↑ Blood Monocyte
AICD

↑ Dendritic Cell Ao
(late stages)
Bcl-2

↑ Dendritic (CD21+)
Cell loss

↑ Aortic endothelial Ao,
(late stages)
Adrenomedulin

↑ Circulating (shed)
endothelial cell

↑ Mucosal (GALT) Ao;
T-/B-cells, epithelia
(primarily late stages)
FasL, Bcl-2

↑ Mucosal (GALT) Ao;
T-/B-cells, epithelia

FIG. 2.   The levels of apoptosis (Ao) seen in experimental septic mice and septic patients, as well as the mediators that affect the onset and frequency of Ao in various immune cell types.

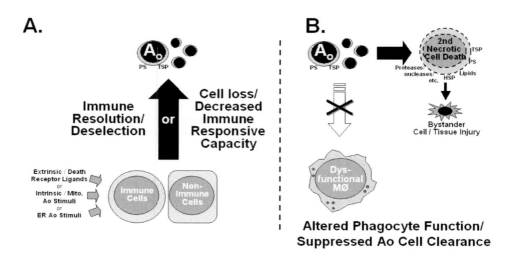

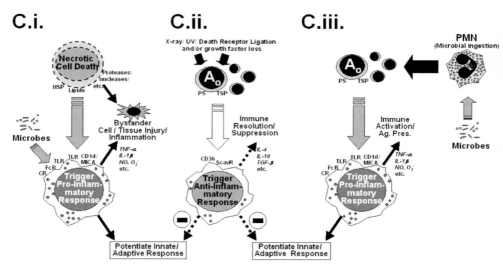

Assuming Normal Phagocyte Function

FIG. 3.   A depiction of several possible mechanisms of immune suppression. (A) Illustrates the simple hypothesis (mechanism) that the immune dysfunction observed is a result of advertant/inadvertent apoptotic (Ao) loss of immune cell potential/capacity resultant from extrinsic and/or intrinsic Ao pathway activation. Here, no consideration is made for Ao cell clearance. (B) Depicts a scheme in which phagocytic function is compromised, so as to block apoptotic cell clearance, subsequently allowing apoptotic cells to move into secondary necrosis, that may in turn produce bystander tissue injury. The scenarios illustrated in C.i.–C.iii. represent the proposed effects that clearance of necrotic (C.i.) and/or apoptotic cell materials (induced by classic Ao stimuli [C.ii.] or ingestion of microbes [C.iii.]) has on the developing macrophage functional phenotype (pro-inflammatory vs. anti-inflammatory/immune suppressive) assuming phagocytic function is normal. CD36, cell differentiation antigen 36; CR, complement receptor(s); CD1d/MICA, non-variant major histocompatability class 1-like antigen family; FcR, immunoglobulin constant region receptor(s); HSP, heat shock protein(s); PS, phosphatidyl serine; ScavR, scavenger receptor(s) which bind PS; TSP, thrombospondin.

mice (CD11c-diptheria toxin receptor transgenic mice) (Scumpia et al 2005). While a little more controversial (because of the capacity of phagocytes to engulf apoptotic material), macrophages have in some cases also been reported to undergo apoptosis during sepsis (Williams et al 1998, Iwata et al 2003). Here again, indirect evidence from Iwata et al (Iwata et al 2003) shows that mice over-expressing Bcl-2 under a myeloid as opposed to a lymphoid restricted fashion, not only produced a survival advantage but also found that adoptive transfer of blood monocytes from these animals to septic rodents improved their survival. This implies that protecting the myeloid compartment from apoptosis is also a valuable asset to the host's immune response to sepsis. These results, however, extend the concept from simply the loss of lymphocytes to include the loss of dendritic cells and myeloid cells as contributors to the septic host's inability to ward off the lethal effects of sepsis.

In contrast, it is worth noting that *in vivo* neutrophils, unlike lymphocytes or the other cell types mentioned above, undergo constitutive induction of apoptosis within 1–2 days normally (Fig. 2). Also unlike the lymphocytes, in response to a septic insult, they react with a decrease in apoptosis, which appears to be linked to a decrease in caspase 9 and caspase 3 activity and a prolonged maintenance of the mitochondrial transmembrane potential (Taneja et al 2004). Studies investigating neutrophil apoptosis during septic peritonitis in mice have revealed that while blood neutrophils react with a decrease in apoptosis, which is regulated by TNFα, after immigration into the peritoneal cavity they exhibit increased apoptosis (Wesche et al 2005). However, in some cases this response may also be detrimental. As an example, experimental haemorrhage also primes neutrophils into delaying apoptosis and increasing their respiratory burst (Ayala et al 2002) in a fashion similar to that seen in trauma patients' blood neutrophils (Jimenez et al 1997). Transfer of these experimentally primed neutrophils to a septic environment increases their recruitment into the lungs and leads to acute lung injury (Ayala et al 2002).

That said, it is now becoming more evident that non-immune cells may also be exhibiting apoptotic changes that were not initially clear because they were not rigorously looked for or were not obvious using the techniques available (Fig. 2). In this respect, increased apoptosis of the gut mucosal epithelial cells (Coopersmith et al 2002, Perl et al 2005), hepatocytes (Kim et al 2000) and to a lesser extent endothelial cells (Mutunga et al 2001) has been reported in clinically comparable models of sepsis (Zhou et al 2004). While the significance of these apoptotic events in sepsis is yet to be clarified, it is tempting to speculate how this potentiated loss of cells might contribute not only to loss of innate host defence/barrier function, but also to organ dysfunction/damage.

What regulates these changes in immune cell apoptosis during sepsis? Interestingly, this appears, at least with respect to the lymphoid compartment, to vary somewhat with the cell and/or tissue type being examined. Also while high doses of endotoxin can induce this process *in vitro* and/or *in vivo*, studies with more clinically comparable models of sepsis indicate that much of the immune cell apoptosis seen occurs independent of the capacity to sense/respond to endotoxin through Toll-like receptor 4 (TLR4) (Wesche et al 2005, Hotchkiss et al 2003). Lymphocyte apoptosis in the thymus appears to be affected by glucocorticoids (Wesche et al 2005), nitric oxide and by the 5a fragment of complement (Guo et al 2000), but not by endotoxin or death receptors (Wesche et al 2005). Alternatively, in the bone marrow and lamina propria B cells (Wesche et al 2005), splenic T cells, intestinal intraepithelial lymphocytes (IELs), and mucosal T and B cells of the Peyer's patches (Chung et al 1998, Ayala et al 2003), apoptosis is mainly death receptor-driven via Fas-FasL activation. Interestingly, evidence of both intrinsic and extrinsic apoptotic pathway activation has been reported in the peripheral blood of septic patients (Hotchkiss et al 2005).

Lymphocyte apoptosis may be associated with immune dysfunction as a result of decreased proliferation and IFNγ release capability. IFNγ is a potent macrophage activator and induces a Th1 response (Docke et al 1997). As seen in apoptotic and necrotic splenocyte adoptive transfer experiments, necrotic and apoptotic cells exert their effects through variation of IFNγ levels. Transfer of apoptotic splenocytes retro-orbitally in CLP mice decreased their survival, whereas adoptive transfer of necrotic splenocytes increased splenocyte IFNγ, and in doing so, improved survival. This survival benefit was blocked in IFNγ deficient mice and in mice treated with an anti-IFNγ antibody. These results are interesting as this adoptive transfer study illustrates the potential impact of apoptotic cells *in vivo* in sepsis and thus points to another mechanism (beside loss/death of functional immune cells; Fig. 3B,C) by which immune suppression might be promulgated in the septic animal (Hotchkiss et al 2003) (Fig. 3Cii). Alternatively, the inability to appropriately clear these dying lymphocytes/cells due to dysfunction in their phagocytic capacities often seen following sepsis and shock (Rana et al 1990, Huber-Lang et al 2002) may allow them to progress to a state of secondary necrosis, producing localized bystander injury in the tissue (Fig. 3B). Such a scenario has been recently put forward by Vandivier et al (2002) as a possible mechanism for tissue inflammation and the enhanced susceptibility to infection seen in cystic fibrosis patients. It remains to be determined whether such defects in macrophage-mediated clearance of apoptotic cells contribute to the changes seen in septic mice.

Intrinsic and extrinsic aspects of the apoptotic process as a therapeutic target

One of the earliest anti-apoptotic approaches considered for sepsis was the inhibition of caspase activation. Caspase inhibitors usually contain fluoromethyl ketones (fmk) or chloromethyl ketones (cmk) that are derivatives of peptides that imitate cleavage sites of known caspase substrates. The caspase-specific inhibitors that have been used include z-DEVD-fmk (caspase 3 and 7) and Ac-YVAD-cmk (caspase 1) (Rouquet et al 1996). It has also been shown that broad spectrum caspase inhibitors such as z-VAD-fmk can prevent lymphocyte apoptosis in sepsis, and in turn, improve septic animal survival by 40–45% (Hotchkiss et al 2003). However, at high doses, caspase inhibitors can have non-specific effects and cause cytotoxicity. In this respect, a different kind of pan-caspase inhibitor called Q-VD-Oph has been studied (Caserta et al 2003), which potently inhibits apoptosis but is less toxic at high doses and may be more efficacious in the clinical setting.

Peptidomimetics represent another potentially useful method of targeting the apoptotic pathway. 'Peptidomimetics' are mimics that have similar structure and functional properties as the native parental peptides. This approach was adopted since the use of biologically active peptides as pharmaceutical compounds has more-or-less failed due to their inability to stay bioavailable and reach their cellular targets. Synthetic mimics, however, can be generated to be more conformationally stable compounds that resist enzyme degradation, can cross cell membranes and target specific proteins (Li et al 2004). We mention this type of approach here, for while it is being studied at present only for its potential pro-apoptotic effect on Bid (Walensky et al 2004) activation as well as via antagonism of IAP (Li et al 2004) in cancer models, it seems possible that peptidomimetics may also be useful in future therapies that modulate anti-apoptotic protein–protein interactions in the case of sepsis. This idea may also be an alternative to gene therapy, which, in the past, has not done well in the clinical setting due to marked inflammatory sequelae and oncogenesis (Lehrman 1999).

With respect to gene therapy, enhancement of anti-apoptotic proteins, such as Bcl-2, has been shown to produce almost complete protection against T cell apoptosis in mice that overexpress Bcl-2. This, in turn, improved their survival after sepsis (Hotchkiss et al 2003). In addition, adoptive transfer of T cells from Bcl2 over-expressing mice into wild-type septic mice also improved their survival (Hotchkiss et al 2003). While this clearly illustrates the important role of the lymphocyte in sepsis in controlling infection, it also illustrates a clear therapeutic target, which might also be exploited to restore lymphocyte numbers during this state.

Yet another target that decreases lymphocyte apoptosis is Akt, a regulator of cell proliferation and death. It has been shown that in mice over-expressing Akt lymphocyte apoptosis is decreased and survival after CLP is improved to 94% (Bommhardt et al 2004). It may be at this level (i.e. the activation of Akt) that treatments such as glucose control with insulin therapy or low-dose steroids have an effect on apoptosis in septic individuals.

Based on the observation of increased Fas expression in the tissues of septic mice (Chung et al 2003, 1998, Wesche-Soldato et al 2005), there has been increasing interest in targeting components of the death receptor/extrinsic pathway in an attempt to ameliorate the effects of sepsis. In this regard, our own studies had initially focused on blocking the pathway at the death receptor itself (Fas). Animals that were treated with Fas fusion protein (FasFP; Amgen Inc., Thousand Oaks, CA), to inhibit the receptor ligation, exhibited a marked survival benefit (Chung et al 2003) and showed reduced hepatic injury while improving total hepatic, intestinal and cardiac blood flow during sepsis (Wesche et al 2005, Chung et al 2001). In addition, the cell survival tyrosine kinase (MET) has been found to sequester Fas on hepatocytes but in a fashion that inhibits Fas self-aggregation and Fas ligand binding, protecting the liver from injury (Wang et al 2002).

Most recently, we have utilized interfering RNA technology to target gene expression of members of the extrinsic death receptor/Fas pathway. Fas and caspase-8 siRNA given 30 min after CLP improved survival by 50% and reduced indices of organ damage and apoptosis in both the liver and spleen (Wesche-Soldato et al 2005). This is in keeping with the findings that both Fas and caspase-8 siRNA have salutary effects in models of fulminant hepatitis (Song et al 2003). The mechanism of this survival benefit in sepsis is still largely unknown; however, our preliminary data suggest that $CD4^+$ and $CD8^+$ T cells, B cells as well as hepatocytes take up Fas siRNA. In the case of the spleen, it appears that lymphocyte apoptosis is reduced by silencing Fas, therefore enabling the host to maintain innate and/or adaptive immune response to septic challenge. With respect to the liver, preliminary results suggest that Fas siRNA reduces not only the expression of Fas on potential target cells in the liver, but also suppresses recruitment of potentially activated cytotoxic lymphocytes. It has been suggested in a model of hepatitis C that Fas ligand-expressing $CD4^+$ T cells can induce chronic hepatic inflammation (Cruise et al 2005), which in the case of sepsis, may be instrumental in initiating multiple organ failure. By the same token, experimental CLP mice lacking $CD8^+$ T cells exhibit improved survival over wild-type (Sherwood et al 2003).

As intriguing as this approach is, several hurdles need to be overcome beyond cell targeting before siRNA can be applied clinically. While we saw little evidence of overt toxicity/off-target effects/inflammation, as we observed no marked induction of IFNα, TNFα or IL6 with either targeted siRNAs or the control constructs, these issues will need further consideration as the delivery systems are changed/modified and/or lipid conjugations of siRNA are added (Wesche-Soldato et al 2005). Probably the biggest hurdle facing the use of siRNA clinically is that of its delivery. While a hydrodynamic-based method (where large volume and rapid rate of injection are critical in the uptake of naked constructs) is easily employed in research, it clearly cannot be used in human therapy. Because naked siRNAs are degraded within seconds following a normal low volume injection (as opposed to hydrodynamic-based delivery), there needs to be a carrier or delivery vehicle that will protect the siRNA. Cationic liposomes encoding anti-TNF siRNA have been studied, and appeared to reduce TNFα levels after endotoxaemia. While this represents a useful alternative method for encapsulating/delivering siRNA, uptake of siRNA was largely limited to vascular endothelial cells following i.v. administration (Sorenson et al 2003). Other investigators have suggested the use of vectors as another mode of targeted siRNA delivery. However, vectorized gene delivery may cause inflammation by itself (Bridge et al 2004).

Conclusions

Despite overwhelming research efforts and clinical trials, there has yet to be a therapy offered that significantly modifies the outcome of sepsis. Even though there have been promising candidates for therapeutic intervention, sepsis manifests itself as multiple processes, making this task difficult. Here we have reviewed several experimental studies that have focused not only on the apoptotic process and its potential pathological roles in sepsis, but have also revealed several targets within the apoptotic pathway, that may be useful going forward in designing individual or adjuvant therapies for this critically ill patient population.

Acknowledgements

This work was supported in part by funds from NIH-RO1s GM53209 and HL73525 (to A.A.), as well as fellowship support from NIH-T32 GM65085 (for R.S.) and GAANN P200A03100 (for D.E.W-S.).

References

Angus DC, Linde-Zwirble WT, Lidicker J, Clermont G, Carcillo J, Pinsky MR 2001 Epidemiology of severe sepsis in the United States: analysis of incidence, outcome, and associated costs of care. Crit Care Med 29:1303–1310

Annane D, Sebille V, Charpentier C et al 2002 Effect of treatment with low doses of hydrocortisone and fludrocortisone on mortality in patients with septic shock. JAMA 288: 862–871

Ayala A, Chung CS, Lomas JL et al 2002 Shock induced neutrophil mediated priming for acute lung injury in mice: divergent effects of TLR-4 and TLR-4/FasL deficiency. Amer J Pathol 161:2283–2294

Ayala A, Lomas JL, Grutkoski PS, Chung CS 2003 Pathological aspects of apoptosis in severe sepsis and shock? Int J Biochem Cell Biol 35:7–15

Barinaga M 1998 Is apoptosis key in Alzheimer's disease? Science 281:1303–1304

Barr PJ, Tomei LD 1994 Apoptosis and its role in human disease. Bio/Technology 12: 487–493

Bommhardt U, Chang KC, Swanson PE et al 2004 Akt decreases lymphocyte apoptosis and improves survival in sepsis. J Immunol 172:7583–7591

Bridge AJ, Pebernard S, Ducraux A, Nicovlaz AL, Iggo R 2004 Induction of an interferon response by RNAi vectors in mammalian cells. Nature Genet 34:263–264

Caserta TM, Smith AN, Gultice AD, Reedy MA, Brown TL 2003 Q-VD-OPh, a broad spectrum caspase inhibitor with potent antiapoptotic properties. Apoptosis 8:345–352

Chung CS, Xu YX, Wang W, Chaudry IH, Ayala A 1998 Is Fas ligand or endotoxin responsible for mucosal lymphocyte apoptosis in sepsis? Arch Surg 133:1213–1220

Chung CS, Yang SL, Song GY et al 2001 Inhibition of Fas signaling prevents hepatic injury and improves organ blood flow during sepsis. Surgery 130:339–345

Chung CS, Song GY, Lomas J, Simms HH, Chaudry IH, Ayala A 2003 Inhibition of Fas/Fas ligand signaling improves septic survival: differential effects on macrophage apoptotic and functional capacity. J Leukoc Biol 74:344–351

Coopersmith CM, Stromberg PE, Dunne WM et al 2002 Inhibition of intestinal epithelial apoptosis and survival in a murine model of pneumonia-induced sepsis. JAMA 287:1716–1721

Cruise MW, Melief HM, Lukens J, Soguero C, Hahn YS 2005 Increased Fas ligand expression of CD4$^+$ T cells by HCV core induces T cell-dependent hepatic inflammation. J Leukocyte Biol 78:412–425

Docke WD, Randow F, Syrbe U et al 1997 Monocyte deactivation in septic patients: restoration by IFN-gamma treatment. Nat Med 3:678–681

Guo R-F, Huber-Lang M, Wang X et al 2000 Protective effects of anti-C5a in sepsis-induced thymocyte apoptosis. J Clin Invest 106:1271–1280

Hotchkiss RS, Tinsley KW, Karl IE 2003 Role of apoptotic cell death in sepsis. Scand J Infect Dis 35:585–592

Hotchkiss RS, Osmon SB, Chang KC, Wagner TH, Coopersmith CM, Karl IE 2005 Accelerated lymphocyte death in sepsis occurs by both the death receptor and mitochondrial pathway. J Immunol 174:5110–5118

Huber-Lang MS, Riedemann NC, Sarma JV et al 2002 Protection of innate immunity by C5aR antagonist in septic mice. FASEB J 16:1567–1574

Iwata A, Stevenson VM, Minard A et al 2003 Over-expression of Bcl-2 provides protection in septic mice by a trans effect. J Immunol 171:3136–3141

Jimenez MF, Watson WG, Parodo J et al 1997 Dysregulated expression of neutrophil apoptosis in the systemic inflammatory response syndrome. Arch Surg 132:1263–1270

Kim Y-M, Kim T-H, Chung H-T, Talanian RV, Yin X-M, Billiar TR 2000 Nitric oxide prevents tumor necrosis factor α-induced rat hepatocyte apoptosis by the interruption of mitochondrial apoptotic signaling through S-nitrosylation of caspase-8. Hepatology 32:770–778

Lehrman S 1999 Virus treatment questioned after gene therapy death. Nature 401:517–518

Li CJ, Friedman DJ, Wang C, Metelev V, Pardee AB 1995 Induction of apoptosis in uninfected lymphocytes by HIV-1 Tat protein. Science 268:429–431

Li L, Thomas RM, Suzuki H, DeBrabander JK, Wang X, Harran PG 2004 A small molecule smac mimic potentiates TRAIL- and TNF-alpha-mediated cell death. Science 305:1471–1474

Liles WC 1997 Apoptosis-role in infection and inflammation. Curr Opin Infect Dis 10:165–170

Mutunga M, Fulton B, Bullock R et al 2001 Circulating endothelial cells in patients with septic shock. Am J Respir Crit Care Med 163:195–200

Perl M, Chung CS, Lomas-Neira J et al 2005 Silencing of Fas- but not caspase-8 in lung epithelial cells ameliorates experimental acute lung injury. Am J Pathol 167:1545–1559

Rana MW, Ayala A, Dean RE, Chaudry IH 1990 Decreased Fc receptor expression on macrophages following simple hemorrhage as observed by scanning immuno electron microscopy. J Leukocyte Biol 48:512–518

Rice TW, Bernard GR 2005 Therapeutic interventions and targets for sepsis. Annual Review Medicine 56:225–248

Rouquet N, Pages JC, Molina T, Briand J, Joulin V 1996 ICE inhibitor YVADcmk is a potent therapeutic agent against in vivo liver apoptosis. Curr Biol 6:1192–1195

Scumpia PO, McAuliffe PF, O'Malley KA et al 2005 CD11c+ dendritic cells are required for survival in murine polymicrobial sepsis. J Immunol 175:3282–3286

Sherwood ER, Lin CY, Tao W et al 2003 B2 microglobulin knockout mice are resistant to lethal intra-abdominal sepsis. Am J Respir Crit Care Med 167:1641–1649

Song E, Lee-S-K, Wang J et al 2003 RNA interference targeting Fas protects mice from fulminant hepatitis. Nat Med 9:347–351

Sorenson DR, Leirdal M, Sioud M 2003 Gene silencing by systemic delivery of synthetic siRNAs in adult mice. J Mol Biol 327:761–766

Taneja R, Parodo J, Jia SH, Kapus A, Rotstein OD 2004 Delayed neutrophil apoptosis in sepsis is associated with maintenance of mitochondrial transmembrane potential and reduced caspase-9 activity. Crit Care Med 32:1460–1469

van den Berghe G, Wouters P, Weekers F et al 2001 Intensive insulin therapy in critically ill patients. N Engl J Med 345:1359–1367

Vandivier RW, Fadok VA, Hoffmann PR et al 2002 Elastase-mediated phosphatidylserine receptor cleavage impairs apoptotic cell clearance in cystic fibrosis and bronchiectasis. J Clin Invest 109:661–670

Walensky LD, Kung AL, Escher I et al 2004 Activation of apoptosis in vivo by a hydrocarbon-stapled BH3 helix. Science 305:1466–1470

Wang X, DeFrances MC, Dai Y et al 2002 A mechanism of cell survival: sequestration of Fas by the HGF receptor Met. Mol Cell 9:411–421

Wesche-Soldato DE, Chung CS, Lomas-Neira J, Doughty LA, Gregory SH, Ayala A 2005 In vivo delivery of caspase 8 or Fas siRNA improves the survival of septic mice. Blood 106:2295–2301

Wesche DE, Lomas-Neira JL, Perl M, Chung CS, Ayala A 2005 Leukocyte apoptosis and its significance in sepsis and shock. J Leukocyte Biol 25:325–337

Williams MA, Withington S, Newland AC, Kelsey SM 1998 Monocyte anergy in septic shock is associated with a prediliction to apoptosis and is reversed by granulocyte-macrophage colony stimulating factor ex vivo. J Infect Dis 178:1421–1433

Zhou M, Simms HH, Wang P 2004 Adrenomedullin and adrenomedullin binding protein-1 attenuate vascular endothelial cell apoptosis in sepsis. Ann Surgery 240:321–330

DISCUSSION

Marshall: Your observation that you can't alter mortality if you give the Fas fusion protein prior to the infectious insult, but you can if you give it 12h later is very exciting for people who have tried to apply biology to clinical practice. It is easy to save a mouse from just about anything if you pretreat, but it is very difficult to pretreat humans! Are there any attempts to try to translate this observation into a clinical trial?

Ayala: This is the challenge. I'm probably one of the worst people to discuss/try to represent the link to industry, because I never manage to set up really good connections. That said, there were several companies who started to go forward with caspase inhibitors (for example, IDUN, Merck, etc.). I don't know the story with Fas fusion protein (which was an Amgen Inc. product). Peptidomimetics are so new that they haven't come to the floor yet. siRNA is in the same state, but it will get its initial trial soon. Several clinical trials are going forward with siRNA against various respiratory viruses.

Piantadosi: If I look at the whole apoptosis picture I see several things. I see cells dying by design—execution—and cells that die accidentally. There are multiple ways for the body to kill the cell. There are multiple receptor and mitochondrial initiation pathways. Can you describe some pros and cons of intervening in upstream versus downstream ways? What might the implications of this be for intentional versus accidental cell death?

Ayala: The value of interfering upstream is that the receptors are much more limited in their expression. Endothelial and epithelial cells are primary places where they are expressed. These death receptors become interesting targets because therapy could be somewhat more cell directed. It will be harder with the intrinsic receptor signalling proteins that are downstream, because we don't know what the effector will be upstream. It may differ according to the tissue.

With respect to how cells die, I think of the apoptotic process versus the necrotic process primarily as landmarks. There are a variety of different forms of cell death that use parts of these signalling systems. Interfering with them may be advantageous or disadvantageous; we don't know. It is easier to go after things where we know there are receptors that exist for them; it will be more difficult if we don't know the downstream events.

Cohen: In those elegant experiments you showed clearly the effect of the various interventions. In the treated groups, which are not dying, what are they not dying of?

Ayala: That's a good question. I can probably answer it most easily in the double-hit insult. The model of sepsis as we use it doesn't have a strong lung component to it. It does have strong liver and cardiac components, and there are other organ systems such as the gut that are injured. The double-hit model seems to add the acute lung injury into the mix. There is this aspect of potentiation of susceptibility. In this system we can say that lung injury is adding something on top of the other organs that tips the scale, and says that they will die more often. When we measure overall mortality, we find that they do. This injury, shock alone, added to sepsis is enough to enhance their death.

Fink: In your CLP model, do you provide antibiotics?

Ayala: No. Richard Hotchkiss does and finds similar results.

Fink: Do you provide source control? Do you have a necrotic dead thing in the abdomen?

Ayala: We don't, but other labs that have studied this do. This will modify it but not change the nature of the response. We have looked at not puncturing the cecum and assessing how the animal responds to this. However, the mortality in these animals is less unless you add another insult on top of the cecal injury. You have to add an infectious stimulus to convert that model to achieve high mortality. By itself it represents a non-lethal response.

Fink: What I am driving at is that if you rig the model so that the animals are going to die of overwhelming infection, because you haven't provided antibiotics and you haven't removed the source of bugs (and the standard of care is to do both), then not having any lymphocytes around is really bad for you. But if you treat the animal the way you would a human, doing an appendectomy or a left hemi-colectomy and provide systemic antimicrobial chemotherapy, then maybe not having any lymphocytes present isn't so bad.

Ayala: I agree with that, at least in part. The experiment has been done by Richard Hotchkiss and colleagues where they use antibiotics. They can show using a mouse lymphocyte Bcl2 overexpression transgenic, that in the CLP model with antibiotics present, the T cell deficiency that is typically encountered in these animals is not observed and their survival is protected (Hotchkiss et al 1999). In an immune-suppressed animal the antibiotics buy it time to use its immune system.

Szabó: I have some questions and problems. The concept that there is either something called apoptosis or something called necrosis is an oversimplification. There are a range of processes. The cells don't know whether they are dying of apoptosis or necrosis; they know they have been subjected to certain kinds of trauma, and then they do different things in response to the injury. The mitochondrial component is a prominent feature of both apoptosis and necrosis. If you subject a thymocyte population to oxidative stress, some of the cells go into apoptosis and some into necrosis. Depending on what kind of parameter you look at—cell membrane permeability or mitochondrial permeability transition or caspase activation—different pharmacological agents might increase one and decrease another. The overall outcome would be different depending on what you look at. It is like the blind man feeling the elephant. I think we are better off just referring to it as 'cell death' because some of the tools we use to investigate cell death are not as sharp as we would like them to be. Let's take one example. You showed that in your CLP model the liver enzymes were elevated. Then you treated the animals with an anti-apoptotic approach, which decreased this elevation. When I was in medical school they taught me that liver enzymes go up because of hepatocyte necrosis. If the cells are truly apoptotic they will be taken up by other cells and the inside will never get out. When you see liver enzymes rising this is a sign of necrosis not apoptosis. Histologically, in these livers only a very limited number of cells show features of apoptosis.

Ayala: I understand what you are saying. Apoptosis as a discussion is meant to be a starting point for how we define death. There is a pretty broad spectrum from pure necrotic to pure apoptotic death. The extent to which the type of cell death seen is apoptotic or necrotic or something in between depends on what stage a cell is in when it dies apoptotically, i.e. early apoptotic, late apoptotic-necrotic, necrotic, etc. However, the type of cell/tissue death seen may also reflect that there are other systems that are failing simultaneously, for example: the systems that handle apoptotic cell clearance may be failing (if you don't clear apoptotic cells they undergo necrosis). Thus, even if an apoptotic stimulus initiates the process of cell death, the overt type of death actually seen (from necrotic to apoptotic) may vary depending on the factors listed above. Perhaps we see some aspects of necrotic injury because the system that is designed to take care of (clear) an apoptotic cell isn't there either.

Gilroy: In the Hotchkiss paper, he gave apoptotic cells at the start of the septic response and found that there was more animal death. But apoptotic cells are immunosuppressive in many respects when they are in an immune system. Aren't you starting off with an immunocompromized animal? If you gave the apoptotic cells half way through the inflammatory response, you might have a better outcome. Did he do those experiments?

Ayala: No, he didn't. That would be a logical conclusion. Depending on the timing, the response should be different.

Radermacher: I assume your mice are not ventilated. You mentioned that the second hit adds to the mortality because of the pulmonary failure. Do they die from hypoxaemia, or do they die because they don't get rid of their CO_2?

Ayala: They develop a relatively consistent lung leak, but the way we measure these things in mice is limited. We do crude protein levels in lavage fluid and wet weight in the animals. We don't have the kind of data we would like.

Fink: To put a summary on this part of the discussion, people are talking about why their experimental animals die. As has already been alluded to, the reason our patients die is twofold. There is a small group of patients who die of haemodynamic collapse acutely. This is uncommon. Then there is a much larger group who die of what has been called 'therapeutic fatigue', which is when the doctors, patient and nurses have had enough. The reason they die on Tuesday and not Thursday is because everyone has decided that Tuesday is the day they will die; this is different than the mice!

Reference

Hotchkiss RS, Swanson PE, Knudson CM et al 1999 Overexpression of Bcl-2 in transgenic mice decreases apoptosis and improves survival in sepsis. J Immunol 162:4148–4156

Modulating neutrophil apoptosis

John C. Marshall, Zeenat Malam and Songhui Jia

Department of Surgery, and the Interdepartmental Division of Critical Care Medicine, St. Michael's Hospital, University of Toronto, Toronto, Canada

Abstract. Polymorphonuclear neutrophils are short-lived phagocytic cells that serve as cardinal early cellular effectors of innate immunity. Both oxidative and non-oxidative mechanisms contribute to microbial killing by the neutrophil. Neutrophil defence mechanisms are potent but non-specific, with the result that inadvertent injury to host tissues commonly accompanies the activation of a neutrophil-mediated response; this bystander injury has been implicated in the tissue injury of sepsis. The capacity for neutrophils to cause injury to host tissues is attenuated by the relatively short *in vivo* lifespan of the neutrophil, a consequence of a constitutively expressed program of apoptosis. That program can be inhibited, and neutrophil survival prolonged, through the interaction of the neutrophil with a variety of mediators of both microbial and host origin. These, in turn, inhibit apoptosis by increasing the expression of anti-apoptotic genes within the neutrophil: interleukin (IL)1β and a novel cytokine-like molecule pre-B cell colony-enhancing factor (PBEF) are central to this inhibitory influence. Conversely, the phagocytosis of a micro-organism activates the apoptotic program, and so contributes to the resolution of acute inflammation. A complex series of interactions between the neutrophil and microorganisms or their products regulates the duration and intensity of an inflammatory response, and so provides an attractive target for therapeutic manipulation.

2007 Sepsis—new insights, new therapies. Wiley, Chichester (Novartis Foundation Symposium 280) p 53–72

Polymorphonuclear neutrophils (PMNs) are cardinal cellular effectors of the innate host response to infection and injury. They are rapidly recruited to sites of local infectious challenge or tissue trauma following the release of chemotactic factors such as interleukin (IL)8, and are activated to kill invading microorganisms and to support regional host defences to contain an infectious challenge. Their arsenals are both potent and non-specific, with the result that bystander injury to host tissues is an inevitable consequence of neutrophil activation (Smith 1994, Weiss 1989).

Neutrophils also comprise the shortest-lived cellular population in the human body. Their half life *in vivo* is a mere six to eight hours (Savill et al 1989); since the normal number of neutrophils per litre of blood is approximately 1.5×10^{10} in health, it follows that approximately 10^{11} neutrophils are released from the bone marrow each day (Athens et al 1961). And a comparable number of neutrophils must be eliminated each day to maintain a stable population of circulating cells. Moreover the removal of apoptotic cells by professional phagocytes serves to activate gene programs within the phagocytosing cell that are anti-inflammatory and reparative in nature (Savill et al 2002); the stable uptake of apoptotic cells is an integral component of the maintenance of normal immune homeostasis (Fadok et al 1998).

This chapter reviews the biology of neutrophil activation, the mechanisms of normal constitutive neutrophil apoptosis, and the intracellular processes responsible for prolonging neutrophil survival in response to inflammatory stimuli.

Antimicrobial defences of the neutrophil

Pathogen recognition and uptake

Both innate and adaptive immune mechanisms facilitate pathogen recognition by the neutrophil. Toll-like receptors (TLRs)—an evolutionarily ancient family of 10 pattern recognition receptors characterized by leucine-rich extracellular domains—comprise a key mechanism through which cells of the innate immune system recognize danger, and rapidly activate a defensive response (Akira et al 2006). Neutrophils express the full repertoire of TLRs with the exception of TLR3 (Hayashi et al 2003), and so are activated by a broad array of danger signals. TLR engagement activates a complex network of intracellular signalling pathways whose ultimate consequence is induction or repression of hundreds, if not thousands, of genes involved in innate immune defences (Calvano et al 2005), fundamentally altering both the cellular microenvironment and the capacity of the cell to respond, function and survive. Exposure of the neutrophil to lipopolysaccharide (LPS), for example, activates PI3 kinase (Yum et al 2001) and induces the nuclear translocation of the transcription factor NF-κB (McDonald et al 1997), processes that in turn prolong neutrophil function by inhibiting a constitutively expressed apoptotic program (Francois et al 2005).

C3H HeJ mice carrying a mutation in TLR4 that renders them hyporesponsive to LPS show impaired fungal challenge clearance following *in vivo* challenge with viable *Candida albicans*. Production of pro-inflammatory cytokines such as IL1 and tumour necrosis factor (TNF) is impaired, and neutrophil recruitment to the site of infections is reduced; on the other hand, candidacidal activity is normal (Netea et al 2002). Thus, while TLR engagement optimizes the cellular milieu to support antimicrobial defences, pathogen uptake and intracellular killing are dependent on other processes. Pathogen uptake requires opsonization of the organism by complement or immunoglobulin, followed by binding to the neutrophil surface through complement receptors including C1qR, CR1 and Mac-1, or receptors for the Fc component of antibody, including FcεRI, FcεRII, FcαR, FcγRI, FcγRIIa and FcγRIIIb (Kobayashi et al 2003). Engagement of these pathogen uptake receptors results in polymerization of intracellular actin and local membrane remodelling to create the phagosomal cup that engulfs and internalizes the pathogen (Lee et al 2003). Maturation of the phagosome follows pathogen engulfment; through dynamic fusion events with potent intracellular secretory vesicles and granules, microbicidal peptides and proteolytic enzymes are concentrated in the mature phagosome.

Pathogen killing

Neutrophils kill ingested microorganisms through both oxygen-independent and oxygen-dependent mechanisms.

Oxygen-independent effectors of pathogen killing are sequestered in cytoplasmic granules—primarily the azurophilic or primary granules, and the specific granules—and include anti-microbial peptides such as defensins, bactericidal permeability-increasing protein (BPI), and lysozyme that increase bacterial permeability by disrupting anionic surfaces (Faurschou & Borregaard 2003). Proteases such as neutrophil elastase and cathepsin G degrade bacterial proteins, while a vacuolar ATPase transports protons into the phagosome, leading to phagosomal acidification, and activating hydrolytic enzymes that function optimally under conditions of low pH (4.5–6.0) (Ishikawa & Miyazaki 2005). Other granule constituents support antimicrobial defences indirectly. Lactoferrin, for example, sequesters iron, an essential cofactor for microbial growth, while BPI and alkaline phosphatase have endotoxin-neutralizing capacity.

Oxygen-dependent killing mechanisms derive from the capacity of the neutrophil to transform molecular oxygen into a series of highly reactive intermediate species including superoxide anion (O_2^-), hydrogen peroxide (H_2O_2), hydroxide anion (OH^-), and hypochlorous acid (HOCl). Interactions between superoxide anion and nitric oxide generate peroxynitrite ($ONOO^-$) (Hampton et al 1998). Reactive intermediates are generated from molecular oxygen through the activity of NADPH oxidase—a protein complex that is assembled at the membrane of the phagosome following neutrophil activation and pathogen uptake. The NADPH oxidase consists of five glycoprotein subunits—cytochrome b558 which is constitutively present in membrane lipid rafts, and four additional subunits that translocate to lipid rafts on cellular activation (Shao et al 2003). The complex transfers electrons from NADPH to oxygen, generating reactive intermediates that, in turn, can oxidize amino acids, lipids and nucleotides. Patients with chronic granulomatous disease (CGD) manifest defective activity of the NADPH oxidase, and have a clinical course characterized by recurrent bacterial infections (Burg & Pillinger 2001).

Following phagocytosis and activation of a cascade of events leading to pathogen degradation, the resulting fragments are transported from early endosomes to late endosomes. Peptides of non-host derivation that are processed through the endosomal pathway are presented as antigens to T cells. Resting neutrophils express major histocompatibility (MHC) class I molecules on their surface, and contain intracellular stores of MHC class II molecules that bind processed exogenous peptides and facilitate their trafficking to the cell surface, a key characteristic of a professional antigen-presenting cell (Ishikawa & Miyazaki 2005). Neutrophils also contain stores of cathepsins B and D, two lysosomal proteases necessary for antigen presentation (Kimura & Yokoi-Hayashi 1996).

In summary, the interaction of the neutrophil with a pathogen or injured tissue evokes a coordinated response that results in the recognition, uptake, and ultimate destruction of the threat. This process not only contains and eliminates a potentially injurious challenge, but also serves to initiate a specific adaptive immune response, and the subsequent biological processes involved in tissue repair and the resolution of inflammation (Serhan & Savill 2005). Key to the successful evolution of these dynamic imperatives is the capacity of the neutrophil to regulate its survival—to persist in an activated state in the face of an acute challenge, but to involute and die once that challenge has been overcome, and to promote the restoration of normal homeostasis. These twin needs are accomplished through activation, inhibition, and restoration of an endogenous program of controlled cell death, or apoptosis.

The normal biology of neutrophil apoptosis

Apoptosis, or programmed cell death, describes a complex and highly regulated series of enzymatic reactions that result in the controlled degradation of a living cell, and its transformation into membrane-limited apoptotic bodies that are phagocytosed and removed by macrophages. In contrast to necrosis, where cellular degradation is unregulated, with the result that intracellular constituents are released into the environment and evoke a local inflammatory response, apoptotic cell death is non-inflammatory. Not only is the removal of apoptotic bodies accomplished without inducing inflammation, but genes that are anti-inflammatory and reparative are activated in the phagocytosing cell (Savill & Fadok 2000).

The biology of normal apoptosis is shown schematically in Fig. 1. The apoptotic program is activated through one of two principal pathways—the extrinsic and the intrinsic. Stimuli from the extracellular environment can induce apoptosis by binding to cell surface death receptors of the CD95/Fas family, a family that

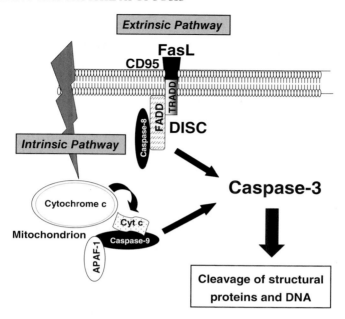

FIG. 1. Apoptosis is initiated by both extrinsic and intrinsic stimuli. The former induce apoptosis through interactions with a receptor of the Fas/CD95 family. Receptor engagement induces oligomerization, and recruits components of the death-inducing signalling complex (DISC), resulting in activational cleavage of caspase 8, which in turn activates caspase 3, leading to the degradation of key cytostructural and nuclear proteins. Activation of the intrinsic pathway results from stimuli that increase mitochondrial permeability, permitting the efflux of cytochrome c into the cytoplasm. Cytochrome c forms a ternary complex with APAF1 and pro-caspase 9—the apoptosome—that results in activational cleavage of caspase 9, which can also activate caspase 3.

includes not only Fas itself, but also the TNF receptor, CD40, and the receptor for nerve growth factor. Engagement of the receptor by its ligand—Fas ligand or TNF, for example—results in receptor trimerization, and the recruitment of adapter proteins such as FADD (Fas-associated death domain) and TRADD (TNF receptor-associated death domain); these interactions create a multi-protein complex known as the DISC (death-inducing signalling complex) that results in autocatalysis and activation of caspase 8. The intrinsic pathway of apoptosis is activated by insults such as ionizing radiation that cause a loss of mitochondrial membrane stability, and that open the mitochondrial transition pore, $\Delta\psi M$. Increased mitochondrial permeability results in the efflux of cytochrome c, which complexes with two cytoplasmic proteins, APAF-1 and pro-caspase 9. This interaction induces cleavage and activation of caspase 9.

Caspases are members of a family of 16 proteolytic enzymes, twelve of which are found in human cells, that are homologous to the prototypic apoptotic gene *Ced-3* of *Caenorhabditis elegans*. The name 'caspase' derives from the fact that each of these is a cysteine protease and cleaves its target proteins adjacent to an aspartic acid residue. Caspases reside in the cell in an inactive form, and are activated either by autocatalysis, or by cleavage by another caspase. The intracellular process of apoptosis is effected through a caspase cascade that culminates with the activation of caspase 3, an enzyme capable of degrading key proteins involved in cell structure and DNA integrity. DNA cleavage into fragments that are multiples of 180 base pairs, producing a characteristic ladder pattern on DNA gel electrophoresis, is the result of the caspase-induced activation of a DNase (Enari et al 1998).

Neutrophils are constitutively apoptotic cells that begin to undergo apoptosis within hours of their release from bone marrow stores, unless that process is subverted through the activation of an anti-apoptotic program (see below). The mechanisms responsible for the constitutive expression of apoptosis are essentially unknown. It has been suggested that interactions between Fas and Fas ligand on the neutrophil surface can spontaneously activate the apoptotic program by activating caspase 8 (Liles et al 1996, Liles & Klebanoff 1995). Alternatively, neutrophils in culture display spontaneous loss of mitochondrial transmembrane potential with activation of caspase 9 (Susin et al 1999, Taneja et al 2004), a state that may be facilitated by the absence of the anti-apoptotic protein Bcl-2 in the mature neutrophil (Iwai et al 1994).

Inhibition of neutrophil apoptosis during inflammation

Although quiescent neutrophils are short-lived, neutrophil activation is associated with prolonged functional survival, enabling the cell to respond to the threat that evoked its activation. Apoptosis is the default state for the neutrophil, and enhanced survival requires the transduction of survival signals, and the transcription of survival genes that block or delay the apoptotic programme.

Cellular mechanisms inhibiting apoptosis

Apoptosis is a tightly regulated process that can be inhibited at multiple steps during its expression. Cleavage of death receptors such as the receptor for TNF from the cell surface results in inhibition of apoptosis in response to environmental stimuli (Smith et al 1997). The activity of the apical caspases of the extrinsic and intrinsic pathways—caspases 8 and 9, respectively—can be inhibited by post-translational modifications. Caspase 8 activity is reduced by either serine/threonine (Alvarado-Kristensson et al 2004) or tyrosine (Cursi et al 2006) phosphorylation. Similarly serine phosphorylation of caspase 9 blocks the formation

TABLE 1 Factors implicated in the inhibition of neutrophil apoptosis

Microbial Products	*Host-derived Mediators*
Endotoxin	Interleukin (IL)1β
Lipoteichoic acid	IL2
Mannan	IL3
Modulins from CONS	IL4
E. coli verotoxin	IL6
Helicobacter pylori surface proteins	IL8
Butyric acid	Tumour necrosis factor
Propionic acid	Interferons
	G-CSF, GM-CSF
Respiratory syncytial virus	Leptin
	Pre-B cell colony enhancing factor
	C5a
	Cathelicidins
Physiological processes	
Transendothelial migration	

of the apoptosome—the complex of pro-caspase 9, cytochrome c, and APAF1—and so inhibits caspase 9-induced apoptosis (Cardone et al 1998, Martin et al 2005). A splice variant of caspase 8, termed caspase 8L (for long), serves as a dominant negative inhibitor of caspase 8 by blocking the recruitment of caspase 8 to FADD (Himeji et al 2002). Finally, a membrane-associated inhibitor of caspase 8, termed FLIP (FLICE-like inhibitory protein) blocks apoptosis by inhibiting the formation of the DISC (Irmler et al 1997, Yang et al 2005).

The intrinsic pathway of apoptosis is inhibited primarily through mechanisms that maintain the normal mitochondrial transmembrane potential, $\Delta\psi M$, and so prevent the efflux of cytochrome c and the assembly of the apoptosome. The Bcl-2 family members, Bcl-2 and Bcl-x_L, serve to inhibit membrane-depolarizing and pro-apoptotic Bcl-2 proteins Bak and Bax (Bouchier-Hayes et al 2005), and so block the intrinsic pathway of apoptosis. Mature neutrophils lack Bcl-2; however, this role is subserved by an additional family member, Mcl-1 (Leuenroth et al 2000). Caspase 9 is serine phosphorylated by Akt, and phosphorylation results in inhibition of catalytic activity (Cardone et al 1998).

Apoptosis can be inhibited by a family of proteins known as inhibitors of apoptosis (IAPs) (Table 1). The eight known members of this family share a baculovirus inhibitory repeat (BIR) domain, so named because of its homology to an anti-apoptotic protein encoded by a baculovirus (Crook et al 1993). The anti-apoptotic mechanisms of IAP family members are complex, and include direct binding to caspases and promotion of protein ubiquitination (Vaux & Silke 2005). Neutrophils express a number of IAPs, including cIAP1, cIAP2, XIAP (Hasegawa et al 2003, O'Neill et al 2004) and survivin (Altznauer et al 2004), their expression being enhanced by anti-apoptotic stimuli such as GM-CSF.

Although the precise mechanisms are unknown, both the Erk/MAP kinase (Gardai et al 2004, Klein et al 2000) and PI3 kinase (Francois et al 2005, Hu & Sayeed 2005) pathways are implicated in signalling for delayed neutrophil apoptosis. Oxidative stress induces, and antioxidants inhibit apoptosis in the neutrophil (Watson et al 1997).

Delayed neutrophil apoptosis in inflammation and clinical sepsis

Microbial products such as endotoxin activate intracellular signalling cascades that prolong neutrophil survival by inhibiting constitutive neutrophil apoptosis. This inhibitory influence is an active process, requiring the transcription and translation of anti-apoptotic proteins. Delayed neutrophil apoptosis in response to a microbial product such as endotoxin or a host-derived anti-apoptotic cytokine such as GM-CSF requires the synthesis and release of IL1β from the neutrophil, and can be prevented by either blocking the transcription of IL1β, or by preventing the binding of IL1β to its receptor (Watson et al 1998). Intriguingly, both LPS and GM-CSF induce the transcription not only of IL1β, but also of the enzyme responsible for activating IL1 by converting pro-IL1 to the mature enzyme; this enzyme—the interleukin 1 converting enzyme—is better known as caspase 1, and was the first identified mammalian homologue of the *C. elegans* gene, *Ced-3*.

The anti-apoptotic activity of IL1, in turn, requires further *de novo* gene expression. Among the genes whose expression is up-regulated in neutrophils by IL1β are heat shock protein 90 (HSP90), Bruton's tyrosine kinase (btk), and pre-colony B cell enhancing factor (PBEF) (Jia et al 2004). PBEF is a highly conserved 52 kDa cytokine-like molecule, first identified as a secreted protein that synergizes with IL1 and stem cell factor to promote the growth and differentiation of pre-B cells (Samal et al 1994). However, PBEF is found in both prokaryotes and eukaryotes (Martin et al 2001), including in invertebrate sponges (Muller et al 1999), suggesting that its biological relevance extends beyond the support of adaptive immunity. Recent work has shown that PBEF exerts multiple influences on cellular energetics, as both an intracellular enzyme and an extracellular cytokine. The predominant intracellular activity of PBEF is as a nicotinamide phosphoribosyl transferase that catalyses the conversion of nicotinamide to nicotinamide mononucleotide (Rongvaux et al 2002), and serves as the rate-limiting step in a pathway of NAD biosynthesis (Bieganowski & Brenner 2004). As an extracellular cytokine-like molecule, PBEF is known to up-regulate pro-inflammatory cytokines in human

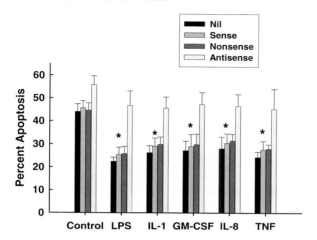

FIG. 2. Prevention of the translation of PBEF by transient transfection of neutrophils with an anti-sense oligonucleotide prevents delayed neutrophil apoptosis in response to a variety of microbial and host-derived stimuli. The anti-sense and non-sense controls have no activity. From (Jia et al 2004).

fetal membranes (Ognjanovic et al 2003). Recently PBEF has also been found to exert activity as an insulin-like molecule, produced by visceral fat, that binds to the insulin receptor, triggering some insulin-like activities, and antagonizing others (Fukuhara et al 2005).

PBEF plays a necessary role in the inhibition of neutrophil apoptosis in response to a wide variety of anti-apoptotic signals, including IL1β (Fig. 2) (Jia et al 2004). PBEF message is maximally up-regulated 10 hours following endotoxin stimulation, and the mechanism of its anti-apoptotic activity is unknown. However, it not only represents a final common pathway to delayed neutrophil apoptosis, but is also highly expressed in neutrophils harvested from critically ill patients with severe sepsis and septic shock (Jia et al 2004).

Delayed neutrophil apoptosis as a therapeutic target in sepsis

Activated neutrophils are cardinal early effectors of innate immune defences, but also an important cause of the inflammatory injury that characterizes sepsis (Smith 1994). Thus neutrophil recruitment and removal at the site of injury or infection must be tightly regulated to optimize host defences whilst minimizing tissue damage (Mayadas & Cullere 2005). Neutrophil-mediated inflammation is terminated primarily through the apoptotic death of the neutrophil. Sustained inflammation results from the targeted disruption of proteins involved in the

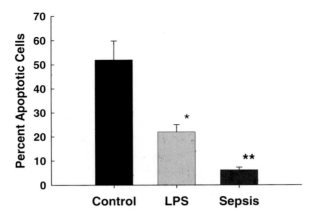

FIG. 3.   Following 24 hours of *in vitro* culture, approximately 50% of neutrophils harvested from healthy volunteers show flow cytometric features of apoptosis. Exposure to endotoxin reduces rates of apoptosis, so that only 20% of cells show the characteristic features. In contrast, neutrophils harvested from the circulation of patients with sepsis show profound inhibition of apoptosis, with only 5 to 10% of cells demonstrating apoptotic features. Adapted from Taneja et al (2004); *$P < 0.05$ vs. control cells; **$P < 0.05$ vs. cells stimulated with endotoxin.

induction of neutrophil apoptosis (Rowe et al 2002), or in the clearance of apoptotic neutrophils (Teder et al 2002, Vandivier et al 2002).

Activated neutrophils induce injury of the lung (Abraham 2003), liver (Ho et al 1996), intestine (Kubes et al 1992) and kidney (Lowell & Berton 1998) in experimental animal models. Their pathological role in human sepsis is less clear, however patients with sepsis exhibit widespread neutrophil infiltration of the lung (Steinberg et al 1994) and distant organs (Goris et al 1985). Moreover, neutrophils harvested from the systemic circulation of patients with sepsis (Jimenez et al 1997, Taneja et al 2004) and from the lungs of patients with the acute respiratory distress syndrome (ARDS) (Matute-Bello & Liles 1997) show profound delays in the normal expression of apoptosis (Fig. 3).

One of the more potent triggers of neutrophil apoptosis is the phagocytosis of microorganisms (Rotstein et al 2000, Watson et al 1996, Yamamoto et al 2002), a stimulus that not only accelerates constitutive apoptosis, but also overcomes the endotoxin-mediated inhibition of apoptosis. Sookhai and colleagues reported that neutrophil-mediated pulmonary lethality in a rodent model of intestinal ischaemia-reperfusion injury could be attenuated by intratracheal instillation of killed *Esherichia coli* (Sookhai et al 2002), suggesting that while microbial products can prolong inflammation, infection itself serves as a physiological stimulus to accelerate its resolution.

Conclusions

Normal interactions between potential pathogens and the host innate immune response are enormously complex. While infection is a threat to the survival of multicellular organisms, the mechanisms that have evolved to counter that threat have frequently involved the incorporation of microbial products into the host genome. Indeed key proteins in innate immunity including heat shock proteins, inhibitor of apoptosis proteins, IL10 and PBEF are all proteins whose origins lie in the prokaryotic or viral world. In its most fully developed form, this interaction is exemplified in the observation that while microbial products inhibit apoptosis, and so permit neutrophils to successfully eradicate viable microorganisms, the final steps of this process—the phagocytosis of the organism—results in the programmed cell death of the neutrophil and the resolution of inflammation.

Acknowledgments

This work was supported in part by a grant from the Canadian Institutes for Health Research.

References

Abraham E 2003 Neutrophils and acute lung injury. Crit Care Med 31:S195–199
Akira S, Uematsu S, Takeuchi O 2006 Pathogen recognition and innate immunity. Cell 124: 783–801
Altznauer F, Martinelli S, Yousefi S et al 2004 Inflammation-associated cell cycle-independent block of apoptosis by survivin in terminally differentiated neutrophils. J Exp Med 199: 1343–1354
Alvarado-Kristensson M, Melander F, Leandersson K, Ronnstrand L, Wernstedt C, Andersson T 2004 p38-MAPK signals survival by phosphorylation of caspase-8 and caspase-3 in human neutrophils. J Exp Med 199:449–458
Athens JW, Haab OP, Raab SO et al 1961 Leukokinetic studies. IV. The total blood, circulating, and marginal granulocyte pools and the granulocyte turnover rate in normal subjects. J Clin Invest 40:989–995
Bieganowski P, Brenner C 2004 Discoveries of nicotinamide riboside as a nutrient and conserved NRK genes establish a Preiss-Handler independent route to NAD+ in fungi and humans. Cell 117:495–502
Bouchier-Hayes L, Lartigue L, Newmeyer DD 2005 Mitochondria: pharmacological manipulation of cell death. J Clin Invest 115:2640–2647
Burg ND, Pillinger MH 2001 The neutrophil: function and regulation in innate and humoral immunity. Clin Immunol 99:7–17
Calvano SE, Xiao W, Richards DR et al 2005 A network-based analysis of systemic inflammation in humans. Nature 437:1032–1037
Cardone MH, Roy N, Stennicke HR et al 1998 Regulation of cell death protease caspase-9 by phosphorylation. Science 282:1318–1321
Crook NE, Clem RJ, Mille LK 1993 An apoptosis-inhibiting baculovirus gene with a zinc finger-like motif. J Virol 67:2168–2174

Cursi S, Rufini A, Stagni V et al 2006 Src kinase phosphorylates Caspase-8 on Tyr380: a novel mechanism of apoptosis suppression. EMBO J 25:1895–1905

Enari M, Sakahira H, Yokoyama H, Okawa K, Iwamatsu A, Nagata S 1998 A caspase-activated DNase that degrades DNA during apoptosis, and its inhibitor ICAD. Nature 391:43–50

Fadok VA, Bratton DL, Konowal A, Freed PW, Westcott JY, Henson PM 1998 Macrophages that have ingested apoptotic cells in vitro inhibit proinflammatory cytokine production through autocrine/paracrine mechanisms involving TGF-beta, PGE2, and PAF. J Clin Invest 101:890–898

Faurschou M, Borregaard N 2003 Neutrophil granules and secretory vesicles in inflammation. Microb Infect 5:1317–1327

Francois S, El Benna J, Dang PM, Pedruzzi E, Gougerot-Pocidal MA, Elbim C 2005 Inhibition of neutrophil apoptosis by TLR agonists in whole blood: involvement of the phosphoinositide 3-kinase/Akt and NF-kappaB signaling pathways, leading to increased levels of Mcl-1, A1, and phosphorylated Bad. J Immunol 174:3633–3642

Fukuhara A, Matsuda M, Nishizawa M et al 2005 Visfatin: a protein secreted by visceral fat that mimics the effects of insulin. Science 307:426–430

Gardai SJ, Whitlock BB, Xiao YQ, Bratton DB, Henson PM 2004 Oxidants inhibit ERK/MAPK and prevent its ability to delay neutrophil apoptosis downstream of mitochondrial changes and at the level of XIAP. J Biol Chem 279:44695–44703

Goris RJ, te Boekhorst TP, Nuytinck JK, Gimbrere JS 1985 Multiple-organ failure. Generalized autodestructive inflammation? Arch Surg 120:1109–1115

Hampton MB, Kettle AJ, Winterbourn CC 1998 Inside the neutrophil phagosome: oxidants, myeloperoxidase, and bacterial killing. Blood 92:3007–3017

Hasegawa T, Suzuki K, Sakamoto C et al 2003 Expression of the inhibitor of apoptosis (IAP) family members in human neutrophils: up-regulation of cIAP2 by granulocyte colony-stimulating factor and overexpression of cIAP2 in chronic neutrophilic leukemia. Blood 101:1164–1171

Hayashi F, Means TK, Luster AD 2003 Toll-like receptors stimulate human neutrophil function. Blood 102:2660–2669

Himeji D, Horiuchi T, Tsukamoto H, Hayashi K, Watanabe T, Harada M 2002 Characterization of caspase-8L: a novel isoform of caspase-8 that behaves as an inhibitor of the caspase cascade. Blood 99:4070–4078

Ho JS, Buchweitz JP, Roth RA, Ganey PE 1996 Identification of factors from rat neutrophils responsible for cytotoxicity to isolated hepatocytes. J Leukoc Biol 59:716–724

Hu Z, Sayeed MM 2005 Activation of PI3-kinase/PKB contributes to delay in neutrophil apoptosis after thermal injury. Am J Physiol Cell Physiol 288:C1171–1178

Irmler M, Thome M, Hahne M et al 1997 Inhibition of death receptor signals by cellular FLIP. Nature 388:190–195

Ishikawa F, Miyazaki S 2005 New biodefense strategies by neutrophils. Arch Immunol Ther Exp (Warsz) 53:226–233

Iwai K, Miyawaki T, Takizawa T et al 1994 Differential expression of bcl-2 and susceptibility to anti-Fas-mediated cell death in peripheral blood lymphocytes, monocytes, and neutrophils. Blood 84:1201–1208

Jia SH, Li Y, Parodo J et al 2004 Pre-B cell colony-enhancing factor inhibits neutrophil apoptosis in experimental inflammation and clinical sepsis. J Clin Invest 113:1318–1327

Jimenez MF, Watson RWG, Parodo J et al 1997 Dysregulated expression of neutrophil apoptosis in the systemic inflammatory response syndrome (SIRS). Arch Surg 132:1263–1270

Kimura Y, Yokoi-Hayashi K 1996 Polymorphonuclear leukocyte lysosomal proteases, cathepsins B and D affect the fibrinolytic system in human umbilical vein endothelial cells. Biochim Biophys Acta 1310:1–4

Klein JB, Rane MJ, Scherzer JA et al 2000 Granulocyte-macrophage colony-stimulating factor delays neutrophil constitutive apoptosis through phosphoinositide 3-kinase and extracellular signal-related kinase pathways. J Immunol 164:4286–4291

Kobayashi SD, Voyich JM, DeLeo FR 2003 Regulation of the neutrophil-mediated inflammatory response to infection. Microbes Infect 5:1337–1344

Kubes P, Hunter J, Granger DN 1992 Ischemia/reperfusion-induced feline intestinal dysfunction: importance of granulocyte recruitment. Gastroenterology 103:807–812

Lee WL, Harrison RE, Grinstein S 2003 Phagocytosis by neutrophils. Microbes Infect 5:1299–1306

Leuenroth SJ, Grutkoski PS, Ayala A, Simms HH 2000 The loss of Mcl-1 expression in human polymorphonuclear leukocytes promotes apoptosis. J Leuk Biol 68:158–166

Liles WC, Klebanoff SJ 1995 Regulation of apoptosis in neutrophils—Fas track to death? J Immunol 155:3289–3291

Liles WC, Kiener PA, Ledbetter JA, Aruffo A, Klebanoff SJ 1996 Differential expression of Fas (CD95) and Fas ligand on normal human phagocytes: Implications for the regulation of apoptosis in neutrophils. J Exp Med 184:429–440

Lowell CA, Berton G 1998 Resistance to endotoxic shock and reduced neutrophil migration in mice deficient for the Src-family kinases Hck and Fgr. Proc Natl Acad Sci USA 95:7580–7584

Martin PR, Shea RJ, Mulks MH 2001 Identification of a plasmid-encoded gene from Haemophilus ducreyi which confers NAD independence. J Bacteriol 183:1168–1174

Martin MC, Allan LA, Lickrish M, Sampson C, Morrice N, Clarke PR 2005 Protein kinase A regulates caspase-9 activation by Apaf-1 downstream of cytochrome c. J Biol Chem 280:15449–15555

Matute-Bello G, Liles WC 1997 Neutrophil apoptosis in acute respiratory distress syndrome. Am Rev Respir Crit Care Med 156:1969–1977

Mayadas TN, Cullere X 2005 Neutrophil beta2 integrins: moderators of life or death decisions. Trends Immunol 26:388–395

McDonald PP, Bald A, Cassatella MA 1997 Activation of the NF-kB pathway by inflammatory stimuli in human neutrophils. Blood 89:3421–3433

Muller WE, Perovic S, Wilkesman J, Kruse M, Muller IM, Batel R 1999 Increased gene expression of a cytokine-related molecule and profilin after activation of Suberites domuncula cells with zenogeneic sponge molecule(s). DNA Cell Biol 18:885–893

Netea MG, Van Der Graaf CA, Vonk AG, Verscheueren I, van der Meer JW, Kullberg BJ 2002 The role of toll-like receptor (TLR) 2 and TLR4 in the host defense against disseminated candidiasis. J Infect Dis 185:1483–1489

O'Neill AJ, Doyle BT, Molloy E et al 2004 Gene expression profile of inflammatory neutrophils: alterations in the inhibitors of apoptosis proteins during spontaneous and delayed apoptosis. SHOCK 21:512–518

Ognjanovic S, Tashima LS, Bryant-Greenwood GD 2003 The effects of pre-B-cell colony-enhancing factor on the human fetal membranes by microarray analysis. Am J Obstet Gynecol 189:1187–1195

Rongvaux A, Shea RJ, Mulks MH et al 2002 Pre-B cell colony-enhancing factor, whose expression is up-regulated in activated lymphocytes, is a nicotinamide phosphoribosyltransferase, a cytosolic enzyme involved in NAD biosynthesis. Eur J Immunol 32:3225–3234

Rotstein D, Parodo J, Taneja R, Marshall JC 2000 Phagocytosis of Candida albicans induces apoptosis of human neutrophils. SHOCK 14:278–283

Rowe SJ, Allen L, Ridger VC, Hellewell PG, Whyte MK 2002 Caspase-1-deficient mice have delayed neutrophil apoptosis and a prolonged inflammatory response to lipopolysaccharide-induced acute lung injury. J Immunol 169:6401–6407

Samal B, Sun Y, Stearns G, Xie C, Suggs S, McNiece I 1994 Cloning and characterization of the cDNA encoding a novel human pre-B-cell colony-enhancing factor. Mol Cell Biol 14:1431–1437

Savill J, Fadok V 2000 Corpse clearance defines the meaning of cell death. Nature 407: 784–788

Savill JS, Wyllie AH, Henson JE, Henson PM, Haslett C 1989 Macrophage phagocytosis of aging neutrophils in inflammation. J Clin Invest 83:865–875

Savill JS, Dransfield I, Gregory C, Haslett C 2002 A blast from the past: clearance of apoptotic cells regulates immune responses. Nat Rev Immunol 2:965–975

Serhan CN, Savill J 2005 Resolution of inflammation: the beginning programs the end. Nat Immunol 6:1191–1197

Shao D, Segal AW, Dekker LV 2003 Lipid rafts determine efficiency of NADPH oxidase activation in neutrophils. FEBS Lett 550:101–106

Smith JA 1994 Neutrophils, host defense, and inflammation: A double-edged sword. J Leuk Biol 56:672–686

Smith MR, Kung H, Durum SK, Colburn NH, Sun Y 1997 TIMP-3 induces cell death by stabilizing TNF-alpha receptors on the surface of human colon carcinoma cells. Cytokine 9:770–780

Sookhai S, Wang JJ, McCourt M, Kirwan W, Bouchier-Hayes D, Redmond HP 2002 A novel therapeutic strategy for attenuating neutrophil-mediated lung injury in vivo. Ann Surg 235:285–291

Steinberg KP, Milberg JA, Martin TR, Maunder RJ, Cockrill BA, Hudson LD 1994 Evolution of bronchoalveolar cell populations in the adult respiratory distress syndrome. Am J Respir Crit Care Med 150:113–122

Susin SA, Lorenzo HK, Zamzami N et al 1999 Mitochondrial release of caspase-2 and -9 during the apoptotic process. J Exp Med 189:381–393

Taneja R, Parodo J, Kapus A, Rotstein OD, Marshall JC 2004 Delayed neutrophil apoptosis in sepsis is associated with maintenance of mitochondrial transmembrane potential (DYM) and reduced caspase-9 activity. Crit Care Med 32:1460–1469

Teder P, Vandivier RW, Jiang D et al 2002 Resolution of lung inflammation by CD44. Science 296:155–158

Vandivier RW, Fadok VA, Hoffmann PR et al 2002 Elastase-mediated phosphatidylserine receptor cleavage impairs apoptotic cell clearance in cystic fibrosis and bronchiectasis. J Clin Invest 109:661–670

Vaux DL, Silke J 2005 IAPs, RINGs and ubiquitylation. Nat Rev Mol Cell Biol 6:287–297

Watson RWG, Redmond HP, Wang JH, Condron C, Bouchier-Hays D 1996 Neutrophils undergo apoptosis following ingestion of Escherichia coli. J Immunol 156:3986–3992

Watson RWG, Rotstein OD, Jimenez M, Parodo J, Marshall JC 1997 Augmented intracellular glutathione inhibits Fas-triggered apoptosis of activated human neutrophils. Blood 89:4175–4181

Watson RWG, Rotstein OD, Parodo J, Bitar R, Marshall JC 1998 The interleukin-1 beta converting enzyme (caspase-1) inhibits apoptosis of inflammatory neutrophils through activation of IL-1b. J Immunol 161:957–962

Weiss SJ 1989 Tissue destruction by neutrophils. N Engl J Med 320:365–376

Yamamoto A, Taniuchi S, Tsuji S, Hasui M, Kobayashi Y 2002 Role of reactive oxygen species in neutrophil apoptosis following ingestion of heat-killed Staphylococcus aureus. Clin exp Immunol 129:479–484

Yang JK, Wang L, Zheng L et al 2005 Crystal structure of MC159 reveals molecular mechanism of DISC assembly and FLIP inhibition. Mol Cell 20:939–949

Yum HK, Arcaroli J, Kupfner J et al 2001 Involvement of phosphoinositide 3-kinases in neutrophil activation and the development of acute lung injury. J Immunol 167:6601–6608

DISCUSSION

Hellewell: I have a question about neutrophil apoptosis in septic patients. Do you think you should be promoting or preventing this?

Marshall: We have to be careful about speculating too much. Like any physiological process, apoptosis has an appropriate context. I don't think these observations can be translated into a single conclusion for a heterogeneous process such as sepsis. Intriguingly, many of the stimuli that inhibit neutrophil apoptosis, induce it in epithelial cells and lymphocytes. The same things that will induce apoptosis in the lymphocyte will inhibit it in the neutrophil. It is highly context dependent.

Choi: You beautifully showed that lipopolysaccharide (LPS) is one of the best inducers of apoptosis in cell culture models. This is why I think broad spectrum caspase inhibitors won't work here. These have been tried in other diseases, and the increase in carcinogenesis in rats could be a real problem. pre-B cell colony-enhancing factor (PBEF) is interesting. Dr Skip Garcia has just identified this from the ventilator induced lung injury model.

Fink: Have you made an antibody to PBEF?

Marshall: There is one commercially available. It has proven very difficult to produce a monoclonal against PBEF, presumably because the protein is quite highly conserved.

Choi: Dr Garcia has identified polymorphism in acute lung injury (ALI) patients, so he is really excited about PBEF.

Fink: Has anyone tried a therapy yet based on PBEF, even with a polyclonal antibody?

Marshall: Not yet. It's a great idea. There is a polyclonal antibody that is commercially available. One of the potential insights that this line of work might provide is to reconcile contradictions in the inflammatory process. LPS is both pro- and anti-apoptotic; TNF is both pro- and anti-apoptotic. TNF induces apoptosis in cancers but is anti-apoptotic in neutrophils. Understanding the complex processes that create scaffolding and signalling structures will be critical to understanding the circumstances under which we want to modulate apoptosis.

Fink: I was struck by one of the numbers you mentioned, which was 10^{11} neutrophils a day. This is a big number, sort of like the cost of the war in Iraq at an hourly rate! When I do a white blood cell count on the patients I take care of, the numbers range from really low (a few thousand) to 30–40 000. It is never a huge number. The differences in the apoptotic rate you showed in the *in vitro* assay were orders of magnitude different. Is it possible that the derangement in apoptosis is actually subserving homeostasis? The bone marrow might not be producing enough of this stuff and the neutrophils could be compensating.

Marshall: That's an excellent question. For that to occur, there would have to be profound inhibition of release or synthesis in bone marrow. I am not aware of anyone having looked at this.

Griffiths: From a clinical perspective, your message was about the mechanisms involved in the recovery of the system from the insult of sepsis.

Singer: Has anyone looked at survival differences? In a patient, does the delay relate to better or worse outcome?

Marshall: Given that a high degree of suppression is so ubiquitous, we have not seen a clear-cut association. There doesn't seem to be a clear association between the inhibition of circulating neutrophil apoptosis and survival.

Singer: The neutrophils we can draw out of a syringe are not the same as the neutrophils that have migrated through the vessel into the parenchyma. Do you know anything about how they behave?

Marshall: The group from Washington have looked at neutrophils from the lungs of patients with acute respiratory distress syndrome (ARDS). One could argue that the ones that are shed from the alveoli aren't the same as those staying in the wall, but they also showed the same changes.

Choi: There are some old data showing that if you take neutrophils from nasal versus bronchoalveolar lavage (BAL), the superoxide production is different. The whole concept is that neutrophils from different sources are different.

Singer: That was my next question. Does a white cell have a certain reservoir? Once it degranulates, is that it? Or can it carry on being active?

Marshall: That's a good question. I don't know the answer.

Fink: I think degranulation is it.

Marshall: But the implication is that the cell lives longer once it has degranulated.

Szabó: What is the result of neutrophil depletion in clinically relevant sepsis models in which antibiotics were used? Does it decrease multiple organ failure? I remember one study that used a neutrophil NADPH oxidase knockout model in mice.

Herndon: That's the smoke inhalation injury model. There's a marked diminution in damage by neutrophil depletion. But subsequent bacterial challenges were not well tolerated.

Singer: Isn't the argument that there are just enough white cells around? In the haematology literature, neutropenia is not a risk factor for worse outcome.

Fink: This brings up an interesting point. Many years ago, the common wisdom was that ARDS in sepsis is a neutrophil-mediated phenomenon. But clinicians who care for cancer patients treated with aggressive chemotherapy were seeing occasional patients with septic shock. Some of these patients didn't have a neutrophil in their body, because of the bone marrow suppression caused by the chemotherapy. Yet some of these patients had florid ARDS.

Choi: This is why we teach the interns in medical schools that neutrophils are not only players but also effectors.

Cohen: Chris Haslett showed this ages ago.

Marshall: A propos of this, the initial stages of ARDS reflect a permeability problem, and if there are abnormalities in the endothelium you don't have to have neutrophils.

Choi: Jim Hogg has published results from a smoking model (Hogg 2006). We all know about smoking and emphysema; he beautifully showed in humans that the ex-smokers had ferocious BAL neutrophilia after giving up. His concept is that whatever stimulated neutrophilia persists even after the stimulus is stopped. This could be extended to sepsis.

Fink: Has anyone looked at the neutrophil compartment in mice that have been manipulated using the strategies that Alfred Ayala talked about, such as Bcl-2 overexpressing mice treated with zymosan? Since there is already an apoptotic defect in the neutrophil compartment, does inhibiting apoptosis make it even worse?

Choi: Scott Worthen published papers a few years ago showing that p38 isoforms are the critical ones for regulating neutrophil cell death and inflammation (Nick et al 1999, Frasch et al 1998). These were landmark papers, because they showed specificity of a cell.

Marshall: Mature neutrophils don't express Bcl-2. It may not be effective.

Fink: They express caspases.

Marshall: In a neutrophil you could inhibit caspase 1 with a pan-caspase inhibitor, and induce neutrophil apoptosis.

Choi: Do they have the other Bcl-2 family members?

Marshall: Yes, they have Bax, Mcl1 and Bad. If we take neutrophils from healthy volunteers, their mitochondrial membrane permeability spontaneously dissipates in culture. If we trigger them with LPS or take neutrophils from patients with sepsis, their mitochondrial transmembrane potential is higher than it is in a normal neutrophil.

Fink: So everything you know about for your garden variety cell, such as a hepatocyte, is turned on its head in the neutrophil.

Ayala: The closest thing I was aware of to the Bcl-2 work was the work of Iwata et al (2003) with a human Bcl myeloid overexpressor. They have observed protection in a model of sepsis with that. We have recapitulated some of this work in our own laboratory, and have found that to really make this work we need antibiotics, or neutrophils hanging around to fight bugs and not endotoxin.

Singer: Is the message I am hearing that the white cell might not be important in the pathophysiology of organ failure, but is important in terms of survival because of bacterial clearance.

Choi: That is too strong. In ARDS, neutrophils in the lung is one of the critical denominators of outcome.

Singer: We were arguing earlier that in terms of the neutropenic patient, where you can't measure the white cells, that they were not so important!

Ayala: This is the exception that proves the rule.

Szabó: There was one paper which used NADPH oxidase knockouts and there was no difference in survival (Nicholson et al 1999).

Choi: They were more susceptible to gp91 phox knockout. Now we know that there are other adaptive proteins that regulate that.

Hellewell: Coming back to this issue of neutropenic patients getting ARDS, I don't remember the studies, but presumably they were looking in the blood. It doesn't mean that the lungs weren't stuffed full of neutrophils.

Choi: That is a good point. Remember that BAL neutrophilia is only a fraction of total neutrophils. The best test for lung neutrophils is MPO.

Hellewell: You don't even need the neutrophils in the air space to cause damage. They can be trapped in the capillaries.

Singer: The point is, they are neutropenic before they become infected.

Hellewell: They are neutropenic because they are immune compromised.

Fink: That is why this is a complicated field. Someone who has an absolute neutrophil count of 500 when they get septic, may get so septic that other pathways of lung injury are activated that are neutrophil-independent. Those data that neutropenia doesn't protect from ARDS are a warning flag, but don't rule out the neutrophil/lung injury hypothesis.

Van den Berghe: If the bone marrow of these patients recovers, they get worse.

Fink: A better example of this is if we treat these patients with white blood cell transfusions, which was a therapeutic strategy 20 years ago, they go from being sick to being sick-unto-death almost instantaneously (Wright et al 1981).

Singer: This is interesting, because our haematologists have a slight penchant for white cell transfusion in certain patients. They don't seem to get obviously sicker.

Fink: They used to!

Griffiths: What happens to these 10^{11} neutrophils? Where are they cleared? Is there any advantage in the system from which they are cleared by not being so loaded?

Marshall: It is hard to know whether there is an advantage. They are cleared in reticuloendothelial beds—the liver and spleen.

Fink: Do the funny shaped nuclei in neutrophils have HMGB1 in them?

Szabó: I don't know. But I know that they don't have PARP.

Fink: If they do have HMGB1 in them, then that's an HMGB load every day that is enormous.

Marshall: It may be cleaved.

Fink: The dogma that has been articulated by Bianchi in Italy is that the fundamental difference between necrosis and apoptosis is that HMGB1 in the nucleus is released in necrosis, and remains bound to the chromatin in apoptosis (Scaffidi et al 2002).

Cavaillon: Where are the macrophages to remove apoptotic neutrophils?

Marshall: They are in the liver, in huge numbers.

Piantadosi: Let's not forget the lung, which has been referred to as the graveyard of neutrophils.

Gilroy: You are assuming that all the cells are cleared in one day. There is some evidence in the literature that there are subpopulations of neutrophils that preferentially go to different sites in the body (Buckley 2006 and references therein). They may not all be cleared at the same time; they may play a surveillance role and persist for longer than 6–8 h.

Marshall: These data come from kinetic studies done in the 1960s with labelled neutrophils, and calculations based on total numbers of neutrophils. The lifespan of the neutrophil means that for this to happen there has to be that degree of turnover. We see numbers that go from 10^{10} to 10^{12}, but given that they are short-lived and that the white cell count remains constant, they have to be turning over.

Hellewell: Another site of removal is the bone marrow. If neutrophils are taken out, labelled with a gamma emitter, and replaced, the bone marrow lights up in whole body scintigraphy.

Ulloa: Our recent studies indicate that splenectomy can improve survival in septic and endotoxaemic mice. We think that the spleen is a major source of immune cells and pro-inflammatory cytokines. I was wondering about the effects of the spleen on neutrophils during sepsis.

Marshall: We try to save the spleen whenever we can.

References

Buckley CD 2006 Identification of a phenotypically and functionally distinct population of long-lived neutrophils in a model of reverse endothelial migration. J Leukoc Biol 79: 303–311

Frasch SC, Nick JA, Fadok VA, Bratton DL, Worthen GS, Henson PM 1998 p38 mitogen-activated protein kinase-dependent and -independent intracellular signal transduction pathways leading to apoptosis in human neutrophils. J Biol Chem 273:8389–8397

Hogg JC 2006 Why does airway inflammation persist after the smoking stops? Thorax 61:96–97

Iwata A, Stevenson VM, Minard A et al 2003 Over-expression of Bcl-2 provides protection in septic mice by a trans effect. J Immunol 171:3136–3141

Nicholson SC, Grobmyer SR, Shiloh MU et al 1999 Lethality of endotoxin in mice genetically deficient in the respiratory burst oxidase, inducible nitric oxide synthase, or both. Shock 11:253–238

Nick JA, Avdi NJ, Young SK et al 1999 Selective activation and functional significance of p38alpha mitogen-activated protein kinase in lipopolysaccharide-stimulated neutrophils. J Clin Invest 103:851–858

Scaffidi P, Misteli T, Bianchi ME 2002 Release of chromatin protein HMGB1 by necrotic cells
    triggers inflammation. Nature 418:191–195
Wright DG, Robichaud KJ, Pizzo PA, Deisseroth AB 1981 Lethal pulmonary reactions associ-
    ated with the combined use of amphotericin B and leukocyte transfusions. N Engl J Med
    304:1185–1189

HMGB1 as a potential therapeutic target

Haichao Wang*†, Wei Li*, Richard Goldstein*†, Kevin J. Tracey† and Andrew E. Sama*

*Department of Emergency Medicine, North Shore University Hospital, New York University School of Medicine and †Feinstein Institute for Medical Research, Manhasset, NY 11030, USA

Abstract. Despite recent advances in antibiotic therapy and intensive care, sepsis remains the most common cause of death in the intensive care units, claiming approximately 225 000 victims annually in the USA alone. The pathogenesis of sepsis is attributable, at least in part, to dysregulated systemic inflammatory responses characterized by excessive accumulation of various proinflammatory cytokines. A ubiquitous nuclear protein, high mobility group box 1 (HMGB1), is released by activated macrophages/monocytes, and functions as a late mediator of lethal endotoxaemia and sepsis. First, circulating HMGB1 levels are elevated in a delayed fashion (after 16–32 h) in endotoxaemic and septic animals. Second, administration of recombinant HMGB1 to mice recapitulates many clinical signs of sepsis, including fever, derangement of intestinal barrier function, lung injury and lethal multiple organ failure. Third, administration of anti-HMGB1 antibodies or inhibitors (e.g. ethyl pyruvate, nicotine, stearoyl lysophosphatidylcholine and Chinese herbs such as *Angelica sinensis*) protects mice against lethal endotoxaemia, and rescues mice from lethal experimental sepsis even when the first doses are given 24 hours after onset of sepsis. Taken together, these experimental data establish HMGB1 as a late mediator of lethal endotoxaemia and sepsis with a wider therapeutic window for the clinical management of lethal systemic inflammatory diseases.

2007 Sepsis—new insights, new therapies. Wiley, Chichester (Novartis Foundation Symposium 280) p 73–91

Innate immune cells (such as macrophages, monocytes and neutrophils) constitute a front line of defence against most microbial infections, and are responsible for killing invading pathogens. If invading pathogens are not effectively eliminated, they can trigger a systemic inflammatory response characterized by the overproduction of various proinflammatory mediators. 'Severe sepsis' refers to an overwhelming systemic inflammatory response to infection, and is defined by signs of organ dysfunction that include abnormalities in body temperature, heart rate, respiratory rate and leukocyte counts. Despite recent advances in antibiotic therapy and intensive care, sepsis is still the most common cause of death in intensive care units, claiming approximately 225 000 victims annually in the USA alone. The pathogenesis of sepsis is attributable, at least in part, to dysregulated systemic inflammatory responses characterized by excessive accumulation of various proinflammatory cytokines (Wang et al 2001).

In response to bacterial toxins (e.g. lipopolysaccharide, LPS), macrophages/monocytes release various proinflammatory cytokines such as tumour necrosis factor (TNF), interleukin (IL)1, interferon (IFN)γ, and macrophage migration inhibitory factor (MIF) (Calandra et al 2000), which individually, or in combination, contribute to the pathogenesis of lethal endotoxaemia or sepsis (Wang et al 2001). Inhibition of the release or activity of individual cytokines can attenuate the development of tissue injury in animal models of endotoxaemia and/or sepsis. For instance, neutralizing antibodies against TNF, the first cytokine elaborated in an inflammatory cascade, reduces lethality in an animal model of endotoxaemic/bacteraemic shock (Tracey et al 1987). However, the early release of TNF makes it difficult to target therapeutically in a clinical setting (Tracey et al 1987), prompting the search for late proinflammatory cytokines that may offer a wider therapeutic window for the treatment of lethal systemic inflammatory diseases.

Recently, we discovered that a ubiquitous protein, high mobility group box 1 (HMGB1), is released by activated macrophages/monocytes (Wang et al 1999, Rendon-Mitchell et al 2003, Chen et al 2004a), and functions as a late mediator of lethal endotoxemia and sepsis (Wang et al 1999, 2004b, 2004c, 2005, Yang et al 2004). In this chapter, we will provide an overview of recent advances in uncovering the extracellular role of HMGB1 as a proinflammatory cytokine, and a late mediator of lethal endotoxaemia and sepsis.

Nuclear HMGB1 as a DNA-binding protein

A non-histone nucleosomal protein was purified from nuclei approximately 30 years ago, and termed 'high mobility group 1' (HMG1) (or high mobility group box 1, HMGB1) based on its rapid mobility on electrophoresis gels (Wang et al 2004c). It is constitutively expressed in quiescent cells, and a large 'pool' of preformed HMGB1 is stored in the nucleus due to the presence of two lysine-rich nuclear localization sequences (Bonaldi et al 2003, Chen et al 2005). As an evolutionarily conserved protein, HMGB1 shares 100% homology (in amino acid sequence) between mouse and rat, and a 99% homology between rodent and human.

HMGB1 contains two internal repeats of positively charged domains ('HMG boxes' known as 'A box' and 'B box') in the N-terminus, and a continuous stretch of negatively charged (aspartic and glutamic acid) residues in the C-terminus (Fig. 1). It is capable of binding chromosomal DNA, and has been implicated in diverse cellular functions, including determination of nucleosomal structure and stability, and binding of transcription factors to their cognate DNA sequences (Muller et al 2004).

1 MGKGDPKK**PRGKMSSYAFFVQTCREEHKKKHPDASVNFSEFSKKCSERWK** **50**
"A Box"

51 **TMSAKEKGKFEDMAKADKARYEREMKTYI**PPKGETKKKFKDPNA**PKRPPS** **100**

101 **AFFLF**CSEYRPKIKGEHPGLSIG**DVAKKLGEMWNNTAADDKQPYEKKAA**K **150**
"*Cytokine Domain*"   *"B Box"*

151 LKEKYEKDIAAYRAKGKPDAAKKGVVKAEKSKKKKEEEEDEEDEEDEEEE **200**
"*RAGE-binding*"

201 EDEEDEDEEEDDDDE **215**

FIG. 1. Amino acid sequence of human HMGB1. The N-terminal portion of HMGB1 comprises two internal repeats of a positively charged domain of about 80 amino acids (termed 'HMG boxes') (shown by bold text). The cytokine-stimulating motif ('Cytokine Domain') of HMGB1 does not overlap with its RAGE-binding site, implicating the potential involvement of other cell surface receptors for HMGB1-mediated inflammatory responses.

Release of HMGB1

Active secretion

In response to exogenous bacterial products (such as endotoxin), macrophage/ monocyte cultures actively release HMGB1 in a time- and dose-dependent manner (Wang et al 1999). The minimal LPS concentrations effective for inducing HMGB1 release are higher than that for inducing early proinflammatory cytokines (e.g. TNF) (Chen et al 2004a), indicating that HMGB1 is released at conditions when LPS levels are relatively high (Table 1).

An innate recognition system consisting of LPS-binding protein (LBP), CD14 and Toll-like receptor 4 (TLR4) enables macrophages/monocytes to sensitively detect bacterial endotoxin, thereby initiating a feed-forwarding cytokine cascade characterized by the sequential release of early (e.g. TNF) and late (e.g. HMGB1) proinflammatory cytokines. The critical role of CD14 in LPS-mediated TNF production is evidenced by the loss of LPS-induced TNF production in CD14-deficient cells (Chen et al 2004a). In contrast, depletion of CD14 expression only partly attenuates LPS-mediated HMGB1 release (Chen et al 2004a), indicating a partial role for CD14 in LPS-induced HMGB1 release (Table 1) (Chen et al 2004a). Despite the fact that CD14 only partly contributes to endotoxin-mediated HMGB1 release, a downstream LPS receptor, TLR4, is still critically important in endotoxin-mediated HMGB1 release, because LPS fails to induce HMGB1 release in TLR4-defective C3H/HeJ murine macrophages (Wang et al 1999).

TABLE 1   Distinct mechanisms underlying endotoxin-induced release of TNF and HMGB1

	TNF	*HMGB1*
Basal expression levels	Low (if any at all) in quiescent macrophages/monocytes	Constitutively expressed in quiescent macrophages/monocytes to maintain a 'pool' of HMGB1 in the nucleus
LPS-induced release	LPS can induce rapid TNF synthesis and secretion (*within 1–2 h*) even at concentrations as low as 1 ng/ml	LPS can induce HMGB1 release (*after 8–16 h*) only at concentrations > 10 ng/ml
Mechanisms of LPS-induced release	(1) CD14-dependent (2) MAP kinase-dependent (3) Secretion via the classical ER–Golgi secretory pathway	(1) Partly CD14-dependent (2) MAPK-independent (3) Acetylation-driven cytoplasmic translocation, followed by cytoplasmic vesicle-mediated release

In addition to exogenous stimuli, endogenous proinflammatory cytokines (such as TNF, IL1β) can also stimulate macrophages, monocytes and pituicytes to actively release HMGB1 (Wang et al 1999). Similarly, IFNγ, an immunoregulatory cytokine known to mediate the innate immune response, dose-dependently induces release of TNF and HMGB1, but not other cytokines such as IL1α, IL1β or IL6 (Rendon-Mitchell et al 2003). The IFNγ-induced HMGB1 release is partially dependent on the induction of TNF, because genetic disruption of TNF expression partially impairs IFNγ-mediated HMGB1 release (Rendon-Mitchell et al 2003). Similarly, inhibition of TNF expression (by gene knockout) or activity (by neutralizing antibodies) partially attenuates LPS-induced HMGB1 release (Chen et al 2004a), indicating a partial role for TNF in LPS-induced HMGB1 release (Table 1). This is not unexpected, because LPS also induces the release of other proinflammatory cytokines (such as IL1β) that individually, or synergistically stimulate(s) macrophages to release HMGB1.

Although bacterial endotoxin activates macrophages to sequentially release early (e.g. TNF) and late (e.g. HMGB1) proinflammatory cytokines, the mechanisms underlying the regulation of early and late cytokines are quite different. TNF is produced in vanishingly small amounts (*if any at all*) in quiescent macrophages, but its synthesis is rapidly up-regulated by LPS, leading to timely secretion via a classical endoplasmic reticulum (ER)–Golgi secretory pathway (Table 1). In contrast to the critical roles of p38 and ERK1/2 MAPK in LPS-induced TNF production, these MAP kinases are not important in LPS-induced HMGB1 release (Chen et al 2004a). Lacking a signal sequence in the N-terminus, HMGB1 cannot be released via the classical endoplasmic ER–Golgi secretory pathway. Instead, activated macrophages/monocytes acetylate HMGB1 at potential nuclear localization sequences, leading to its cytoplasmic translocation and subsequent release into the extracellular milieu (Table 1) (Gardella et al 2002).

Passive leakage

In addition to its active release from innate immune cells, HMGB1 can also be released passively from necrotic or damaged cells (Scaffidi et al 2002, Degryse et al 2001). HMGB1 released by necrotic cells is capable of inducing an inflammatory response, thereby transmitting the 'injury' signal to neighbouring immune cells (Scaffidi et al 2002). For instance, HMGB1 is released quickly after tissue ischaemia/reperfusion injury (Tsung et al 2005), thereby functioning as an inflammatory mediator of tissue injury. However, HMGB1 is not released by apoptotic cells (Scaffidi et al 2002), which disintegrate themselves without setting off an inflammatory response.

Systemic accumulation

The kinetics of HMGB1 accumulation *in vivo* has been studied in murine models of endotoxaemia and sepsis (induced by cecal ligation and puncture, CLP). Serum HMGB1 is first detectable 8 h after the onset of lethal endotoxemia and experimental sepsis, increases to plateau levels from 16–32 h, and remains elevated for at least 72 h (Wang et al 1999, Yang et al 2004). The late appearance of HMGB1 parallels with the onset of animal lethality from endotoxaemia or sepsis, and distinguishes itself from TNF and other early proinflammatory cytokines (Wang et al 2001). In septic patients, serum HMGB1 levels are elevated, and are significantly higher in non-surviving septic patients as compared to survivors (Wang et al 1999).

In an animal model of haemorrhagic shock, circulating HMGB1 levels are significantly increased, and agents (e.g. adrenomedullin and adrenomedullin-binding protein) capable of attenuating systemic HMGB1 accumulation confer protection against haemorrhagic injury (Cui et al 2005). Similarly, serum HMGB1 levels increase significantly in a patient with haemorrhagic shock, and return toward basal levels as the clinical condition improves (Ombrellino et al 1999). The mechanisms of HMGB1 release in the absence of infection remain elusive, but are possibly attributable to active release from immune cells, as well as passive leakage from damaged and dying cells (Wang et al 2001). Therefore, HMGB1 might be a critical molecule that allows innate immune cells to respond to both infection and injury, thereby triggering a rigorous inflammatory response.

HMGB1 binding of cell surface receptors

Once released, extracellular HMGB1 binds to the receptor for advanced glycation end products (RAGE), and the Toll-like receptor 4 (TLR4), and activates MAP kinase- and NF-κB-dependent signalling pathways (Li et al 2003, Park et al 2003a). As a member of the immunoglobulin superfamily of cell surface molecules, RAGE can bind a diverse group of ligands including advanced glycation end products (AGEs) and HMGB1. Engagement of RAGE with HMGB1 activates mitogen-activated protein kinase (MAPK) and NF-κB (Huttunen & Rauvala 2004), and induces production of various proinflammatory cytokines. The important role of RAGE in HMGB1-induced cytokine production has been supported by the notion that disruption of RAGE expression partially attenuates HMGB1-induced production of proinflammatory cytokines (Kokkola et al 2005).

Accumulating evidence supports the potential involvement of other cell surface receptors (e.g. TLR2 and/or TLR4) in HMGB1-mediated activation of innate immune cells (Park et al 2003b,Yu et al 2004). Consistently, TLR4-defective (C3H/HeJ) mice are more resistant to HMGB1-mediated ischaemic injury (Tsung et al 2005), supporting an important role for TLR4 in HMGB1-mediated inflammatory responses.

Extracellular HMGB1 as a proinflammatory cytokine

Induction of proinflammatory cytokines

HMGB1 stimulates macrophages, monocytes, and neutrophils to release proinflammatory cytokines (Fig. 2) (e.g. TNF, IL1, IL6, IL8 and MIP1) (Andersson et al 2000, Li et al 2003, Park et al 2003a). MAP kinases play important roles in HMGB1-mediated cytokine production, because recombinant HMGB1 induces phosphorylation of p38 and JNK MAP kinases (Li et al 2003), the inhibition of which abrogates HMGB1-mediated production of proinflammatory cytokines (Park et al 2003a). Similarly, in response to HMGB1 stimulation, human microvascular endothelial cells increase the expression of intracellular adhesion molecule 1 (ICAM1), vascular adhesion molecule 1 (VCAM1), proinflammatory cytokines (e.g. TNF), and chemokines (e.g. IL8) (Fiuza et al 2003), suggesting that HMGB1 can propagate an inflammatory response in the endothelium during infection or injury.

Intratracheal administration of HMGB1 induces lung neutrophil infiltration, local production of proinflammatory cytokines (e.g. IL1 and TNF), and acute lung

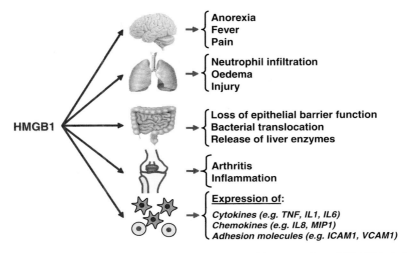

FIG. 2. HMGB1 mediates proinflammatory responses. Administration of HMGB1 via intre-cerebroventricular, intratracheal, intraperitoneal and intraarticular routes induces marked inflammatory responses, and activates various innate immune cells.

injury (Fig. 2) (Abraham et al 2000, Ueno et al 2004). Intracerebroventricular application of HMGB1 induces brain TNF and IL6 production, and sickness behaviours such as anorexia and taste aversion (Agnello et al 2002). Focal administration of HMGB1 near the sciatic nerve induces unilateral and bilateral low threshold mechanical allodynia (Chacur et al 2001). Finally, intraperitoneal injection of HMGB1 increases ileal mucosal permeability, leading to bacterial translocation to mesenteric lymph nodes (Sappington et al 2002). Considered together, these studies indicate that accumulation of HMGB1 can amplify the cytokine cascade, and mediate injurious inflammatory responses.

Although excessive HMGB1 may be pathogenic, low levels of HMGB1 might still be beneficial. For instance, HMGB1 is capable of attracting stem cells (Palumbo et al 2004), and may be needed for tissue repair and regeneration. A recent study demonstrated that HMGB1 facilitates myocardial cell regeneration after myocardial infarction, and consequently improves myocardial function (Limana et al 2005). Therefore, like other proinflammatory cytokines, there may be protective advantages of extracellular HMGB1 when released at low amounts (Li et al 2006).

Innate recognition of bacterial CpG-DNA

An innate recognition consisting of HMGB1 and TLR9 has recently been implicated in the innate recognition of CpG motif-containing bacterial DNA. First,

HMGB1 colocalizes with TLR9 and CpG-DNA in cytoplasmic vesicles of macrophage cultures (Ivanov et al 2006). Second, recombinant HMGB1 efficiently augments CpG DNA-driven cytokine production in macrophage cultures. Finally, depletion of HMGB1 expression significantly impairs CpG DNA-induced production of TNF, IL6 and IL12, as well as inducible nitric oxide synthase (iNOS) (Ivanov et al 2006). It thus appears that innate immune cells have evolved a mechanism to utilize HMGB1 to detect low levels of bacterial DNA, thereby initiating a rigorous inflammatory response.

Extracellular HMGB1 as a late mediator of lethal endotoxemia and sepsis

Suppression of HMGB1 activities

The important role of HMGB1 as a late mediator of lethal endotoxemia and sepsis (induced by CLP) has been established using HMGB1-specific neutralizing antibodies (Fig. 3). Administration with a single dose of HMGB1-specific antibodies

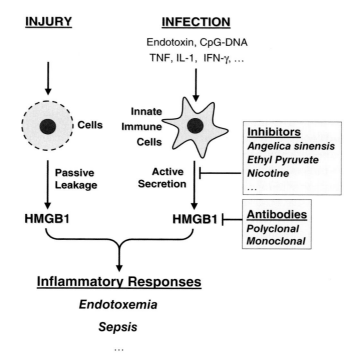

FIG. 3.   Schematic summary of recent developments in pharmacological inhibition of the HMGB1 release and action. In addition to HMGB1-specific antibodies, a number of HMGB1 inhibitors have been shown to be protective in animal models of endotoxaemia and sepsis.

30 min before an LD_{100} dose of LPS did not significantly improve animal survival rate (Wang et al 1999). Additional doses of HMGB1-specific antibodies (+12, +36 h post endotoxemia) dose-dependently improve animal survival (from 0% to 70%, $P < 0.05$) (Wang et al 1999).

Although endotoxaemia is useful to investigate the complex cytokine cascades, more clinically relevant animal models are necessary to investigate the pathogenic role of HMGB1 in lethal sepsis. One well-characterized, standardized animal model of sepsis is induced by CLP. In light of the late and prolonged kinetics of HMGB1 accumulation in experimental sepsis (Yang et al 2004), we reasoned that it might be possible to rescue mice from lethal sepsis even if HMGB1-specific antibodies are administered after the onset of sepsis. The first dose of the HMGB1-specific antibodies were given 24 h after the onset of sepsis, a time point at which mice developed clear signs of sepsis (including lethargy, diarrhoea, piloerection). Repeated administration of HMGB1-specific antibodies beginning 24 h *after* the onset of sepsis (followed by two additional doses at +24, +36 h post sepsis) significantly increased animal survival rate from ~30% to ~70% ($P < 0.05$), indicating a pathogenic role for HMGB1 in experimental sepsis (Fig. 3) (Yang et al 2004).

Suppression of HMGB1 release

The discovery of HMGB1 as a late mediator of lethal systemic inflammation has initiated a new field of investigation for the development of experimental therapeutics. The search for potential therapeutic agents capable of inhibiting HMGB1 release has been fruitful. An increasing number of agents (ethyl pyruvate, stearoyl lysophosphatidylcholine, nicotine, anti-IFNγ antibodies, green tea and Chinese herbs) have shown efficacy in inhibiting bacterial endotoxin-induced HMGB1 release, and protecting animals against lethal endotoxaemia and sepsis (Ulloa et al 2002, Wang et al 2004b, 2004a, Yan et al 2004, Chen et al 2005, 2006, Yin et al 2005).

Acetylcholine and nicotine. For instance, acetylcholine, a neurotransmitter of the vagus nerve, has recently been shown to attenuate LPS-induced production of various proinflammatory cytokines (Borovikova et al 2000). Nicotine, a selective cholinergic agonist of acetylcholine, inhibits LPS-induced HMGB1 release, and confers protection against lethal endotoxaemia and sepsis (Wang et al 2004b), indicating that agents capable of inhibiting HMGB1 release may hold potential in the treatment of lethal sepsis.

Lysophosphatidylcholine (LPC). Stearoyl LPC has recently been suggested to be protective against experimental sepsis by stimulating neutrophils (*but not macrophages*) to destroy ingested bacteria in an H_2O_2-dependent mechanism (Yan et al 2004).

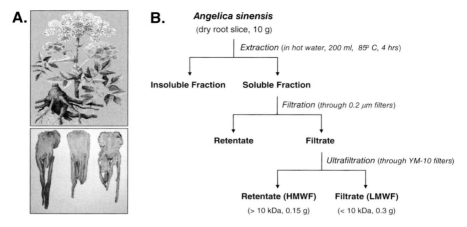

FIG. 4. *Angelica sinensis.* The genus name *Angelica* comes from the Greek word *angelikós,* meaning angelic, whereas the species name *sinensis* is a Latin word derived from the Greek *Sĩnai,* meaning Chinese people. *Angelica sinensis* is a fragrant perennial herb with a branched taproot (Panel A, top). Slices of *Angelical sinensis* root (Panel A, bottom) were extracted in hot water, and the water-soluble fraction was cleared sequentially by centrifugation and filtration (through 0.2μm filter). The clear filtrate was subsequently size-fractionated into a low (<10 kDa) and high (>10 kDa) molecular weight fraction.

However, it also confers protection against lethal endotoxaemia (Yan et al 2004), implying that it may exert protective effects through additional bactericidal-independent mechanisms (Wang et al 2004a). We discovered that repeated administration of stearoyl (but not caproyl or lauroyl) LPC, significantly attenuated systemic HMGB1 accumulation in endotoxemia and sepsis (Chen et al 2005). Together, the parallel capacity of stearoyl LPC to simultaneously enhance neutrophils' bactericidal activities (Yan et al 2004) and attenuate systemic HMGB1 levels, strengthens the notion that the pathogenesis of sepsis is attributable to both invading pathogens, and excessive accumulation of 'late' proinflammatory cytokines (such as HMGB1).

Chinese herbs. A Chinese herb, Dang Gui (also known as Dong Quai, or *Angelica sinensis*) is often referred to as the female ginseng because of its clinical use for gynecological disorders such as abnormal, painful menstruation (dysmenorrhea) (Fig. 4) (Wang et al 2006). We discovered that a low (<10 kDa) molecular weight fraction of *A. sinensis* extract significantly attenuated endotoxin-induced HMGB1 release, and protected mice against lethal endotoxemia (Wang et al 2006). Furthermore, in an animal model of sepsis induced by CLP, delayed administration of *A. sinensis* extract beginning 24 h after CLP rescues mice from lethal sepsis (Wang et al 2006). In light of our observation that delayed administration of *A. sinensis* extract significantly attenuated systemic accumulation of HMGB1 (but not TNF or nitric oxide), we propose that *A. sinensis* rescues mice from lethal sepsis partly by attenuating systemic HMGB1 accumulation. At present, there are not many pro-inflammatory mediators that can be targeted late in the course of experimental sepsis to rescue mice from lethality. For instance, anti-MIF antibodies are protective only if administered within 8 h of the onset of sepsis (Calandra et al 2000). With continuous increase in the consumption of botanical supplements in the USA, it might be beneficial to explore the therapeutic potential of *A. sinensis* in the clinical management of human sepsis and other inflammatory diseases in future studies.

Conclusions

Despite recent advances in antibiotic therapy and intensive care, sepsis remains a widespread problem in critically ill patients. The high mortality of sepsis is in part mediated by bacterial endotoxin, which stimulates macrophages/monocytes to sequentially release early (e.g. TNF, IL1 and IFNγ) and late (e.g. HMGB1) pro-inflammatory cytokines. Our discovery of HMGB1 as a late mediator of lethal systemic inflammation has initiated a new field of investigation for development of experimental therapeutics. The downstream or 'late' action of HMGB1 is a marked departure from the early activities of TNF and other classical proinflammatory cytokines. With limited efficacy from available treatment for septic patients (e.g. the 'early goal directed therapy', and the use of activated protein C), other agents capable of inhibiting late-acting, clinically accessible mediators (such as HMGB1) are needed for the clinical management of lethal systemic inflammatory diseases.

Acknowledgements

The studies summarized in this review were supported in part by the National Institutes of Health, National Institute of General Medical Science (R01GM063075, R01GM070817 to HW).

References

Abraham E, Arcaroli J, Carmody A, Wang H, Tracey KJ 2000 HMG-1 as a mediator of acute lung inflammation. J Immunol 165:2950–2954

Agnello D, Wang H, Yang H, Tracey KJ, Ghezzi P 2002 HMGB1, a DNA-binding protein with cytokine activity, induces brain TNF and IL-6 production, and mediates anorexia and taste aversion. Cytokine 18:231–236

Andersson U, Wang H, Palmblad K et al 2000 High mobility group 1 protein (HMG-1) stimulates proinflammatory cytokine synthesis in human monocytes. J Exp Med 192:565–570

Bonaldi T, Talamo F, Scaffidi P et al 2003. Monocytic cells hyperacetylate chromatin protein HMGB1 to redirect it towards secretion. EMBO J 22:5551–5560

Borovikova LV, Ivanova S, Zhang M et al 2000 Vagus nerve stimulation attenuates the systemic inflammatory response to endotoxin. Nature 405:458–462

Calandra T, Echtenacher B, Roy DL et al 2000 Protection from septic shock by neutralization of macrophage migration inhibitory factor. Nat Med 6:164–170

Chacur M, Milligan ED, Gazda LS et al 2001 A new model of sciatic inflammatory neuritis (SIN): induction of unilateral and bilateral mechanical allodynia following acute unilateral peri-sciatic immune activation in rats. Pain 94:231–244

Chen G, Li J, Ochani M et al 2004a Bacterial endotoxin stimulates macrophages to release HMGB1 partly through CD14- and TNF-dependent mechanisms. J Leukoc Biol 76:994–1001

Chen G, Li J, Qiang X et al 2005 Suppression of HMGB1 release by stearoyl lysophosphatidyl-choline: an additional mechanism for its therapeutic effects in experimental sepsis. J Lipid Res 46:623–627

Chen X, Li W, Wang H 2006 More tea for septic patients?—Green tea may reduce bacterial endotoxin-induced release of high mobility group box 1 and other proinflammatory cytokines. Med Hypotheses 66:660–663

Cui X, Wu R, Zhou M et al 2005 Adrenomedullin and its binding protein attenuate the proin-flammatory response after hemorrhage. Crit Care Med 33:391–398

Degryse B, Bonaldi T, Scaffidi P et al 2001 The high mobility group (HMG) boxes of the nuclear protein HMG1 induce chemotaxis and cytoskeleton reorganization in rat smooth muscle cells. J Cell Biol 152:1197–1206

Fiuza C, Bustin M, Talwar S et al 2003 Inflammation-promoting activity of HMGB1 on human microvascular endothelial cells. Blood 101:2652–2660

Gardella S, Andrei C, Ferrera D et al 2002 The nuclear protein HMGB1 is secreted by mono-cytes via a non-classical, vesicle-mediated secretory pathway. EMBO Rep 3:955–1001

Huttunen HJ, Rauvala H 2004 Amphoterin as an extracellular regulator of cell motility: from discovery to disease. J Intern Med 255:351–366

Ivanov S, Dragoi A-M, van Essen D et al 2006 HMGB1 is a cofactor for TLR9 in mediating cellular responses to immunostimulatory DNA. Blood (submitted)

Kokkola R, Andersson A, Mullins G et al 2005 RAGE is the major receptor for the proinflam-matory activity of HMGB1 in rodent macrophages. Scand J Immunol 61:1–9

Li J, Kokkola R, Tabibzadeh S et al 2003 Structural basis for the proinflammatory cytokine activity of high mobility group box 1. Mol Med 9:37–45

Li W, Sama AE, Wang H 2006 Role of HMGB1 in cardiovascular diseases. Curr Opin Phar-macol 6:130–135

Limana F, Germani A, Zacheo A et al 2005 Exogenous high-mobility group box 1 protein induces myocardial regeneration after infarction via enhanced cardiac C-Kit+ cell prolifera-tion and differentiation. Circ Res 97:e73–83

Muller S, Ronfani L, Bianchi ME 2004 Regulated expression and subcellular localization of HMGB1, a chromatin protein with a cytokine function. J Intern Med 255:332–343

Ombrellino M, Wang H, Ajemian MS et al 1999 Increased serum concentrations of high-mobility-group protein 1 in haemorrhagic shock [letter]. Lancet 354:1446–1447

Palumbo R, Sampaolesi M, De Marchis F et al 2004 Extracellular HMGB1, a signal of tissue damage, induces mesoangioblast migration and proliferation. J Cell Biol 164:441–449

Park JS, Arcaroli J, Yum HK et al 2003a Activation of gene expression in human neutrophils by high mobility group box 1 protein. Am J Physiol Cell Physiol 284:C870–879

Park JS, Svetkauskaite D, He Q et al 2003b Involvement of TLR 2 and TLR 4 in cellular activa-tion by high mobility group box 1 protein (HMGB1). J Biol Chem 279:7370–7377

Rendon-Mitchell B, Ochani M, Li J et al 2003 IFN-γ induces high mobility group Box 1 protein release partly through a TNF-dependent mechanism. J Immunol 170:3890–3897

Sappington PL, Yang R, Yang H et al 2002 HMGB1 B box increases the permeability of Caco-2 enterocytic monolayers and causes derangements in intestinal barrier function in mice. Gastroenterology 123:790–802

Scaffidi P, Misteli T, Bianchi ME 2002 Release of chromatin protein HMGB1 by necrotic cells triggers inflammation. Nature 418:191–195

Tracey KJ, Fong Y, Hesse DG et al 1987 Anti-cachectin/TNF monoclonal antibodies prevent septic shock during lethal bacteraemia. Nature 330:662–664

Tsung A, Sahai R, Tanaka H et al 2005 The nuclear factor HMGB1 mediates hepatic injury after murine liver ischemia-reperfusion. J Exp Med 201:1135–1143

Ueno H, Matsuda T, Hashimoto S et al 2004 Contributions of high mobility group box protein in experimental and clinical acute lung injury. Am J Respir Crit Care Med 170:1310–1316

Ulloa L, Ochani M, Yang H et al 2002 Ethyl pyruvate prevents lethality in mice with established lethal sepsis and systemic inflammation. Proc Natl Acad Sci USA 99:12351–12356

Wang H, Bloom O, Zhang M et al 1999 HMG-1 as a late mediator of endotoxin lethality in mice. Science 285:248–251

Wang H, Yang H, Czura CJ, Sama AE, Tracey KJ 2001 HMGB1 as a late mediator of lethal systemic inflammation. Am J Respir Crit Care Med 164:1768–1773

Wang H, Czura CJ, Tracey KJ 2004a Lipid unites disparate syndromes of sepsis. Nat Med 10:124–125

Wang H, Liao H, Ochani M et al 2004b Cholinergic agonists inhibit HMGB1 release and improve survival in experimental sepsis. Nat Med 10:1216–1221

Wang H, Yang H, Tracey KJ 2004c Extracellular role of HMGB1 in inflammation and sepsis. J Intern Med 255:320–331

Wang H, Li W, Li J et al 2006 The aqueous extract of a popular herbal nutrient supplement, Angelica sinensis, protects mice against lethal endotoxemia and sepis. J Nutr 136:360–365

Yan JJ, Jung JS, Lee JE et al 2004 Therapeutic effects of lysophosphatidylcholine in experimental sepsis. Nat Med 10:161–167

Yang H, Ochani M, Li J et al 2004 Reversing established sepsis with antagonists of endogenous high-mobility group box 1. Proc Natl Acad Sci USA 101:296–301

Yin K, Gribbin E, Wang H 2005 Interferon-gamma inhibition attenuates lethality after cecal ligation and puncture in rats: implication of high mobility group box 1. Shock 24:396–401

Yu M, Li J, Yang L et al 2004 HMGB1 signals through Toll-like receptor 2. Shock 21 [suppl 2]:14

DISCUSSION

Hellewell: Could you say something about how HMGB1 acts on cells?

Wang: So far this protein uses multiple cell surface receptors, including RAGE, Toll-like receptor 2 (TLR2) and TLR4 to induce the production of various chemokines and cytokines in many kinds of cells.

Radermacher: You mainly mentioned CLP models and lipopolysaccharide (LPS) challenges. You mentioned the analogy to green tea, which is a very good peroxynitrite scavenger. Have you ever looked at nitrosative stress and oxygen radical stress in your models? Is blockade of the molecule as efficient in models more like ischaemia/reperfusion?

Wang: We haven't look at this yet in detail. Many antioxidants can probably attenuate formation of many free radicals. We don't have any idea whether the formation of free radicals leads to the subsequent release of HMGB1.

Fink: I can address this question partially. Alan Tsung and Tim Billiar and others, including me, published a recent paper showing in a mouse model of partial hepatic ischaemia/reperfusion that anti-HMGB1 antibodies are remarkably protective (Tsung et al 2005). In another paper, pre-treatment of mice with a tiny dose of HMGB1 prior to ischaemia/reperfusion was found to protect them (Izuishi et al 2006). It is a complicated story.

Szabó: I remember seeing that if you put HMGB1 on cells, it induces the release of TNF. You said this could be a mechanism to explain the pathophysiological role of HMGB1. But we know that *in vivo*, in sepsis, TNF comes first and HMGB1 comes later. From the *in vivo* situation it is unlikely that HMGB1 is triggering the TNF; it is probably the other way around. If you just take a cell and put HMGB1 on top of it, do you see any cell death? Do you see suppression of respiration? Do the cells have trouble dealing with this HMGB1 load? Or if you inject the HMGB1 into animals, is there any sickness?

Wang: So far we have only used HMGB1 to stimulate innate immune cells such as macrophages and monocytes. We first did this because we had these cells in the lab. We were looking to understand whether HMGB1 kills cells by necrosis and apoptosis, and we found that it couldn't kill cells by itself. The direct cytokine-stimulating activity of HMGB1 may not be the major cause for the pathogenesis of experimental sepsis. Recombinant HMGB1 protein has to be given in large amounts to kill animals. However, if you give a small amount of LPS and HMGB1 protein together, it can kill animals very effectively. This is more relevant, because HMGB1 can be released actively from innate immune cells and passively from injured cells, and orchestrate a rigorous inflammatory response particularly in synergy with bacterial products (such as LPS or CpG-DNA).

Szabó: Does it correlate with the severity of sepsis?

Wang: There are some unpublished results on this.

Fink: The human data from the GeNIMS study raise more questions than they answer. There is a difference between survivors and non-survivors in HMGB1 levels, which are higher in the non-survivors. But there are people, who go home feeling fine with persistently high levels of HMGB1, and 30–60 days later the HMGB1 levels are still high. It is unclear what is going on. It could be refractoriness or tolerance to HMGB1, or the stuff that we are measuring in a Western blot may not be biologically reactive.

Choi: I was intrigued by the binding to chromatin. Is there any cross-talk with HDACs? Why did you choose that band?

Wang: We looked at all the bands, and could only identify a few.

Fink: Are other bands important?

Wang: Yes. One of the bands turned out to be the macrophage migration inhibitory factor, MIF.

Marshall: Which was the one at 42 kDa? This was very strong.

Wang: The N-terminal segment of this 42 Da band is blocked perhaps by acetylation, so we don't know what this is

Fink: The histone deacetylase question is very important. A few years ago, Bianchi reported that the export phenomenon from the nucleus involves the hyperacetylation of some key lysine residues on HMGB1 (Bonaldi et al 2003). The regulation of HMGB1 secretion is a twofold process. First of all, HMGB1 is going back and forth between the cytosol and the nucleus. The nuclear localization sequence involves these lysine residues. When HMGB1 gets hyperacetylated, it can't get back into the nucleus any more and accumulates in the cytosol. Then there is some other signal, because it doesn't have a leader sequence, that tells it to get out of the cell. We recently published data showing the way that it gets out of the cell is by being packaged in exosomes (Liu et al 2006). The immunohistochemistry pictures of Hi-Chao Wang showed that it is not diffuse cytosolic staining, but in little balls, which we think are exosomes.

Choi: What regulates this may be a critical factor in knowing the mechanism of function. It makes it so inefficient for a cell for these molecules to go into the nucleus, do their thing and come out. What regulates going out of the cell? There may be another class of proteins that does this.

Fink: Absolutely. This group is familiar with the danger signal hypothesis of Polly Matzinger. The idea is that the immune system doesn't work by recognizing self versus non-self, but rather safe versus dangerous. The notion is that there are a whole host of danger signals that are normal intracellular proteins. When they get outside the cell, other cells (particularly innate immune cells) can recognize that.

Choi: You mentioned HSP70. In the cell it is cytoprotective, but when it is extracellular, it does a lot of bad things.

Ulloa: We are publishing a review (Ulloa & Messmer 2006) where we proposed that HMGB1 can be a friend or a foe, because it can induce both protective and detrimental effects. Extracellular HMGB1 appears to represent an immunological marker selected by the innate immune system to recognize tissue damage and initiate reparative responses. For example, HMGB1 induces myocardial regeneration after infarction (Limana et al 2005). However, extracellular HMGB1 also acts as a potent pro-inflammatory cytokine that contributes to the pathogenesis of diverse inflammatory and infectious disorders. In this sense, HMGB1 is a successful therapeutic target in experimental models of ischaemia/reperfusion, acute respiratory distress syndrome, rheumatoid arthritis, sepsis and cancer. A critical challenge will be to identify the molecular bases for such a different potential.

Thiemermann: You mentioned that some anti-inflammatory strategies prevent HMGB1 release, while others, such as COX-2 inhibitors, do not. I'd like to ask more specifically about two other strategies which interest me. These are inhibitors of NF-κB and lysophosphatidylcholine (LPC).

Wang: The only NF-κB inhibitor we have tested is MG132. This was done with macrophage cell cultures, which did not inhibit bacterial endotoxin-induced HMGB1 release. There was a paper last year showing that stearoyl lysophosphatidylcholine can stimulate neutrophils to destroy ingested bacteria by producing hydrogen peroxide (Yan et al 2004). In an animal model for sepsis, CLP, stearoyl lysophosphatidylcholine does show some partial attenuation of HMGB1 release.

Cavaillon: Considering the synergy of HMGB-1 with LPS, can we fit this with a specific receptor? Which one seems most relevant to synergize with the LPS receptor? You mentioned RAGE. Is there another ligand for RAGE that synergizes with LPS? Then you mentioned TLR4. This can't lead to a synergy with LPS. You also mentioned TLR2, which can synergize with LPS-induced signalling. Can you put together a story?

Wang: That's a tough one, and we do not have a clear answer yet. Depending on the environment, it is likely that HMGB1 can bind to different cell surface receptors to trigger inflammatory response. In addition, it may bind and facilitate recognition of other ligands (such as CpG-DNA) by their receptors, thereby mediating a synergistic effect.

Piantadosi: I was curious about the interaction with TLR2 and 4. If this is important in terms of the contribution to either cell death or organ failure, you should see secondary innate responses as a result of this interaction. Is there any evidence for that?

Fink: There is *in vitro*. If we add HMGB1 to macrophages, TNF is released.

Piantadosi: If you take an animal that has had CLP or exposure to live bacteria to the point of HMGB1 release, do you see a secondary phase of responses?

Ulloa: One of the problems is that the experiments are done in macrophages that never saw TNF.

Piantadosi: It could be as simple as further up-regulation of NF-κB in the secondary response, if this is important.

Ulloa: The experiment would be to have macrophages with TNF, remove this TNF and add HMGB1. This would be similar to the situation in animals.

Evans: The structure of HMGB1 is very unusual in that it has this highly acidic C-terminus. Are there any structure–function studies with the molecule, such as mutation of specific residues? One might imagine that HMGB1 has a non-specific effect: when it is released, it can interact with lots of different things. Or is there really a specific interaction with a limited range of receptors?

Fink: All the pro-inflammatory activity resides in the B box portion of the molecule.

Ulloa: The B box is completely outside of the Raid binding site. The Raid binding site also has pro-inflammatory activity.

Van den Berghe: Is HMGB1 acetylated in humans?

Fink: No one knows.

Wang: Bonaldi et al (2003) have found that a portion of the HMGB1 released by human monocytes is acetylated.

Piantadosi: Do other HMGB proteins do the same kind of thing? There is a whole family of them.

Wang: The closest member is HMGB2, which has an amino acid sequence with very high homology to HMGB1. At present, we haven't looked at this, but a group from Japan have used recombinant or native HMGB2. They couldn't see any cytokine activity or tissue injury after intratracheal administration of HMGB2 into mice (Ueno et al 2004).

Singer: What other effects on non-immune cells does HMGB1 have? Has it been given to hepatocytes or endothelial cells?

Wang: Although this protein is present in all kinds of cells, there are several organs in which its expression is very low, such as brain, eye and testis. It may be a protective mechanism by which these critical organs prevent an injurious inflammatory response in case these tissues are injured and HMGB1 is passively released.

Singer: So it doesn't have a direct toxic effect when it is released from white cells?

Fink: No. If you add exogenous HMGB1 to endothelial cells in culture, you activate them and trigger cytokine and chemokine release. If you add exogenous HMGB1 to gut epithelial cells in culture you get hyperpermeability, iNOS induction, NF-κB activation and so forth. If you inject rodents with recombinant HMGB1 you up-regulate iNOS in the liver and cause hepatocellular enzyme leak.

Singer: Is this physiopathological, or pharmacological?

Fink: Who knows?

Ulloa: It is interesting to remember that HMGB1 appears to have a critical physiological role in neuronal differentiation. Also called amphoterin, HMGB1 is expressed in the cellular membrane of neurons and it appears to be involved in neurite outgrowth and neuronal differentiation (Merenmies et al 1991). There are several publications suggesting that HMGB1 has some homology with β-amyloid, can form amyloid fibrils, and it may contribute to Alzheimer's disease (Kallijarvi et al 2001).

Thiemermann: You mentioned so many of the effects of HMGB1 *in vitro* and *in vivo*. I would like to know how many of the effects are dependent on NF-κB because most of the things you just mentioned are driven by activation of NF-κB.

Wang: I don't have an answer to this.

Fink: RAGE signalling is through NF-κB and a bit through ERK1 and ERK2. TLR signalling is through NF-κB. The three known receptors for HMGB1 all have NF-κB as a node in the downstream signalling cascade, so it is probably important.

Radermacher: When you inject NF-κB into rodents it produces the same kinds of cascades as HMGB1. When you take your concentration measurements in the patients and try to extrapolate the amount necessary for producing such a picture in a rodent, do you reproduce the same difference in orders of magnitude for the nitric oxide production between rodents and humans? Or, in other words, is a rodent less sensitive to HMGB1 than a human?

Fink: The way the rodent experiments have been done is to give a bolus dose of HMGB1 intraperitoneally or intravenously Presumably, in response to an infection or LPS it is released more continuously. We haven't done the calculation of what the expected level would be, and we haven't measured what the level is when we give recombinant HMGB1.

Griffiths: Is it possible to produce anti-HMGB1 antibodies?

Ulloa: We have published a review indicating that endogenous antibodies against HMGB1 are found in the serum of patients with pulmonary hypertension, rheumatoid arthritis drug-induced autoimmunity, systemic lupus erythematosus and other autoimmune diseases. Even in the absence of infection, HMGB1 can be released from necrotic cells, injured tissues or activated immune cells, and function as an immunogen in a variety of critical inflammatory and infectious disorders (Ulloa & Tracey 2005).

References

Bonaldi T, Talamo F, Scaffidi P et al 2003 Monocytic cells hyperacetylate chromatin protein HMGB1 to redirect it towards secretion. EMBO J 22:5551–5560

Izuishi K, Tsung A, Jeyabalan G et al 2006 Cutting edge: high-mobility group box 1 preconditioning protects against liver ischemia-reperfusion injury. J Immunol 176:7154–7158

Kallijarvi J, Haltia M, Baumann MH 2001 Amphoterin includes a sequence motif which is homologous to the Alzheimer's β-amyloid peptide (Aβ), forms amyloid fibrils in vitro, and binds avidly to Aβ. Biochemistry 40:10032–10037

Limana F, Germani A, Zacheo A et al 2005 Exogenous high-mobility group box 1 protein induces myocardial regeneration after infarction via enhanced cardiac C-kit+ cell proliferation and differentiation. Circ Res 97:73–83

Liu S, Stolz DB, Sappington PL et al 2006 HMGB1 is secreted by immunostimulated enterocytes and contributes to cytomix-induced hyperpermeability of Caco-2 monolayers. Am J Physiol Cell Physiol 290:C990–999

Merenmies J, Pihlaskari R, Laitinen J, Wartiovaara J, Rauvala H 1991 30-kDa heparin-binding protein of brain (amphoterin) involved in neurite outgrowth. Amino acid sequence and localization in the filopodia of the advancing plasma membrane. J Biol Chem 266: 16722–16729

Tsung A, Sahai R, Tanaka H et al 2005 The nuclear factor HMGB1 mediates hepatic injury after murine liver ischemia-reperfusion. J Exp Med 201:1135–1143.

Ueno H, Matsuda T, Hashimoto S et al 2004 Contributions of high mobility group box protein in experimental and clinical acute lung injury. Am J Respir Crit Care Med 170:1310–1316

Ulloa L, Messmer D 2006 HMGB1 as a friend and foe. Cytokine Growth Factors Rev 17:189–201

Ulloa L, Tracey KJ 2005 The cytokine profile: a code for sepsis. Trends Mol Med 11:56–62

Yan JJ, Jung JS, Lee JE et al Therapeutic effects of lysophosphatidylcholine in experimental sepsis. Nat Med 10:161–167

Poly (ADP-ribose) polymerase activation and circulatory shock

Csaba Szabó

Department of Surgery, UMD NJ-New Jersey Medical School, Newark, NJ 07103, USA

Abstract. Sepsis is associated with increased production of reactive oxidant species. Oxidative and nitrosative stress can lead to activation of the nuclear enzyme poly (ADP-ribose) polymerase (PARP), with subsequent loss of cellular functions. Activation of PARP may dramatically lower the intracellular concentration of its substrate, NAD thus slowing the rate of glycolysis, electron transport and subsequently ATP formation. This process can result in cell dysfunction and cell death. In addition, PARP enhances the expression of various pro-inflammatory mediators, via activation of NF-κB, MAP kinase and AP-1 and other signal transduction pathways. Preclinical studies in various rodent and large animal models demonstrate that PARP inhibition or PAR deficiency exerts beneficial effects on the haemodynamic and metabolic alterations associated with septic and haemorrhagic shock. Recent human data also support the role of PARP in septic shock: In a retrospective study in 25 septic patients, an increase in plasma troponin level was related to increased mortality risk. In patients who died, significant myocardial damage was detected, and histological analysis of heart showed inflammatory infiltration, increased collagen deposition, and derangement of mitochondrial criptae. Immunohistochemical staining for poly(ADP-ribose) (PAR), the product of activated PARP was demonstrated in septic hearts. There was a positive correlation between PAR staining and troponin I; and a correlation of PAR staining and LVSSW. Thus, there is significant PARP activation in animal models subjected to circulatory shock, as well as in the hearts of septic patients. Based on the interventional studies in animals and the correlations observed in patients we propose that PARP activation may be, in part responsible for the cardiac depression and haemodynamic failure seen in humans with severe sepsis. Interestingly, recent studies reveal that the protective effects of PARP inhibitors are predominant in male animals, and are not apparent in female animals. Oestrogen, by providing a baseline inhibitory effect on PARP activation, may be partially responsible for this gender difference.

2007 Sepsis—new insights, new therapies. Wiley, Chichester (Novartis Foundation Symposium 280) p 92–107

Introduction: the poly(ADP-ribose) polymerase activation suicide pathway

Poly(ADP-ribose) polymerase (PARP) is a protein-modifying and nucleotide-polymerizing enzyme which is abundantly present in the nucleus (see Ueda & Hayaishi 1985, Jagtap & Szabó 2005 for review). PARP consists of the DNA-binding N-terminal domain, the central automodification domain and the C-terminal catalytic domain. The DNA-binding domain utilizes two zinc fingers, which recognize breaks in double-stranded DNA. The central, highly conserved domain can be auto-poly-ADP-ribosylated by PARP. The C-terminal catalytic domain is involved in the synthesis of poly(ADP-ribose) polymer. Recent work identifies several isoforms of PARP. For the current review, 'PARP' generally refers to the firstly identified, common isoform (which is now also termed PARP-1).

The obligatory trigger of PARP activation is DNA single strand breaks, which can be induced by a variety of environmental stimuli and free radical/oxidants, most notably hydroxyl radical and peroxynitrite (see below). In response to DNA damage, PARP becomes activated and, using NAD^+ as a substrate, catalyses the building of homopolymers of adenosine diphosphate ribose units. NAD^+ levels regulate an array of vital cellular processes. NAD^+ serves as a cofactor for glycolysis and the tricarboxylic acid cycle, thus providing ATP for most cellular processes. NAD^+ also serves as the precursor for NADP, which acts as a cofactor for the pentose shunt, for bioreductive synthetic pathways, and is involved in the maintenance of reduced glutathione pools. The observation that activation of PARP can lead to massive NAD^+ utilization, and changes in the cellular NAD^+ levels led Berger to propose that consumption of NAD^+ due to DNA damage and activation of PARP can affect cellular energetics and function (Berger et al 1986). In the 1980s, a variety of *in vitro* studies demonstrated that rapid depletion of NAD^+ due to PARP activation lead to cellular ATP depletion and functional alterations of the cell, with eventual cell death. An additional important pathway related to PARP and inflammation goes through the regulation of various inflammatory signal transduction pathways such as AP-1, nuclear factor κB (NF-κB) and MAP kinases, which are regulated by PARP such that PARP inhibition or PARP deficiency is associated with the inhibition of the production of various pro-inflammatory cytokines and chemokines (e.g. Hassa & Hottinger 2002, Hasko et al 2002, Veres et al 2003).

The initial studies on the role of PARP were performed using pharmacological inhibitors of PARP. More recent studies, using cells from PARP knockout animals confirmed the role of the PARP pathway in oxidant-mediated cell injury (overviewed in Virag & Szabó 2002). The mode of cell death by PARP overactivation has been clarified: PARP activation-related cell death is related to the triggering of cell necrosis (rather than apoptosis), which occurs because of the severe energetic crisis of the cell. Pharmacological inhibition of PARP shifts the necrotic cell population into the normal, as well as the apoptotic population, as determined by flow cytometry studies in thymocytes exposed to peroxynitrite or hydrogen peroxide (Virag et al 1998).

Triggers of DNA single-strand breakage and PARP activation in circulatory shock

DNA single-strand breakage is an obligatory trigger of activation of PARP. Peroxynitrite is a labile, toxic oxidant species produced from the reaction of superoxide and nitric oxide (NO). This species, as well as hydroxyl radicals, are the key pathophysiologically relevant triggers of DNA single-strand breakage (overviewed in Virag & Szabó 2002). Endogenous production of peroxynitrite and other oxidants has been shown to lead to DNA single-strand breakage and PARP activation. For example, in immunostimulated macrophages and smooth muscle cells—which simultaneously produce NO and superoxide, and thus peroxynitrite from endogenous sources—DNA single-strand breakage has been demonstrated, and the time course of the strand breakage was shown to parallel the time course of NO and peroxynitrite production (Zingarelli et al 1996). In mammalian cells the process of DNA single-strand breakage by peroxynitrite may not only be a direct result of peroxynitrite interacting with nuclear DNA, but, may also be related, at least in part, to a secondary, endogenous production of oxidants (Virag et al 1998).

There is much evidence that the peroxynitrite–PARP axis plays a role in various forms of systemic inflammation/circulatory shock. These conditions are associated with the enhanced formation of oxyradicals and with the expression of a distinct inducible isoform of NOS, resulting in overproduction of NO. NO and superoxide react to form peroxynitrite, which can be demonstrated in various organs and tissues in animals or humans suffering from various forms of systemic inflammation and shock. In isolated cells and tissues, peroxynitrite is capable of mimicking many of the pathophysiological alterations associated with shock (endothelial and epithelial dysfunction, vascular hyporeactivity and cellular dysfunction), and these alterations are, in part, related to PARP activation (overviewed in Szabó 1996).

The vascular contractile failure associated with circulatory shock is closely related to overproduction of NO within the blood vessels. Expression of the inducible NO synthase within the vascular smooth muscle cells has been implicated in the pathogenesis of vascular hyporeactivity during various forms of shock (overviewed in Szabó 1995). There are also data that suggest that the vascular hyporeactivity may be related to peroxynitrite generation, rather than NO *per se* (Szabó et al 1995). The role of the PARP pathway in vascular alterations associated with circulatory shock has been demonstrated in studies in anaesthetized rats, where inhibition of PARP with 3-aminobenzamide and nicotinamide were able to reduce the suppression of the vascular contractility of the thoracic aorta in *ex vivo* experiments (Szabó et al 1996, Zingarelli et al 1996, Tasatargil et al 2005). Similarly, in a murine model of caecal ligation and puncture, inhibition of PARP with 3-aminobenzamide improved microvascular contractility (Osman 1998). In another study in pigs injected with *Escherichia coli* endotoxin, pretreatment with 3-aminobenzamide eliminated the LPS-induced rise in pulmonary and total respiratory resistance, indicating that PARP activation plays an important role in the changes of lung mechanics associated with endotoxin-induced acute lung injury (Albertini et al 2000).

Peroxynitrite production has been suggested to contribute to endothelial injury in various pathophysiological conditions. Peroxynitrite can impair the endothelium-dependent relaxations (Villa et al 1994, Szabó et al 1997). Data, demonstrating protective effects of 3-aminobenzamide against the development of endothelial dysfunction in vascular rings obtained from rats with endotoxic shock (Szabó et al 1997) suggested that DNA strand breakage and PARP activation occur in endothelial cells during shock and that the subsequent energetic failure reduces the ability of the cells to generate NO in response to acetylcholine-induced activation of the muscarinic receptors on the endothelial membrane. Indeed, several lines of *in vitro* data demonstrate DNA injury, PARP activation and consequent cytotoxicity in endothelial cells exposed to hydroxyl radical generators, or in response to peroxynitrite (e.g. Junod et al 1989, Kirkland 1991).

NO (or a related species, such as peroxynitrite) plays a pathogenetic role in the cellular energetic changes and the related organ dysfunction associated with endotoxic shock. Peroxynitrite-induced activation of the PARP pathway has also been implicated in the pathophysiology of the cellular energetic failure associated with endotoxin shock by demonstration of increased DNA strand breakage, decreased intracellular NAD^+ and ATP levels and mitochondrial respiration in peritoneal macrophages obtained from rats subjected to endotoxin (Zingarelli et al 1996). This cellular energetic failure was reduced by pretreatment of the animals with the PARP inhibitors 3-aminobenzamide or nicotinamide (Zingarelli et al 1996). Importantly, a recent study, using clinical samples has confirmed the crucial importance of PARP activation in the pathogenesis of mitochondrial respiration and vascular dysfunction associated with sepsis. Human umbilical vein endothelial cells were incubated with serum from healthy controls, patients with septic shock, and critically ill patients who were not septic. Endothelial cell mitochondrial respiration was significantly depressed by septic serum, which was abolished by pretreatment with the PARP inhibitor 3-aminobenzamide (Boulos et al 2003).

In an endotoxic shock model in the rat, inhibition of PARP with 1,5-dihydroxy-isoquinoline resulted in a small protective effect (Wray et al 1998), whereas the PARP inhibitor PJ34 resulted in significant protection against liver and kidney dysfunction in endotoxic shock in the rat (Jagtap et al 2002, Soriano et al 2002). 5-aminoisoquinolinone, a water-soluble, potent PARP inhibitor, significantly reduced the circulating aspartate aminotransferase, alanine aminotransferase and γ-glutamyltransferase levels (indicators of liver injury and dysfunction) in haemor-rhagic shock (McDonald et al 2000).

PARP activation appears to play a significant role in the renal failure associated with various forms of shock: both pharmacological inhibition of PARP and genetic inactivation of PARP provides significant protection against the shock-associated increases in circulating blood urea nitrogen (BUN) and creatinine levels in various forms of shock (Jagtap et al 2002, McDonald et al 2000). Similarly, the acute respiratory distress syndrome and lung dysfunction associated with circulatory shock of various aetiologies is markedly attenuated by PARP inhibition or PARP deficiency (Liaudet et al 2002, Shimoda et al 2003). Finally, there is a clear and pronounced protection by PARP inhibition against the shock-induced intestinal epithelial permeability changes as well. Both in endotoxic shock in rats and mice, inhibition of PARP activation by 3-aminobenzamide or by PJ34 protects against the intestinal hyperpermeability, and so does genetic depletion of PARP in hemor-rhagic shock (Jagtap et al 2002, Liaudet et al 2000). Similar protective effects of PARP inhibitors have been reported in splanchnic occlusion shock models (Cuzzocrea et al 1997, DiPaola et al 2005). Finally, the endotoxin- or sepsis-induced depression of the myocardial contractility is dependent on PARP activa-tion (Pacher et al 2002, Goldfarb et al 2002).

The role of PARP activation in the pathogenesis of haemorrhagic shock was investigated in detail in a murine model, by comparing the response to haemor-rhage and resuscitation in wild-type and PARP-deficient mice (Liaudet et al 2000). Animals were bled to a mean blood pressure of 45 mmHg and were subsequently resuscitated after 45 min with isotonic saline. There was a massive activation of PARP, detected by poly(ADP-ribose) immunohistochemistry, which localized to the areas of the most severe intestinal injury, i.e. the necrotic epithelial cells at the tip of the intestinal villi, and co-localized with tyrosine nitration, an index of per-oxynitrite generation. A similar pattern of intestinal PARP activation was detected in shock induced by cecal ligation and puncture in rats, as well as in splanchnic occlusion-reperfusion shock (Soriano et al 2002). PARP-deficient mice were also protected from the rapid decrease in blood pressure after resuscitation and showed an increased survival time, as well as reduced pulmonary neutrophil sequestration (Liaudet et al 2000). In a large animal model of haemorrhagic shock, treatment with 3-aminobenzamide significantly ameliorated the fall in blood pressure, cardiac output and stroke work; slightly increased left atrial pressure during resuscitation; and significantly prolonged survival (Szabó et al 1998). Thus, it is likely that PARP activation and associated cell injury (necrosis or pre-necrosis) plays a crucial role in the intestinal injury, cardiovascular failure, and multiple organ damage associated with endotoxic and septic shock, as well as resuscitated hemorrhagic shock. The sum of these organ-protective effects may be responsible for the finding that pharmacological inhibition of PARP, either with 3-aminobenzamide or with the novel potent PARP inhibitors 5-iodo-6-amino-1,2,-benzopyrone or PJ34 improves survival rate in mice challenged with high dose endotoxin or in various rodent and large animal models of sepsis. In addition to the pharmacological studies, several investigations compared the survival times of wild-type and PARP-deficient mice in response to high dose endotoxin, and compared the degree and nature of liver damage in the two experimental groups. In one study, all PARP deficient animals survived high-dose (20 mg/kg) LPS-mediated shock, which killed 60% of wild-type animals (Kuhnle et al 1999). Similar results were obtained by another independent group (Oliver et al 1999). In yet another study, the effect of PARP inhibition or PARP deficiency was tested in the cecal ligation and puncture (CLP) model of sepsis, a polymicrobial systemic inflammation/shock model that is considered by many investigators clinically more relevant than the endotoxin models. In the CLP model, too, absence of functional PARP provided a significant survival benefit (Soriano et al 2002). Similar findings have been reported in a pneumonia-induced sepsis and gut injury model (Lobo et al 2005).

One of the remaining questions is whether PARP activation is also effective in human septic shock. This question can only be addressed directly, in Phase II or Phase III clinical trials using ultrapotent novel PARP inhibitors. (Such inhibitors have recently entered clinical trials for various cardiovascular and oncological indications [Southan & Szabó 2003, Jagtap & Szabó 2005], but it is not known whether or not sepsis or septic shock trials have began as of early 2006). In the absence of direct clinical studies, observational studies can be conducted and correlations can be drawn. In collaboration with Dr Garcia Soriano at the University of Sao Paulo, we have recently conducted such a study in order to analyse the cardiac alterations in septic patients (Soriano et al 2006). In this study, a total of 25 patients were enrolled. During the 28 days of follow-up, 12 patients died (48%). All patients were mechanically ventilated and received catecholamines. The two groups had similar APACHE II Scores (non survivors 26 ± 2, survivors 24 ± 5; NS). CPK, CKMB, echocardiography analysis, cardiac output and vascular resistance did not show any significant difference at any time point during the study. Analysis of the patients' systemic inflammatory response was conducted by measuring plasma levels of CRP. On the first day, the CRP levels were similar in the two groups studied. However, on day 3 the survivors presented a decrease in CRP, while the non-survivors maintained elevated CRP plasma levels.

Clinical heart damage was assessed by plasma troponin, which showed a significant difference in the first day of study: the survivor group presented 0.53 ± 0.13 ng/ml, while the non-survivor group presented 2.31 ± 1.01 ng/ml ($P < 0.05$). Data on day 3 showed a persistent difference, in troponin serum levels between survivors and non-survivor group. There was a significant degree of cardiac dysfunction in the patients, as detected by left ventricular stroke work index. Non-survivors presented a more severe degree of cardiac depression, compared to survivors. The difference on stroke work data became more apparent from day 3 to 6. End-diastolic volume from the left ventricle was obtained using data from pulmonary catheter and echocardiography. Using left ventricle size and ejection fraction from echocardiography and systolic volume from pulmonary catheter data, we calculated left ventricular end-diastolic volume. These data showed that the surviving septic patients presented an increase in end-diastolic volume, while non-survivors did not present with this pattern. There were no differences in catecholamine requirements in the surviving and non-surviving groups. Histological myocardial damage, as assessed by haematoxylin/eosin staining, conducted in the hearts of the non-surviving patients, demonstrated an increased number of inflammatory cells in the heart tissue. Picro Sirius-Red staining for collagen also showed an increased amount of collagen in the interstitium. These histological findings may be related to cardiac rigidity and inability to dilate in order to adapt for sepsis.

There was evidence of nuclear staining for poly(ADP-ribose) (PAR), the product of activated PARP, in the nuclei of the myocytes from septic patients, as well as in tissue-infiltrating mononuclear cells. There was a strong correlation between the PAR staining densitometry and troponin I and a similar, highly significant correlation between PAR staining densitometry and LVSWI.

Thus, in this study, surviving and non-surviving patients presented with no differences in severity of illness, as shown by their APACHE II score. This finding highlights that there was no difference in the initial disease severity between groups, which would have determined the ultimate progression of the disease, and the ultimate survival. Analysis of patients' systemic inflammatory response was conducted by measuring plasma levels of CRP. On the first day, the CRP levels were similar in the two groups studied. However, on day 3, non-survivors tended to maintain elevated CRP plasma levels, when compared to survivors, indicative of a persistent inflammatory response. In order to investigate if there is a direct damage to the heart in the patients, we measured biochemical markers, haemodynamics with pulmonary catheter and trans-thoracic echocardiography. We found a significant difference in troponin levels between survivors and non-survivors on the first day of the study and the results suggested that an increase in troponin may be associated with a poorer outcome. We found that the minimum LVSWI negatively correlated to the maximum troponin recorded: the decrease in LVSWI that is seen in septic shock occurs during a process of myocardial stress or damage, which probably resolves with an improvement in left ventricular function in patients who survive. Importantly, the immunostaining for PAR showed positive staining in tissue sections from the hearts of septic patients, consistent with PARP activation in these hearts. The results showed a good correlation among cardiac function, serum biomarker troponin I and PARP activation in these hearts. These data are consistent with the preclinical data presented in the first section of the current overview, implicating PARP activation as a final common effector in various types of tissue injury including systemic inflammation, circulatory shock and ischaemia/reperfusion. As noted earlier, direct studies with PARP inhibitors are needed to test the causative effect of PARP in human sepsis. Nevertheless, it is important to highlight that in the current study there was a good correlation between PAR staining and haemodynamic and biochemical data. If PARP were activated following death and the time-lag for the organs processed, we would have expected no correlation but a flat line for PAR staining in spite of differences in troponin or cardiac function. Thus, it is unlikely that the PARP activation we see in septic hearts in the current study is a processing artifact, but, rather it likely represents a pathophysiological process operative in the septic patients.

Gender differences in PARP activation and the effects of PARP inhibitors

Recent studies reveal a marked gender difference in the systemic inflammatory response with respect to its regulation by PARP (Mabley et al 2005). The response is preferentially down-regulated by PARP in male animals. Female mice produce less tumour necrosis factor (TNF)α and MIP-1α in response to systemic inflammation induced by endotoxin, than male mice, and are resistant to endotoxin-induced mortality. Pharmacological inhibition of PARP is effective in reducing inflammatory mediator production and mortality in male, but not in female mice. Ovarectomy partially reverses the protection seen in female mice. Endotoxin-induced PARP activation in circulating leukocytes is reduced in male, but not female animals by pharmacological PARP inhibition. Pretreatment of male animals with 17-β-oestradiol prevents endotoxin-induced hepatic injury, and reduces poly(ADP-ribosyl)ation *in vivo*. In male, but not female animals, endotoxin treatment results in an impairment of the endothelium-dependent relaxant responses, which is prevented by PARP inhibition (Mabley et al 2005).

Gender differences with respect to PARP were also reported in reperfusion injury: in animal models of stroke (Hagberg et al 2004, McCullough et al 2005) and thoracoabdominal aortic aneurysm surgery (TAAA) (Hauser et al 2006). For example, McCullough and colleagues demonstrated that male mice are preferentially protected against stroke in the absence of functional PARP-1 or by pharmacological PARP inhibition (as opposed to female animals, in which PARP inhibition offered no benefit to the outcome of ischaemic stroke) (McCullough et al 2005). Similarly, in a porcine model of TAAA surgery utilizing swine of both sexes a post-hoc analysis revealed, that the noradrenaline infusion time was statistically significantly reduced by PARP inhibition when all animals were analysed, and the difference remained significant in the male-only subgroup. However, no difference was seen in the female subgroup *without* versus *with* PARP inhibition (Hauser et al 2006).

Recent studies demonstrate gender differences in sensitivity of cells to oxidative injury *in vitro* (Du et al 2004). As far as the mechanism of the gender difference in the protective effect of PARP inhibitors is concerned, there are a number of studies that point towards the role of oestrogen (Mabley et al 2005). *In vitro* oxidant-induced PARP activation is reduced in cultured cells placed in female rat serum, as compared to male serum. Oestrogen, however, does not directly inhibit the enzymatic activity of PARP *in vitro*. Instead of a direct enzymatic inhibitory effect, PARP and estrogen receptor alpha form a complex, which binds to DNA *in vitro*, and the DNA-binding of this complex is enhanced by oestrogen. Thus, oestrogen may anchor PARP to oestrogen receptor α and to the DNA and prevent its recognition of DNA strand breaks and hence its activation.

Conclusions

Strategies aimed at limiting free radical and oxidant-mediated cell/organ injury include agents which catalyse detoxification of superoxide or peroxynitrite, or inhibit the induction or activity of the inducible NO synthase. Less attention has been directed to strategies that interfere with intracellular cytotoxic pathways initiated by nitrogen- or oxygen-derived free radicals or its toxic derivatives. Direct and indirect experimental evidence presented in this review supports the view that peroxynitrite-induced DNA strand breakage and PARP activation importantly contribute to the pathophysiology of various forms of inflammation and shock. As discussed above, PARP inhibition exerts two main protective effects in shock and inflammation. The first one is related to preservation of cellular energetic status, and protection against cell necrosis or pre-necrosis (cytopathic hypoxia), while the second one is related to down-regulation of various pro-inflammatory pathways in the absence of functional PARP. Thus pharmacological inactivation of PARP represents a novel, therapeutically viable strategy to limit cellular injury and improve the outcome of a variety of shock and systemic inflammatory conditions.

A gender difference has also been shown in the susceptibility of patients to systemic inflammatory response and septic shock (Schroder et al 1998). Pharmacological inhibitors of PARP move towards clinical testing for a variety of indications, (Jagtap & Szabó 2005). As circulatory shock, stroke and myocardial infarction predominantly develop in men, or in postmenopausal women, the gender difference with respect to the efficacy of PARP inhibition, does not discourage the clinical testing of the therapeutic effect of PARP inhibitors in both males and females. However, we believe that careful analysis should be conducted: potential gender differences in the up-coming clinical trials should be examined.

References

Albertini M, Clement MG, Lafortuna CL 2000 Role of poly-(ADP-ribose) synthetase in lipopolysaccharide-induced vascular failure and acute lung injury in pigs. J Crit Care 15:73–83

Berger SJ, Sudar DC, Berger NA 1986 Metabolic consequences of DNA damage: DNA damage induces alterations in glucose metabolism by activation of poly (ADP-ribose) polymerase. Biochem Biophys Res Commun 134:227–232

Boulos M, Astiz ME, Barua RS 2003 Impaired mitochondrial function induced by serum from septic shock patients is attenuated by inhibition of nitric oxide synthase and poly(ADP-ribose) synthase. Crit Care Med 31:353–358

Cuzzocrea S, Zingarelli B, Costantino G et al 1997 Beneficial effects of 3-aminobenzamide, an inhibitor of poly (ADP-ribose) synthetase in a rat model of splanchnic artery occlusion and reperfusion. Br J Pharmacol 121:1065–1074

Di Paola R, Mazzon E, Xu W et al 2005 Treatment with PARP-1 inhibitors, GPI 15427 or GPI 16539, ameliorates intestinal damage in rat models of colitis and shock. Eur J Pharmacol 527:163–171

Du L, Bayir H, Lai Y et al 2004 Innate gender-based proclivity in response to cytotoxicity and programmed cell death pathway. J Biol Chem 279:38563–38570

Goldfarb RD, Marton A, Szabó E 2002 Protective effect of a novel, potent inhibitor of poly(adenosine 5′-diphosphate-ribose) synthetase in a porcine model of severe bacterial sepsis. Crit Care Med 30:974–980

Hagberg H, Wilson MA, Matsushita H et al 2004 PARP-1 gene disruption in mice preferentially protects males from perinatal brain injury. J Neurochem 90:1068–1075

Hasko G, Mabley JG, Nemeth ZH, Pacher P, Deitch EA, Szabó C 2002 Poly(ADP-ribose) polymerase is a regulator of chemokine production: relevance for the pathogenesis of shock and inflammation. Mol Med 8:283–289

Hassa PO, Hottiger MO 2002 The functional role of poly(ADP-ribose)polymerase 1 as novel coactivator of NF-kappaB in inflammatory disorders. Cell Mol Life Sci 59:1534–1553

Hauser B, Gröger M, Ehrmann U et al 2006 The PARP-1 inhibitor INO-1001 facilitates hemodynamic stabilization without affecting DNA repair or cell senescence in porcine thoracic aortic cross-clamping/induced ischemia and reperfusion. Shock 25:633–640

Jagtap P, Szabó C 2005 Poly(ADP-ribose) polymerase and the therapeutic effects of its inhibitors. Nat Rev Drug Discov 4:421–440

Jagtap P, Soriano FG, Virag L 2002 Novel phenanthridinone inhibitors of poly (adenosine 5′-diphosphate-ribose) synthetase: potent cytoprotective and antishock agents. Crit Care Med 30:1071–1082

Junod AF, Jornot L, Petersen H 1989 Differential effects of hyperoxia and hydrogen peroxide on DNA damage, polyadenosine diphosphate-ribose polymerase activity, and nicotinamide adenine dinucleotide and adenosine triphosphate contents in cultured endothelial cells and fibroblasts. J Cell Physiol 140:177–185

Kirkland JB 1991 Lipid peroxidation, protein thiol oxidation and DNA damage in hydrogen peroxide-induced injury to endothelial cells: role of activation of poly(ADP-ribose)polymerase. Biochim Biophys Acta 1092:319–325

Kuhnle S, Nicotera P, Wendel A 1999 Prevention of endotoxin-induced lethality, but not of liver apoptosis in poly(ADP-ribose) polymerase-deficient mice. Biochem Biophys Res Commun 263:433–438

Liaudet L, Soriano FG, Szabó E 2000 Protection against hemorrhagic shock in mice genetically deficient in poly(ADP-ribose)polymerase. Proc Natl Acad Sci USA 97:10203–10208

Liaudet L, Pacher P, Mabley JG 2002 Activation of poly(ADP-Ribose) polymerase-1 is a central mechanism of lipopolysaccharide-induced acute lung inflammation. Am J Respir Crit Care Med 165:372–377

Lobo SM, Orrico SR, Queiroz MM 2005 Pneumonia-induced sepsis and gut injury: effects of a poly-(ADP-Ribose) polymerase inhibitor. J Surg Res 129:292–297

Mabley JG, Horvath EM, Murthy KG et al 2005 Gender differences in the endotoxin-induced inflammatory and vascular responses: potential role of poly(ADP-ribose) polymerase activation. J Pharmacol Exp Ther 315:812–820

McCullough LD, Zeng Z, Blizzard KK, Debchoudhury I, Hurn PD 2005 Ischemic nitric oxide and poly (ADP-ribose) polymerase-1 in cerebral ischemia: male toxicity, female protection. J Cereb Blood Flow Metab 25:502–512

McDonald MC, Mota-Filipe H, Wright JA 2000 Effects of 5-aminoisoquinolinone, a water-soluble, potent inhibitor of the activity of poly (ADP-ribose) polymerase on the organ injury and dysfunction caused by haemorrhagic shock. Br J Pharmacol 130:843–850

Oliver FJ, Menissier-de Murcia J, Nacci C 1999 Resistance to endotoxic shock as a consequence of defective NF-kappaB activation in poly (ADP-ribose) polymerase-1 deficient mice. EMBO J 18:4446–4454

Osman J 1998 Poly-ADP ribosyl synthetase inhibition reverses vascular hyporeactivity in septic mice. Crit Care Med 26:A134

Pacher P, Cziraki A, Mabley JG 2002 Role of poly(ADP-ribose) polymerase activation in endotoxin-induced cardiac collapse in rodents. Biochem Pharmacol 64:1785–1791

Schroder J, Kahlke V, Staubach KH, Zabel P, Stuber F 1988 Gender differences in human sepsis. Arch Surg 133:1200–1205

Shimoda K, Murakami K, Enkhbaatar P 2003 Effect of poly(ADP ribose) synthetase inhibition on burn and smoke inhalation injury in sheep. Am J Physiol Lung Cell Mol Physiol 285: L240–249

Soriano FG, Liaudet L, Szabó E 2002 Resistance to acute septic peritonitis in poly(ADP-ribose) polymerase-1-deficient mice. Shock 17:286–292

Soriano FG, Nogueira AC, Caldini EG et al 2006 Potential role of PARP activation in the pathogenesis of myocardial contractile dysfunction associated with human septic shock. Crit Care Med 34:1073–1079

Southan GJ, Szabó C 2003 Poly(ADP-ribose) polymerase inhibitors. Curr Med Chem 10: 321–340

Szabó C 1995 Alterations in nitric oxide production in various forms of circulatory shock. New Horizons 3:2–32

Szabó C 1996 The pathophysiological role of peroxynitrite in shock, inflammation, and ischemia-reperfusion injury. Shock 6:79–88

Szabó C, Salzman AL, Ischiropoulos H 1995 Endotoxin triggers the expression of an inducible isoform of nitric oxide synthase and the formation of peroxynitrite in the rat aorta in vivo. FEBS Lett 363:235–238

Szabó C, Zingarelli B, Salzman AL 1996 Role of poly-ADP ribosyltransferase activation in the vascular contractile and energetic failure elicited by exogenous and endogenous nitric oxide and peroxynitrite. Circ Res 78:1051–1063

Szabó C, Cuzzocrea S, Zingarelli B 1997 Endothelial dysfunction in a rat model of endotoxic shock. Importance of the activation of poly (ADP-ribose) synthetase by peroxynitrite. J Clin Invest 100:723–735

Szabó A, Hake P, Salzman AL 1998 3-Aminobenzamide, an inhibitor of poly (ADP-ribose) synthetase, improves hemodynamics and prolongs survival in a porcine model of hemorrhagic shock. Shock 10:347–353

Tasatargil A, Dalaklioglu S, Sadan G 2005 Inhibition of poly(ADP-ribose) polymerase prevents vascular hyporesponsiveness induced by lipopolysaccharide in isolated rat aorta. Pharmacol Res 51:581–586

Ueda K, Hayaishi O 1985 ADP-ribosylation. Annu Rev Biochem 54:73–100

Veres B, Gallyas F Jr, Varbiro G 2003 Decrease of the inflammatory response and induction of the Akt/protein kinase B pathway by poly-(ADP-ribose) polymerase 1 inhibitor in endotoxin-induced septic shock. Biochem Pharmacol 65:1373–1382

Villa LM, Salas E, Darley-Usmar VM 1994 Peroxynitrite induces both vasodilatation and impaired vascular relaxation in the isolated perfused rat heart. Proc Natl Acad Sci USA 91:12383–12387

Virag L, Szabó C 2002 The therapeutic potential of poly(ADP-ribose) polymerase inhibitors. Pharmacol Rev 54:375–429

Virag L, Salzman AL, Szabó C 1998 Poly(ADP-ribose) synthetase activation mediates mitochondrial injury during oxidant-induced cell death. J Immunol 161:3753–3759

Wray GM, Hinds CJ, Thiemermann C 1998 Effects of inhibitors of poly(ADP-ribose) synthetase activity on hypotension and multiple organ dysfunction caused by endotoxin. Shock 10:13–19

Zingarelli B, O'Connor M, Wong H 1996 Peroxynitrite-mediated DNA strand breakage activates poly-adenosine diphosphate ribosyl synthetase and causes cellular energy depletion in macrophages stimulated with bacterial lipopolysaccharide. J Immunol 156:350–358

DISCUSSION

Thiemermann: There is evidence that the role of PARP protein in the regulation of the activation of transcription factors involved in the inflammatory response is independent of the catalytic activity of PARP. Thus, my question is, does the catalytic activity of the protein play a role? The anti-inflammatory effects are pronounced in the knockout animals, but often much weaker in studies with PARP inhibitors *in vivo* (*see* Ha et al 2002).

Szabó: It depends on who you read. Many studies have attempted to figure this out. In some studies, the effect of PARP deficiency couldn't be reproduced by the effect of the PARP inhibitors. In other studies, both of these approaches have the same kind of effect, but most of the time the PARP deficiency has a more pronounced effect than the PARP inhibition. It depends on the cell system, on the nature of the stimuli (in our hands both PARP inhibition and PARP deficiency work at the same rate when we look at chemokine production, but in many cases only PARP deficiency works when we look at NF-κB activation in cells exposed to high glucose) (Hasko et al 2002). In some cases it is the presence or absence of the enzyme, while in other cases, the catalytic activity of the enzyme matters. I don't think anyone understands it exactly.

Thiemermann: You showed in isolated thymocytes from PARP knockout animals that there was an increase in the number of cells with apoptosis, while the number of cells with necrosis was reduced. At the end of your talk you mentioned the role of PARP in releasing apoptosis-inducing factor (AIF). We did a study in a rat model of myocardial ischaemia and reperfusion, which involved flow cytometric analysis of the cardiac myocytes located in the area of the heart that had been subjected to ischaemia/reperfusion. In this experiment, we found an increase in both apoptosis and necrosis. When we used a highly specific PARP inhibitor we found a reduction in necrosis, which was expected, but we also found a significant reduction in the number of apoptotic cardiac myocytes.

Szabó: Similar results have been found in studies by Zingarelli and colleagues. Probably, *in vivo*, there are more things going on, with interactions between pathways and positive feedback cycles. The ultimate end result is that there are positive feedback cycles between PARP and other pathways of injury. *In vivo*, this system may be interrupted, and all these positive feedback cycles are therefore disrupted. One of the outcomes of this could be that the apoptotic features are reduced. By the way, AIF translocation doesn't mean apoptosis: it can be translated in both apoptosis and necrosis. It is just a mitochondrial type of injury or cell death.

Radermacher: I was impressed by your data on heart function in septic patients. To some extent this replicates the role that has been ascribed to iNOS in heart function in these patients. People are saying that depression of the systolic function is an adaptive phenomenon in order to allow for ventricular dilatation to maintain the stroke volume. Have you looked at diastolic relaxation in these patients? There is a clear effect on systolic contractility, but I didn't see volumetric measures.

Szabó: I don't think we have these data. This was the best correlation we got from all the parameters. I didn't say it is a causal effect; we don't have all the data for these patients and this is a preliminary study. But it was interesting to see the correlation.

Singer: I'll defend the hibernation concept. There was a paper from Cliff Deutschman's group which nicely showed in an animal model that there are various metabolic markers of hibernation which can be replicated in a septic rat model (Levy et al 2005). With your human data, there was horrible looking histology. This reminds me of a wise cardiac pathologist, years ago, called Mike Davies, who said he could always spot the patient who had received inotropes, because there were holes in the myocardium. Therefore, how much of what you are seeing is iatrogenic injury?

Szabó: We don't have a control group because all these patients are on inotrophic agents. You have to give them something. Yes, some of this could be iatrogenic, and yes, the end result is that these hearts don't really look normal.

Singer: I was surprised that females don't get any PARP induction in the animal model. Don't you think this is a bit hard to explain? Presumably, females get DNA breaks.

Szabó: Yes it is interesting, isn't it. But data are accumulating to show this in several models. There are two papers showing the same gender difference in stroke (Hagberg et al 2004, McCullough et al 2005). When female animals that have had a stroke were treated with PARP inhibitors, there was no protection, but there was a very significant beneficial effect in the males.

Singer: Have you looked at pre- and post-menopausal women?

Szabó: We haven't done this in humans yet. In the animals we have used ovar-ectomized animals, which are behaving effectively as post-menopausal rats. They start to behave more like the males, so the effect is probably something to do with oestrogen. Oestrogen could be doing some baseline PARP inhibition.

Van den Berghe: In critical care patients, men produce more oestradiol. There is enhanced aromatase activity that causes metabolism of testosterone into oestra-diol. The women and men have equal levels of oestradiol in the post-menopausal or elderly population.

Griffiths: There's no difference in overall mortality.

Szabó: Isn't it true that you see more males in intensive care units (ICUs) than females? And aren't the females that you see in ICUs usually post-menopausal?

Fink: Most of the patients are in an age group that they would have to be post-menopausal. There have been a couple of retrospective studies that have been adequately powered to look at trauma and burn patients to see whether there is a gender-related outcome difference. As far as I know, those studies have yielded negative results.

Van den Berghe: That is because the pituitary has been shut down.

Fink: I'm not arguing against the gender–inflammation linkage. The best data are from the multiple sclerosis literature, where women have spontaneous remission during the third trimester of pregnancy. Oestrodial levels peak during the third trimester and this autoimmune disease sometimes goes away at least for a while. Do mitochondrial strand breaks activate PARP in the mitochondria?

Szabó: We are looking at this. The first question is whether there is PARP in the mitochondria or not. There is one paper suggesting that there is (Du et al 2003). We have just finished a study where we did some mass spectral analysis. We isolated mitochondria and exposed them to hydrogen peroxide. We did 2D gels and cut out some spots, which were then analysed by mass spectrometry. There are about five proteins that are polyADP-ribosylated in this system. This was all done in a system that consists of mitochondria only. These five proteins are all in the matrix or the inner membrane, and they are all known to be susceptible to oxidative damage. But I don't know whether the activation mechanism is the same.

Griffiths: Two slightly linked questions. What is the consequence of the PARP knockout in the long term? Do you know what happens to PARP function in the elderly?

Szabó: There is only one PARP1 knockout where I know that data are available. It doesn't knock out all PARP function, just 95% of it. These knockouts seem fine as far as lifespan. On the other hand PARP1 and PARP2 double knockouts are lethal.

Fink: Unless they have a defect in the enzymes that are required for homologous recombination of double-strand breaks, and then they get cancer.

Szabó: They also seem to develop more tumours if you put them on oral carcinogens. But without carcinogens, there is no increase in spontaneous tumour incidence in PARP1 knockout mice, when compared to wild-type animals. If you make double knockouts that lack both PARP1 and PARP2, it results in embryonic lethality, and so we don't know if they would develop more cancers over their life. Why the double knockouts are not viable, we don't know yet: there could be many reasons underlying it, including genetic instability.

Griffiths: What about ageing?

Szabó: We did some studies on this. We got some improvement in the cardiovascular function by PARP inhibitors in aged animals (Pacher et al 2004).

Piantadosi: Whether or not mitochondrial PARP is involved in mitochondrial DNA repair is an unanswered question. Mitochondria don't have those other repair enzymes. They can do basic excision repair but that is probably about it. Mitochondria solve the problem by identifying the intact genome and replicating it. Some endonuclease probably gets rid of the bad genome.

Cohen: Aren't there some conditions such as XLP (X-linked lymphoproliferative disease) which are associated with DNA strand breaks? Would this be a good model for looking to see whether this is active and whether your inhibitors would be beneficial?

Szabó: I don't think anyone has looked at this.

References

Du L, Zhang X, Han YY et al 2003 Intra-mitochondrial poly(ADP-ribosylation) contributes to NAD+ depletion and cell death induced by oxidative stress. J Biol Chem 278:18426–18433

Ha HC, Hester LD, Snyder SH 2002 Poly(ADP-ribose) polymerase-1 dependence of stress-induced transcription factors and associated gene expression in glia. Proc Natl Acad Sci USA 99:3270–3275

Hagberg H, Wilson MA, Matsushita H et al 2004 PARP-1 gene disruption in mice preferentially protects males from perinatal brain injury. J Neurochem 90:1068–1075

Hasko G, Mabley JG, Nemeth ZH, Pacher P, Deitch EA, Szabo C 2002 Poly(ADP-ribose) polymerase is a regulator of chemokine production: relevance for the pathogenesis of shock and inflammation. Mol Med 8:283–289

Levy RJ, Piel DA, Acton PD et al 2005 Evidence of myocardial hibernation in the septic heart. Crit Care Med 33:2752–2756

McCullough LD, Zeng Z, Blizzard KK, Debchoudhury I, Hurn PD 2005 Ischemic nitric oxide and poly (ADP-ribose) polymerase-1 in cerebral ischemia: male toxicity, female protection. J Cereb Blood Flow Metab 25:502–512

Pacher P, Vaslin A, Benko R et al 2004 A new, potent poly(ADP-ribose) polymerase inhibitor improves cardiac and vascular dysfunction associated with advanced aging. J Pharmacol Exp Ther 311:485–491

Choosing the right substrate

Xavier Leverve, Cécile Batandier and Eric Fontaine

INSERM E-0221 Bioénergétique Fondamentale et Appliquée, Université Joseph Fourier, BP 53X, 38041 Grenoble, France

Abstract. Carbohydrate and fatty acids are major energetic substrates, although amino acid oxidation also permits ATP synthesis. Among several major metabolic differences between lipids and carbohydrate (activation, transport, effect of insulin, etc.), two are of particular importance when considering energy metabolism of critically ill patients: the yield of ATP synthesis and the response to uncoupling. (I) Oxidative phosphorylation yield is higher when NADH is the electron donor (three coupling sites: complex 1, 3 and 4) as compared to $FADH_2$ (two coupling sites: complex 3 and 4). Since the ratio $NADH/FADH_2$ is higher for glycolysis as compared to β-oxidation, the stoichiometry of ATP synthesis to oxygen consumption is also higher. Lipid oxidation provides more ATP than carbohydrate, but it requires more oxygen per mole of ATP synthesized. (II) The ratio of NADH oxidation versus $FADH_2$ oxidation depends on the proton motive force, and lowering proton motive force by uncoupling favours $FADH_2$ oxidation, i.e. lipids versus carbohydrate. In conclusion, lipid oxidation provides a high rate of ATP synthesis even during a mild uncoupling state, but at a high rate of oxygen consumption. If oxygen availability is limited, the major metabolic adaptation to increase the efficiency is represented by a switch from lipid oxidation to glucose oxidation.

2007 Sepsis—new insights, new therapies. Wiley, Chichester (Novartis Foundation Symposium 280) p 108–127

Energy metabolism in humans, like in all mammals, is fully supported by the complete oxidation of two major substrate families: carbohydrates and lipids. Amino acids released after protein breakdown are also good oxidative substrates. However, after deamination they enter the pathway of carbohydrate oxidation. Interestingly, the metabolism of these two families of substrates exhibits several similarities, while some major differences explain the advantage of maintaining these two different pathways throughout evolution. In specific physiological situations as well as during illnesses, lipids and/or glucose oxidation have both advantages and drawbacks, and choosing the right substrate might confer a substantial advantage.

If we consider cellular energy metabolism, these two substrates exhibit similarities and differences in the regulation of: catabolic pathways (Azzone et al 1985) (glycolysis and β-oxidation), ATP synthesis rate and efficiency (Brand 1990), mitochondrial oxidative phosphorylation and reactive oxygen species production (Fitton et al 1994) and mitochondrial permeability transition pore and its consequence to the commitment to apoptosis (Fontaine et al 1996). Clinical studies have shown that interfering with carbohydrate or lipid metabolism in critically ill patients has important consequences in outcome and morbidity.

Glucose versus fatty acids and the regulation of rate versus efficiency in ATP synthesis

Except for nutrients and waste products, any metabolite will always have a precursor and a product resulting from its metabolism. Hence the entire network *in vivo* is endless, a feature that contrasts with *in vitro* experiments, where the networks studied are limited to the experimental conditions. This must be kept in mind when considering discrepancies occurring between *in vivo* and *in vitro* experiments, especially when investigating the effect of substrate supply. Indeed, the substrate supply is precisely set *in vitro*, while *in vivo* there is large possibility of self-regulation. In addition, all the regulatory factors involved in the pathway of glucose or lipid oxidation will further complicate the comparison between *in vitro* and *in vivo*. The difference between *in vitro* and *in vivo* conditions regarding glucose or lipid as a preferred substrate for oxidation and ATP synthesis is a good example. When carbohydrates (glucose) and lipids (octanoate) are given simultaneously to isolated cells (hepatocytes), lipid oxidation will be preferred by the system and pyruvate oxidation will be powerfully inhibited. This is due to the negative feedback effect of acetylCoA, provided from β-oxidation, on pyruvate dehydrogenase, preventing the formation of acetylCoA from carbohydrate oxidation. However, during the same competition between lipids and glucose as oxidative substrate the opposite is observed *in vivo*. In this situation glucose is preferred over lipids to be oxidized first because of insulin, which activates several steps of glycolysis (e.g. cellular transport, phosphorylation, etc.) while it inhibits acetylCoA entry into the mitochondrial matrix, preventing its oxidation. The competition between the two major metabolites, as substrates for ATP synthesis, results in an opposite picture *in vivo* as compared to *in vitro*.

The mitochondrial oxidative phosphorylation pathway is another good example of a potential discrepancy between *in vivo* and *in vitro* conditions. In intact cells (a situation that might be called '*in vivo*' for mitochondrial metabolism) mitochondrion substrate supply controls both nature and rate of metabolism since the outer membrane is probably more selective than classically believed, and the inner mitochondrial membrane is non-permeable to substrate and highly charged, indicating that substrate supply to matrix is selective and regulated. Moreover, the upstream cytosolic metabolism also plays a crucial role in the control of substrate concentration and therefore competition as oxidative substrates. By contrast, in isolated mitochondria, saturating concentrations of selected substrate(s) completely blunt any control at this level. This is illustrated by the difference in the mitochondrial metabolism of glucose and fatty acids, and the rate and efficiency of oxidative phosphorylation.

Studies on respiratory chain and oxidative phosphorylation are based on well-defined conditions such as state 4 (non-phosphorylating conditions in the presence of oligomycin) or state 3 (phosphorylating conditions in the presence of saturating ADP concentrations), which never occur *in vivo*. Indeed, in intact cells the status of mitochondrial oxidative phosphorylation is always between states 4 and 3, and the varying ATP demand will affect not only the respiratory rate as such but also the protonmotive force, the redox equilibria and the phosphate potential. Most data on the proton leak across the inner membrane or on the slippage between the redox reactions and the vectorial proton pumping have been obtained from state 4 respiratory rate measurement (Azzone et al 1985, Brand 1990, Fitton et al 1994, Fontaine et al 1996, Luvisetto et al 1991, Murphy & Brand 1987, Ouhabi et al 1991, Pietrobon & Caplan 1985, Pietrobon et al 1983, Rigoulet et al 1998, Schmehl et al 1995, van Dam et al 1990, Zoratti et al 1986) and have been extrapolated to the oxidative phosphorylation efficiency *in situ*. It should be kept in mind that the high mitochondrial membrane potential reached in state 4 ($\Delta p = -180$ millivolts, a value approximately fivefold higher than the potential applied to the plasma membrane), never occurs *in vivo* (Fontaine et al 1997).

The nature of the respiratory substrates modulates oxidative phosphorylation efficiency

The mitochondrial inner membrane ordinarily possesses an intrinsically low permeability to ions and solutes. Such a property allows energy conservation in the form of a proton electrochemical potential difference, which is required for ATP synthesis and for transport of several charged molecules including adenine nucleotides, Pi, Ca^{2+} and some respiratory substrates. Nevertheless, the permeability of the inner membrane can be modulated by exogenous compounds such as protonophoric uncouplers (Luvisetto et al 1991, 1987, Zoratti et al 1986), by activation of the uncoupling proteins, or by opening of the permeability transition pore (PTP) (Bernardi 1999). The relevance of the nature of the respiratory substrates (i.e. NADH-related substrates *versus* succinate) is often underestimated, and the standard substrate for *in vitro* mitochondrion studies is almost invariably succinate used in combination with rotenone, a condition that provides electrons directly to complex II. It must be emphasized that this situation never occurs *in vivo* under physiological conditions. Mitochondrial complex I has a prominent regulatory role not only on the oxidative phosphorylation pathway, but also on several other mitochondrial functions such as the permeability transition and the production of reactive oxygen species. This major regulatory role is of course completely erased in the presence of rotenone. Hence, it appears that according to the nature of the respiratory substrate different effects of mitochondrial uncoupling and of PTP regulation can be obtained.

Modulation of oxidative phosphorylation by respiratory substrates

The nature of the cellular substrates (e.g. fatty acids versus carbohydrates) affects the stoichiometry of oxidative phosphorylation by affecting the ratio between NADH, H^+ and $FADH_2$. NADH oxidation involves three sequential coupling sites (complexes I, III and IV), while only two coupling sites are involved in $FADH_2$ oxidation (complexes III and IV). Hence, the yield of ATP synthesis is lowered by approximately 40% when $FADH_2$ is oxidized, as compared to NADH. At variance from carbohydrate metabolism, fatty-acid β-oxidation results in the formation of equimolar amounts of NADH and $FADH_2$. Hence, the stoichiometry of ATP synthesis to oxygen consumption is lower when lipids rather than carbohydrates are oxidized. Because the mitochondrial inner membrane is impermeable to NADH, a shuttle system is required to carry the reducing power into the mitochondrial matrix. Two shuttle systems are involved in this exchange: the malate/aspartate shuttle, which depends on mitochondrial transmembrane electrical potential ($\Delta\mu_H^+$), and the glycerol 3-phosphate/dihydroxyacetonephosphate shuttle, which does not. While the former system provides electrons to complex I (i.e. as NADH), the latter supplies electrons directly to complex II. Thus, by adjusting the flux through these two shuttles the yield of oxidative phosphorylation, that is, the cellular metabolism of oxygen and ATP, can be regulated. One of the major effects of thyroid hormones on mitochondrial energy metabolism is achieved through this mechanism because these hormones affect transcription of the mitochondrial glycerol 3-phosphate dehydrogenase (Kalderon et al 1992, Muller & Seitz 1994), which regulates the flux through the glycerol 3-phosphate/ dihydroxyacetone-phosphate shuttle.

Adjustment of the ratio between oxidation rate and ATP synthesis

Changing the yield of oxidative phosphorylation, that is, the ratio between ATP synthesized and atoms of oxygen consumed (ATP/O), is an important mechanism for the regulation of cellular oxygen consumption and ATP synthesis. The decrease in ATP/O should not be necessarily considered as a negative event leading to a decrease of efficiency because it may reflect the existence of separate adaptive mechanisms for the modulation of oxygen consumption and ATP synthesis. This in turn may have important consequences on several mitochondrial functions linked to one of the three relevant forces implicated: protonmotive force, redox potential and phosphate potential. The efficiency of ATP synthesis is highly regulated and several mechanisms may affect it: the nature of the substrates provided to the respiratory chain (Brand 1990); the slipping of the coupling between redox reactions and proton pumping (Fitton et al 1994); and the proton leak across the inner mitochondrial membrane (Leverve et al 1986). Each of these mechanisms has some relevance in physiology.

From the above, it appears that glucose oxidation has a more efficient oxidative metabolism (5.19 Kcal/L oxygen, with a J_{CO2}/J_{O2} ratio $= 1$) as compared to fatty acids (4.81 Kcal/L oxygen, J_{CO2}/J_{O2} ratio $= 0.7$ for palmitate). Hence, although palmitate does contain more energy per gram of substrate (9.69 Kcal/g) as compared to glucose (481 Kcal/g), it consumes more oxygen to produce one ATP. This could mean that, when oxygen is unlimited lipids are the most appropriate substrate for high and sustained ATP supply. This is exactly the case for aerobic sustained muscle exercise either for specific physiological activity (heart contraction, diaphragm and intercostal muscle contraction) or for sustained muscle activity (marathon running). Conversely, if oxygen is a limiting factor, as it could be in physiological conditions such as exposure to high altitude or exhausting effort, as well as in several diseases with low oxygen delivery/consumption, glucose oxidation appears to be a better choice because of the higher efficiency of ATP synthesis. These different features for glucose or fatty acid as energy suppliers are illustrated in several *in vivo* conditions both in animal models and humans. For instance, it has been shown that high fat diet (80% of energy intake) was responsible for a large enhancement of running endurance as well as training capacity in rats as compared to normal high carbohydrate diet (Koubi et al 1991). Moreover, in an *in vivo* pig model of heart energy metabolism (Korvald et al 2000), lipid oxidation (provided by intralipid/heparin infusion) was responsible for a lower efficiency (+30–40% oxygen consumption/heart workload). Even more interestingly, Hochachka and co-workers have shown in very elegant work (McClelland et al 1998) that, while heart energy supply in healthy men was provided from lipid oxidation at sea level, it was mostly coming from glucose oxidation when these individuals were acclimatized to high altitude. This indicates that the nature of substrate is an adjustable parameter according the best choice: high rate of ATP synthesis (lipid oxidation is preferred) or highest oxidative efficiency (glucose is preferred). Recently it was shown that altered lipid metabolism at the level of fatty acid translocase (FAT-CD39 deficiency) does not compromise heart energy metabolism after ischaemia.

Of course, all the regulating factors that can affect the ratio between glucose and lipid oxidation (insulin and insulin resistance and other hormones, cytokines,

AMP kinase, etc.) are important players in this field of the regulation of 'rate versus efficiency', which is a key factor for metabolic adaptation.

The nature of cellular substrates interferes with the metabolic consequences of uncoupling

Despite the low permeability of the inner membrane, proton leaks across the membrane do occur, and result in uncoupling of oxygen consumption from ATP synthesis, energy being dissipated as heat. Uncoupling through proton leaks permits dissociaton of the rate of oxidation from that of phosphorylation, and thus decreases the yield of oxidative phosphorylation. This mechanism is similar to uncoupling through uncoupling proteins. The discovery of the physiological function of brown fat in mammals, related to the presence of uncoupling protein 1 (UCP1), has opened a new era in our understanding of the regulation of oxidative phosphorylation by describing a role for energy waste. Several other UCPs have been recently described (see reviews by Klingenberg, and Rial and co-workers), and some of these (UCP2 and UCP3) have been found in most tissues including white adipose tissue, muscle, macrophages, spleen, thymus and Kupffer's cells (Bouillaud et al 2001, Ricquier & Bouillaud 2000).

Irrespective of the molecular mechanism(s), the metabolic consequences of a protonophoric leak (uncoupling) can be classified into three categories: (1) those related to the change in oxidation rate and redox state; (2) those related to the change in protonmotive force; and (3) those related to the change in ATP synthesis and phosphate potentials. In isolated mitochondria incubated in the presence of saturating concentrations of respiratory substrates, uncouplers invariably decrease $\Delta\mu H^+$, redox and phosphate potentials and consequently increase respiratory rate. By contrast, in intact cells these forces are involved in a complex metabolic network that may significantly affect the outcome of uncoupling on the very same parameters. We have investigated the effect of uncoupling in intact liver cells in the presence of different substrates (Sibille et al 2001, 1995) by adding the protonophore 2,4-dinitrophenol (DNP) and by determining the resulting effects on respiration and glucose production from dihydroxyacetone (DHA, a carbohydrate entering the pathway at the triose phosphate and allowing a concomitant determination of gluconeogenesis and glycolysis) with a further addition of octanoate. We found that, when uncoupling was achieved without octanoate, it resulted in a profound decrease of both $\Delta\mu H^+$ and of cytosolic and mitochondrial ATP/ADP ratios, while the rate of respiration was not increased. On the other hand, in the presence of octanoate the large increase in respiration was associated with limited effects on $\Delta\mu H^+$ and ATP/ADP ratios. Hence, the metabolic consequences of uncoupling in intact liver cells are variable and critically depend on the metabolic state of the cells (see Fig. 1). In the presence of a large supply of fatty acids and oxygen, the

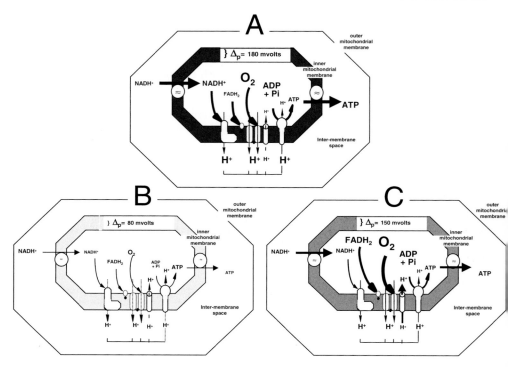

main effect of uncoupling is a dramatic increase of oxygen consumption as well as energy waste. The active mitochondrial β-oxidation sustains a very high rate of mitochondrial respiration and a high membrane potential, while ATP synthesis can be at least partially maintained because of this high respiratory chain activity. Because fatty acid oxidation results in a higher proportion of $FADH_2$ relative to carbohydrate oxidation, the effect of octanoate during uncoupling may be related, in part at least, to its ability to bypass complex I. Conversely, when glycolysis is the unique pathway for substrate supply to the respiratory chain the decreased mitochondrial membrane potential resulting from uncoupling strongly affects the mitochondrial redox potential since the malate/aspartate shuttle, which depends on maintenance of $\Delta\mu H^+$, is not able to sustain a highly reduced redox potential in the matrix. Hence, under these conditions, uncouplers do not affect significantly the respiratory rate, because the supply of reducing equivalents to complex I becomes limiting. The main effect of uncoupling would become a striking decrease of mitochondrial membrane potential and ATP:ADP ratio, with an overall decrease of the cell's metabolic activity. It is not surprising that uncoupling by UCP1 results in a huge increase in the rate of fatty acid oxidation, oxygen consumption and heat

FIG. 1.   Schematic view of oxidative phosphorylation and its uncoupling. (A) Coupled oxidative phosphorylation. The cellular use of oxygen in oxidative phosphorylation pathway is a
highly compartmentalized pathway occurring in the mitochondrial inner membrane. This
pathway consists of successive transductions of potentials from the chemical energy contained
in the nutrient to phosphate potential (ATP/ADP.Pi), which is the energy source for the different biological works. The chemical energy, supplied as reducing equivalent (NADH at
complex I and $FADH_2$ at complex II) is first converted in membrane potential (Δp) by the
respiratory chain, which links redox reaction to proton extrusion from the matrix to the inter-
membrane space. This leads to a very high electrochemical gradient ($-180\,mV$) permitting ATP
synthesis from ADP plus Pi. It must be noted that such high electrochemical gradient has other
functions than ATP synthesis such as Ca^{2+} uptake and substrate transport. The inner membrane
is impermeable to $NADH/NAD^+$ and to ATP/ADP, therefore these compounds must be
translocated by carrier systems: malatate–aspartate shuttle and adenine nucleotide translocase.
These metabolite exchanges across the mitochondrial membrane are electrogenic and therefore
depend on an electrochemical gradient. The gradient favours the entry of reducing equivalent
in the matrix and the transport of ATP into cytosol. Hence, the net result is the higher the
electrochemical gradient, the higher the matricial $NADH:NAD^+$ ratio, allowing a high concentration of respiratory substrate NADH. Similarly, the higher the gradient the higher the
export of ATP, helping maintain a low ATP:ADP.Pi ratio in the matrix (facilitating ATP synthesis) and a high ATP:ADP.Pi ratio in the cytosol (facilitating ATP hydrolysis and energy
utilization). (B) Uncoupling with carbohydrates. By permitting the protons to freely re-enter
into the matrix, the uncoupling process (via uncoupling protein for instance), creates a 'futile
cycling', dissipating energy into heat at the expense of oxygen consumption and water production. In the presence of carbohydrate as exogenous source of energy, reduced substrates are
supplied to the respiratory chain as NADH, and energy dependent import of NADH is
required. Due to the uncoupling, the electrochemical gradient collapses, impairing the active
transport of NADH. Therefore a sufficiently high reducing state in the matrix may not be sustained. In these conditions the net result is a collapse of Δp and the ATP:ADP.Pi ratio, while
oxygen consumption is low, despite the uncoupling state. (C) Uncoupling with fatty acids. In
the presence of fatty acids, the metabolic effects of uncoupling are different. In this case the
production of $FADH_2$ in the matrix by the β-oxidation permits to supply substrates directly to
complex II, even when the electrochemical gradient is collapsed. High levels of substrate supply
to the respiratory chain allow a high activity as evidenced by the very large increase in oxygen
consumption. This high respiration activity permits maintenance, to some extent, of the electrochemical gradient and therefore some ATP synthesis is maintained. In this case the main
effect of uncoupling is an increase in oxygen consumption and heat production.

production in brown fat, where the large storage of triglycerides is associated with
a large number of mitochondria with high oxidative capacity. Conversely in Kupffer
cells, which have a poor metabolism of fatty acids, uncoupling is rather expected
to result in a decreased mitochondrial membrane potential rather than in significant effects on the rate of respiration and on heat production. Thus, depending on
substrate oxidation and heat production, uncoupling in intact cells may have very
different effects on mitochondrial depolarization and on its consequences on cell
energy status. Hence, on one hand uncoupling might be a very efficient way of
decreasing oxygen concentration by reducing it to water, but on the other hand,

by decreasing mitochondrial membrane potential and ATP/ADP ratio, uncoupling may affect all cellular pathways related to these potentials.

Production of reactive oxygen species linked to a reverse electron flux at the first complex of the respiratory chain

Reactive oxygen species (ROS) production is involved in many physiological and pathological events (Droge 2002, Thannickal & Fanburg 2000), but the nature and the location of its production under physiological conditions in the respiratory chain remains unclear. Classically, two production sites are recognized in the respiratory chain: complex I and complex III (Boveris & Chance 1973), and the production of ROS at these sites is mostly revealed by inhibitor additions, namely rotenone for site I and antimycin for site III (for review see Turrens 1997). A reverse electron flux through the respiratory chain complex I has long been recognized (Chance & Hollunger 1961, Hinkle et al 1967) and a production of ROS linked to this pathway was also shown (Korshunov et al 1998, 1997, Kushnareva et al 2002, Kwong & Sohal 1998, Liu et al 2002, Vinogradov & Grivennikova 2001, Votyakova & Reynolds 2001). However, because of the experimental conditions required to demonstrate this ROS production (i.e. isolated mitochondria with lowered natural antioxidant capacity; Korshunov et al 1998, 1997), its physiological relevance is questioned. We have recently provided data showing the reverse flux-related ROS production (Fig. 2A) occurred in liver cells, which were not previously depleted in antioxidant capacity (Batandier et al 2002, 2006). The highest ROS production linked to a reverse electron flux through complex I (i.e. inhibited by rotenone) was observed with succinate alone (Fig. 2B) and, as expected, there was no reverse flux with glutamate alone, rotenone being responsible for an increased ROS production linked to the forward electron flux (Fig. 2C). Interestingly, the combination of glutamate/malate/succinate, a more physiological condition since substrates are supplied simultaneously to sites 1 and 2 as is the case in intact cells, are also responsible for ROS production linked to a reverse electron flux through complex I. Hence, according to the ratio of electron supply upstream or downstream of complex I (as it may occur when different ratio of $NADH+H+$ / $FADH_2$ are provided) different flux of ROS linked to a reverse electron flux at complex I may occur.

Nature of the respiratory substrates, regulation of PTP and commitment to cell death

The PTP is a proteinaceous high conductance inner membrane channel whose molecular identity remains debated. Because PTP opening *in vitro* leads to a sudden increase in permeability to solutes with molecular masses up to 1500 Da,

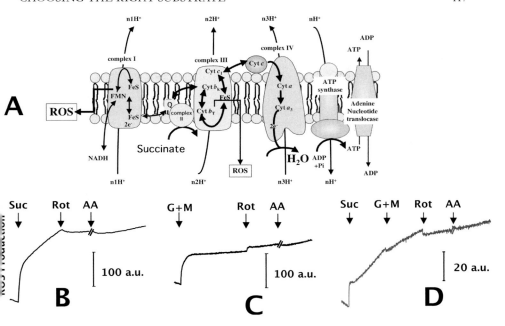

FIG. 2.   ROS production in mitochondria incubated with either succinate or glutamate/malate as respiratory substrates. (A) Schematic view of electron transfer through respiratory chain and ROS production with succinate as single electron donor. When succinate is oxidized by suc-cinodehydrogenase, two electrons are first transferred to the quinone pool, leading to reduced quinone, and then transferred one by one to complex III. During this process, the transitory formation of semiquinone may lead to the formation of the superoxide anion. Electrons flow downstream to oxygen providing a protonmotive force, leading to ATP synthesis. From the current knowledge, it appears that all steps involved in electron transfer at the level of respira-tory chain are reversible with the notable exception of cytochrome oxidase. Hence complex I electron transfer is also reversible, and with succinate as single respiratory substrate, the proton motive force generated by the downstream electron flux allows a simultaneous reversible flux through complex I permitting the reduction of NAD to NADH. Therefore, at complex I both forward and reverse electron fluxes are linked to superoxide formation. (B,C,D) Mitochondria isolated from rat liver (1 mg protein) were incubated with substrates or inhibitors in 2.0 ml medium (30 °C) containing 250 mM sucrose, 0.1 mM EGTA, 20 mM Tris-HCl (pH 7.4), 2.5 mM Pi and 1 mM $MgCl_2$. Hydrogen peroxide (ROS) production was assessed by homovanillic acid/horse radish peroxidase. Where indicated, substrates or inhibitors were added: (B) 2.5 mM succinate (Suc); (C) 2.5 mM glutamate and 1.25 mM malate (G+M); and (D) 2.5 mM succinate (Suc), 2.5 mM glutamate and 1.25 mM malate (G+M+S), and 1 µM rotenone (Rot) and 0.125 µM antimycin A (AA). Spontaneous fluorescence of antimycin A was subtracted and curves were rescaled after its addition. One typical experiment is presented.

LEVERVE ET AL

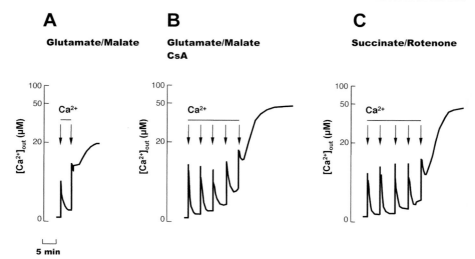

A Glutamate/Malate

B Glutamate/Malate CsA

C Succinate/Rotenone

FIG. 3. Effect of respiratory substrates and CsA on the Ca^{2+} retention capacity of skeletal muscle mitochondria. The incubation medium contained 250 mM sucrose, 10 mM Pi-Tris, 5 μM EGTA-Tris, 10 mM Tris-MOPS, 1 μM Calcium Green-5N. Final volume 2 ml, pH 7.3, 25 °C. Respiratory substrates were 5 mM glutamate-Tris, 2.5 mM malate-Tris (panel A and B), or 5 mM succinate-Tris plus 2 μM rotenone (panel C). In panel B the medium was supplemented with 1 μM CsA. Experiments were started by the addition of 0.3 mg of mitochondria (not shown). Where indicated, 10 μM Ca^{2+} pulses were added (arrows).

it is followed by membrane depolarization, and this channel must be closed in order for oxidative phosphorylation to proceed. The PTP open–closed transitions are modulated by a variety of physiological factors but matrix Ca^{2+} appears to be the single most important PTP inducer. Although long suspected as a mechanism of cell dysfunction, only recently has the occurrence of PTP opening *in vivo* been directly assessed by measuring the diffusion of fluorescent probes that do not cross the inner membrane unless PTP opens (Petronilli et al 1999, 2001). Both transient and long lasting PTP opening have been documented, and their role in cell pathophysiology is being actively addressed. Transient PTP openings in intact cells may serve the physiological function of providing mitochondria with a fast Ca^{2+} release channel, yet relatively long lasting pore opening may eventually lead to the release of mitochondrial pro-apoptotic factors such as cytochrome c into the cytoplasm (Petronilli et al 1999, 2001). Involvement of the PTP in the commitment to cell death is also supported by the protective effects exerted by two PTP inhibitors, cyclosporin A (CsA) (Crompton 1999) and bongkrekic acid (BA) (Pastorino et al 1996), in several models. In a recent study of skeletal muscle mitochondria it was found that PTP opening *in vitro* is dramatically affected by the substrates used for energization in the sense that much higher Ca^{2+} loads are required to open the pore when electrons are provided to complex II rather than to complex I (Fontaine et al 1998), and an example is depicted in the experiments of Fig. 3. Skeletal muscle mitochondria energized with glutamate plus malate were loaded with a train of Ca^{2+} pulses (Fig. 3A). Mitochondria took up and retained Ca^{2+} until the load reached a threshold at which mitochondria underwent fast Ca^{2+} release that was accompanied by depolarization and swelling (data not shown). As expected, Fig. 3B shows that the Ca^{2+} load required to induce Ca^{2+} release was dramatically increased by CsA, proving that the PTP was involved in the release process. It must be noted that when mitochondria were energized by succinate in the presence of rotenone (Fig. 3C) the Ca^{2+} load required to induce PTP opening was similar to that required to open the PTP when mitochondria were energized by glutamate plus malate in the presence of CsA (Fig. 3B).

References

Azzone GF, Zoratti M, Petronilli V, Pietrobon D 1985 The stoichiometry of H+ pumping in cytochrome oxidase and the mechanism of uncoupling. J Inorg Biochem 23:349–356

Batandier C, Fontaine E, Keriel C, Leverve XM 2002 Determination of mitochondrial reactive oxygen species: methodological aspects. J Cell Mol Med 6:175–187

Batandier C, Guigas B, Detaille D et al 2006 The ROS production induced by a reverse-electron flux at respiratory-chain complex 1 is hampered by metformin. J Bioenerg Biomembr 38: 33–42

Bernardi P 1999 Mitochondrial transport of cations: channels, exchangers and permeability transition. Physiol Rev 79:1127–1155

Bouillaud F, Couplan E, Pecqueur C, Ricquier D 2001 Homologues of the uncoupling protein from brown adipose tissue (UCP1): UCP2, UCP3, BMCP1 and UCP4. Biochim Biophys Acta 1504:107–119

Boveris A, Chance B 1973 The mitochondrial generation of hydrogen peroxide. General properties and effect of hyperbaric oxygen. Biochem J 134:707–716

Brand MD 1990 The proton leak across the mitochondrial inner membrane. Biochim Biophys Acta 1018:128–133

Chance B, Hollunger G 1961 The interaction of energy and electron transfer reactions in mitochondria. I. General properties and nature of the products of succinate-linked reduction of pyridine nucleotide. J Biol Chem 236:1534–1543

Crompton M 1999 The mitochondrial permeability transition pore and its role in cell death. Biochem J 341(Pt 2):233–249

Droge W 2002 Free radicals in the physiological control of cell function. Physiol Rev 82:47–95

Fitton V, Rigoulet M, Ouhabi R, Guerin B 1994 Mechanistic stoichiometry of yeast mitochondrial oxidative phosphorylation. Biochemistry 33:9692–9698

Fontaine EM, Moussa M, Devin A et al 1996 Effect of polyunsaturated fatty acids deficiency on oxidative phosphorylation in rat liver mitochondria. Biochim Biophys Acta 1276: 181–187

Fontaine EM, Devin A, Rigoulet M, Leverve XM 1997 The yield of oxidative phosphorylation is controlled both by force and flux. Biochem Biophys Res Commun 232:532–535

Fontaine E, Eriksson O, Ichas F, Bernardi P 1998 Regulation of the permeability transition pore in skeletal muscle mitochondria. Modulation by electron flow through the respiratory chain complex i. J Biol Chem 273:12662–12668

Hinkle PC, Butow RA, Racker E, Chance B 1967 Partial resolution of the enzymes catalyzing oxidative phosphorylation. XV. Reverse electron transfer in the flavin-cytochrome beta region of the respiratory chain of beef heart submitochondrial particles. J Biol Chem 242:5169–5173

Kalderon B, Hertz R, Bar-Tana J 1992 Effect of thyroid hormone treatment on redox and phosphate potentials in rat liver. Endocrinology 131:400–407

Korshunov SS, Skulachev VP, Starkov AA 1997 High protonic potential actuates a mechanism of production of reactive oxygen species in mitochondria. FEBS Lett 416:15–18

Korshunov SS, Korkina OV, Ruuge EK, Skulachev VP, Starkov AA 1998 Fatty acids as natural uncouplers preventing generation of O2.- and H2O2 by mitochondria in the resting state. FEBS Lett 435(2-3):215–218

Korvald C, Elvenes OP, Myrmel T 2000 Myocardial substrate metabolism influences left ventricular energetics *in vivo*. Am J Physiol Heart Circ Physiol 278:H1345–1351

Koubi HE, Desplanches D, Gabrielle C, Cottet-Emard JM, Sempore B, Favier RJ 1991 Exercise endurance and fuel utilization: a reevaluation of the effects of fasting. J Appl Physiol 70:1337–1343

Kushnareva Y, Murphy AN, Andreyev A 2002 Complex I-mediated reactive oxygen species generation: modulation by cytochrome c and NAD(P)+ oxidation-reduction state. Biochem J 368(Pt 2):545–553

Kwong LK, Sohal RS 1998 Substrate and site specificity of hydrogen peroxide generation in mouse mitochondria. Arch Biochem Biophys 350:118–126

Leverve XM, Verhoeven AJ, Groen AK, Meijer AJ, Tager JM 1986 The malate/aspartate shuttle and pyruvate kinase as targets involved in the stimulation of gluconeogenesis by phenylephrine. Eur J Biochem 155:551–556

Liu Y, Fiskum G, Schubert D 2002 Generation of reactive oxygen species by the mitochondrial electron transport chain. J Neurochem 80:780–787

Luvisetto S, Pietrobon D, Azzone GF 1987 On the nature of the uncoupling effect of fatty acids. Biochemistry 26:7332–7338

Luvisetto S, Conti E, Buso M, Azzone GF 1991 Flux ratios and pump stoichiometries at sites II and III in liver mitochondria. Effect of slips and leaks. J Biol Chem 266:1034–1042

McClelland GB, Hochachka PW, Weber JM 1998 Carbohydrate utilization during exercise after high-altitude acclimation: a new perspective. Proc Natl Acad Sci USA 95:10288–10293

Muller S, Seitz HJ 1994 Cloning of a cDNA for the FAD-linked glycerol-3-phosphate dehydrogenase from rat liver and its regulation by thyroid hormones. Proc Natl Acad Sci USA 91:10581–10585

Murphy MP, Brand MD 1987 Variable stoichiometry of proton pumping by the mitochondrial respiratory chain. Nature 329:170–172

Ouhabi R, Rigoulet M, Lavie JL, Guérin B 1991 Respiration in non-phosphorylating yeast mitochondria. Roles of non-ohmic proton conductance and intrinsic uncoupling. Biochim Biophys Acta 1060:293–298

Pastorino JG, Simbula G, Yamamoto K, Glascott PA Jr, Rothman RJ, Farber JL 1996 The cytotoxicity of tumor necrosis factor depends on induction of the mitochondrial permeability transition. J Biol Chem 271:29792–29798

Petronilli V, Miotto G, Canton M et al 1999 Transient and long-lasting openings of the mitochondrial permeability transition pore can be monitored directly in intact cells by changes in mitochondrial calcein fluorescence. Biophys J 76:725–734

Petronilli V, Penzo D, Scorrano L, Bernardi P, Di Lisa F 2001 The mitochondrial permeability transition, release of cytochrome c and cell death. Correlation with the duration of pore openings in situ. J Biol Chem 276:12030–12034

Pietrobon D, Caplan SR 1985 Double-inhibitor and uncoupler-inhibitor titrations. 2. Analysis with a nonlinear model of chemiosmotic energy coupling. Biochemistry 24:5764–5776

Pietrobon D, Zoratti M, Azzone GF 1983 Molecular slipping in redox and ATPase H+ pumps. Biochim Biophys Acta 723:317–321

Ricquier D, Bouillaud F 2000 The uncoupling protein homologues: UCP1, UCP2, UCP3, StUCP and AtUCP. Biochem J 345:161–179

Rigoulet M, Leverve X, Fontaine E, Ouhabi R, Guérin B 1998 Mol Cell Biochem 184:35–52

Schmehl I, Luvisetto S, Canton M, Gennari F, Azzone GF 1995 Quantitative analysis of some mechanisms affecting the yield of oxidative phosphorylation: dependence upon both fluxes and forces. FEBS Lett 375:206–210

Sibille B, Filippi C, Piquet MA et al 2001 The mitochondrial consequences of uncoupling intact cells depend on the nature of the exogenous substrate. Biochem J 355:231–235

Sibille B, Keriel C, Fontaine E, Catelloni F, Rigoulet M, Leverve XM 1995 Octanoate affects 2,4-dinitrophenol uncoupling in intact isolated rat hepatocytes. Eur J Biochem 231:498–502

Thannickal VJ, Fanburg BL 2000 Reactive oxygen species in cell signaling. Am J Physiol Lung Cell Mol Physiol 279:L1005–1028

Turrens JF 1997 Superoxide production by the mitochondrial respiratory chain. Biosci Rep 17:3–8

Vinogradov AD, Grivennikova VG 2001 The mitochondrial complex I: progress in understanding of catalytic properties. IUBMB Life 52(3-5):129–134

Votyakova TV, Reynolds IJ 2001 DeltaPsi(m)-Dependent and -independent production of reactive oxygen species by rat brain mitochondria. J Neurochem 79:266–277

van Dam K, Shinohara Y, Unami A, Yoshida K, Terada H 1990 Slipping pumps or proton leaks in oxidative phosphorylation. The local anesthetic bupivacaine causes slip in cytochrome c oxidase of mitochondria. FEBS Lett 277:131–133

Zoratti M, Favaron M, Pietrobon D, Azzone GF 1986 Intrinsic uncoupling of mitochondrial proton pumps. 1. Non-ohmic conductance cannot account for the nonlinear dependence of static head respiration on delta microH. Biochemistry 25:760–767

DISCUSSION

Singer: The story with lipids and statins is interesting. There is evidence of HMG CoA reductase deficiency in sepsis, and there is also HMG CoA reductase present in mitochondria. Can you put these together?

Leverve: This is the pathway of cholesterol synthesis, and I was actually talking about fatty acid oxidation. The phospholipid composition of the mitochondrial membrane plays a key role in the regulation of oxidative phosphorylation. We have been working on a rodent model of polyunsaturated fatty acid deficiency, and we found that it affected the efficiency of oxidative phosphorylation as indicated by a decrease in ATP/O (Piquet et al 1996). This means that the composition of the membrane is important for this efficiency. There is no cholesterol in the inner membrane of mitochondria and inner membrane fluidity is strongly dependent on the cardiolipin. However, for the plasma membrane, you are right: cholesterol has a key role.

Singer: How do you equate what you have shown with what Greet Van den Berghe has shown, where she drives glucose into the cell?

Leverve: I think this fits perfectly. High glucose is a kind of inflammatory signal, which probably works by increasing the oxidative stress at the level of respiratory chain and but also inhibits the first step (glucose-6-phosphate dehydrogenase) of the pentose phosphate shuttle. It is clear that high glucose results in oxidative stress, which results in insulin resistance. It is also clear that glucose oxidation and NADH production and oxidation has a probable role in the commitment to apoptosis. If the system is slightly uncoupled, there is a switch from glucose oxidation to lipid oxidation, but this will result in an increase in oxygen consumption per mole of ATP produced. I don't know whether this can explain all Greet's results, but this is in agreement.

Radermacher: You mentioned the Korvald et al (2000) paper and the switch to preferential carbohydrate oxidation under hypoxic conditions. Sepsis is mainly the other way round: the tissue has abundant oxygen. Does this mean that there is a switch to lipid oxidation? What happens under hyperoxic conditions?

Leverve: If patients aren't in a condition of limited oxygenation, then respiratory quotient will be close to 0.7, which means lipid oxidation. This might be linked to several things, and one which is very important is the recycling of substrate through the glucose-lactate cycle as described by Cori almost a century ago. When two lactates are converted to glucose in the gluconeogenic pathway, the required energy is provided from fatty acid oxidation in the liver. Hence any increase in the so-called 'futile' cyclings, such as alanine/glucose or lactate/glucose, actually represents an increased lipid oxidation to fuel the system. When patients have to cope with hypoxia, they change the respiratory quotient from 0.7 (lipid oxidation with low oxygen consumption/ATP synthesis efficiency) to close to 1 (highest oxidative phosphorylation efficiency). I don't have any data on efficiency in hyperoxia, but I'd imagine that in this condition you would have side effects due to the fact that hyperoxia stimulates the inflammatory response. In cancer or septic patients, the respiratory quotient is often closer to 0.7 than to 1.

Griffiths: In a ventilated septic patient they are producing a lot of membrane-produced lactate from the Na^+/K^+ pump in the septic muscle. In the absence of contraction that muscle isn't breaking down glycogen to produce lactate in any other way. This lactate shuttles to the liver. Does this account for the increased lipid oxidation in the liver?

Leverve: For red blood cells the question is simple since they do not contain mitochondria. The cycling lactate/glucose turnover between red blood cells and liver results in increasing lipid oxidation in liver. Of course, in muscle the situation is different since these cells can indeed oxidize lactate after its conversion to pyruvate. What you say is very important because in sepsis the activation of Na$^+$/K$^+$ ATPase activity will result in enhancement of glycolysis and lactate release. This lactate release has nothing to do with any hypoxic condition; it is just the result of enhancement of Na$^+$/K$^+$ ATPase activity. This will result in lipid oxidation in the liver.

Griffiths: In a non contracting skeletal muscle the glucose is coming from the blood, not from glycogen breakdown.

Fink: I think it is more complicated than just activation of the Na$^+$/K$^+$ ATPase. There's a lot of evidence that inflammatory cytokines activate signalling through HIF-1 and convert cells to a glycolytic phenotype independent of oxygen tension. They spin glycolysis just because they have the machinery to do it. They have more of the enzymes that are involved in the glycolytic pathway.

Leverve: I agree. However I still think the lactate release linked to Na$^+$/K$^+$ ATPase is a very important phenomenon. There is a paper from the Lausanne group and us (Novel-Chate et al 2001) showing that ouabain is able to decrease the production of lactate. This means that by blocking the Na$^+$/K$^+$ ATPase you also decrease the glycolytic flux strongly as it has been shown in septic patients (Levy et al 2005). There is another important mechanism, which is the hexokinase binding to the voltage-dependent anion channel (VDAC). Normally, hexokinase is highly sensitive to the concentration of its product glucose-6-phosphate (G6P). This is an important mechanism because otherwise high glucose would deplete the cells of ATP, since all glucose would be used to G6P synthesis. For this reason there is a strong inhibitory effect of G6P on its own production. This is true for hexokinase, which is soluble in the cytosol: when this enzyme binds to the VDAC it becomes insensitive to its product. Hence, a huge flux of glycolysis may occur since there is no control anymore at the first step of phosphorylation of glucose.

Fink: I know about as much about metabolism as my next door neighbour, who is an attorney. But I have been introduced to the Warburg hypothesis, which is that cancer cells and fetal cells do metabolism differently. They are glycolytic machines. This is one of the reasons why studying immortalized cell lines as a model for normal biology can lead to misleading results. Immortalized cell lines have a different sort of metabolism. Our data suggest that when you take cells and expose them to inflammatory cytokines, they look like cancer cells. They develop a fetal phenotype. Is this some sort of protective adaptive mechanism?

Leverve: I may have some data that would lead to a hypothesis on this very important issue. Complex I plays probably a key role in the commitment to apoptosis (Chauvin et al 2001, Detaille et al 2005). If cells can bypass complex I, the probability of opening the mitochondrial PTP with a given amount of Ca^{2+} is much lower. To try to survive and avoid apoptosis, cancer cells might also avoid an electron flux through complex I. The cost of this is that the efficiency of the system is decreased, but allows the cells to avoid a dangerous pathway that may lead to apoptosis. To support this we have data showing that the more the cells are resistant to chemotherapy, the less they have complex I working (De Oliveira et al 2006). In sepsis the same kind of event could be happening.

Singer: On that point, we are giving succinate. You can either go through oxidation of fat or through succinate to feed through complex II. The more complex I inhibition in our septic model, the more we can boost things through complex II.

Leverve: That is exactly the mechanism I am describing: if you block complex I you also block this effect. How much Ca^{2+} do you need to open the PTP with glutamate compared with succinate? The ratio was $1:6$, so sixfold more Ca^{2+} is needed to open the PTP with succinate as opposed to glutamate (Fontaine et al 1998).

Szabó: You showed the inhibition of GAP-DH by reactive oxygen species (ROS). We have been looking for this in the literature, but I haven't been able to find any published reports for NADH inhibition in sepsis.

Fink: We have looked for it too without success.

Szabó: In sepsis there is nothing. In diabetes it is only *in vitro* models where anyone has looked at this. It is a good story and I like it, but there's a lack of evidence for it *in vivo* (so far).

Leverve: Actually I was referring to the data published by the group of Michael Brownlee and I don't have personal data on this specific point.

Szabó: But if you have increased ROS then you'd expect GAP-DH would be inhibited the same, but this doesn't seem to be the case.

Fink: It was a good story and was fashionable some years ago, but I don't think it is real.

Van den Berghe: It may be real in diabetes patients. Personally, I don't think that ROS-related inhibition of GAP-DH activity is the mechanism.

Piantadosi: I have a more conventional view of the way uncoupling works, and the way complexes I and II work. Like Mitch Fink said, one of the responses that cells use under stress is to up-regulate glucose transport. They take up glucose and this is phosphorylated immediately. The hexokinase on the cell membrane is activated by cell stress. Thus the cell traps the glucose as phosphoglucose. In addition, the glycolytic pathway is not just anaerobic. It is an aerobic process, and we all use aerobic glycolysis when we begin to exercise, for example. As far as the uncoupling issue is concerned, we shouldn't be confused about the term: it refers to the efficiency of ATP production, often given as P:O ratio. You call it 'uncoupling' when this ratio falls. Uncoupling strictly means that energy isn't conserved. In the UCP1 example you gave, very little ATP is made if any when this is protein expressed, because its presence dissipates the $\Delta\Psi$. Conventionally, uncoupling indicates increased heat generation and not differences in fuel utilization. For example, in the case of succinate you only get about two ATPs for the three you get with pyruvate. This is not uncoupling but a difference in the efficiency of ATP production due to the point of carbon entry into the chain.

Leverve: If you consider a cell (or an organism) in steady state, with no net accumulation of any metabolite, substrate or proteins, etc. (this is the case for a human being, whose body mass doesn't change and at rest without any physical activity involving net work), the final thermodynamic yield will be zero because all energy will be dissipated in heat. Even if the system is fully coupled in terms of respiration and ATP synthesis, it will only generate heat. So when you uncouple such a system *in vivo*, because of the dissipation of $\Delta\Psi$ you increase the respiratory rate, which will increase the heat production. But in terms of the ratio of heat production per mole of oxygen consumed there is no difference between the coupled system and the uncoupled system since at the end in the absence of net work, all energy will be finally converted to heat. This is why, when we speak of efficiency, mostly it is *in vitro*, where there is accumulation of ATP so there is chemical work.

Piantadosi: I want to clarify this point. The proton gradient is coupled to ATP production. The reason you don't get heat is because you conserve the energy in the third phosphate bond. Without that energy conservation there is a huge increase in heat production. This is a key point in terms of the coupling process.

Fink: So there is more heat production when you uncouple?

Piantadosi: Yes, uncoupling gives a lot more heat production for any level of oxygen uptake. This is easily measurable.

Singer: There is some middle ground. There is an argument that there can be 'mild' uncoupling.

Piantadosi: I don't like that term because it does not specify a different function from standard uncoupling.

Singer: It is talked about as a way of decreasing ROS production. It is more on the membrane potential.

Piantadosi: You are not effectively uncoupling there, because the ROS production is tiny and you get about the same amount of ATP for each substrate molecule. In fact, it is also possible to get more ROS under certain conditions. We know of four UCPs: 1–4. UCP1 clearly uncouples and generates heat, but humans use the other UCPs which can be genetically knocked out with no increase in heat production or loss of ATP. There are very small differences, however, in ROS production across the inner membrane. The point is to be specific about the use of the term uncoupling, we don't want to redefine it to mean something to do with the carbon flux independent of the heat and ATP production—i.e. energy conservation.

Leverve: This is an important point. When you have a patient on the bed all the energy is converted to heat, as long as its own mass is not changed and he or she is not doing net physical work. This is the basis of indirect calorimetry where we use oxygen instead of heat production. Do you agree?

Piantadosi: Not exactly.

Leverve: The ATP level is constant. This means that each ATP molecule that has been synthesized should break down at a steady state rate. Then, according to the thermodynamics principle, the thermodynamic yield of life, as humans, is zero unless we are doing some physical (climbing) or metabolic (growth) net work. This means that the efficiency of the whole system is zero. The only thing that changes is the way you go from oxygen to heat.

Fink: Doesn't making proteins or beating your heart count as work?

Leverve: Of course it is work, but ultimately completely converted to heat since in a steady state the content is stable: no net accumulation or consumption. Again, this is the basis of the use of indirect calorimetry. The major difference between uncoupling and coupling *in vivo* is a huge increase in respiration. Of course, there is heat dissipation, but again the ratio between oxygen consumption and heat production is not different in the coupled or uncoupled state.

Piantadosi: I don't argue with the fact that once energy is used it is no longer stored. But the cell maintains 3 mM ATP and even more creatine phosphate.

Leverve: We don't store ATP.

Fink: There are some inherited disorders of mitochondrial function. The symptoms of these diseases are largely neurological and musculoskeletal. But it is not multiple organ system failure.

Van den Berghe: If you stress the individual, it is different.

Fink: These people have dysfunctional mitochondria, and they manifest it by not being able to play football or think properly, depending on the syndrome.

Griffiths: I remember a young man with a profound mitochondrial myopathy who was a psychology graduate and he would present at clinic with a lactate of 15. He had difficulty running up the stairs, but otherwise he was normal except for a very low maximal oxygen consumption!

Piantadosi: But these patients are more susceptible to organ failure after stress.

Fink: But they don't have it at baseline. They have compensated in some way.

Singer: Patients with complex I deficiencies up-regulate complex II. Their phenotype changes to compensate.

Szabó: This doesn't prove anything. You are selectively trying to focus on something in the mitochondria. In a septic patient several things go wrong at the same time. People ask me about the PARP pathway, and how it is possible that PARP is doing this and that. My response is that we are not dealing with a normal cell, but rather one that has all kinds of problems. Being exposed to all sorts of oxidants is not the same thing as feeding an animal with rotenone.

Piantadosi: If what doesn't kill you makes you stronger, this should be true of mitochondrial phenotypes. They are not all the same. When mitochondria are stressed, the cell figures out how to adapt. MnSOD up-regulation is a nice example of this: it will go up 10-fold within the day after lipopolysaccharide (LPS) exposure.

This is an integral mitochondrial protein that responds when mitochondria adapt. CO will do the same if used properly.

Fink: We wasted about three months trying to kill freshly isolated hepatocytes from rats by growing them under oxygen and glucose deprivation, trying to mimic hepatic ischaemia. They are like cockroaches after a nuclear bomb: you can't kill those guys. These little cells are loaded with mitochondria and are supposed to be ox-phos machines. Yet we could only kill 30% of them after 18 h of oxygen–glucose deprivation.

Singer: Did you look at their activity?

Piantadosi: What work did you make them do?

Fink: Not much. We fed them lipid-soluble red dye. Its uptake was one of the assays for viability.

Van den Berghe: Perhaps if you load them with glucose the damage will occur.

Fink: We didn't try that.

Van den Berghe: We found that the Glut transporters are changed in humans or animals that are sick. The normal glucose physiology no longer applies because the gates are wide open.

Fink: So we should try to feed them glucose first.

References

Chauvin C, De Oliveira F, Ronot X, Mousseau M, Leverve X, Fontaine E 2001 Rotenone inhibits the mitochondrial permeability transition-induced cell death in U937 and KB cells. J Biol Chem 276:41394–41398

De Oliveira F, Chauvin C, Ronot X, Mousseau M, Leverve X, Fontaine E 2006 Effects of permeability transition inhibition and decrease in cytochrome c content on doxorubicin toxicity in K562 cells. Oncogene 25:2646–2655

Detaille D, Guigas B, Chauvin C et al 2005 Metformin prevents high-glucose-induced endothelial cell death through a mitochondrial permeability transition-dependent process. Diabetes 54:2179–2187

Fontaine E, Eriksson O, Ichas F, Bernardi P 1998 Regulation of the permeability transition pore in skeletal muscle mitochondria. Modulation by electron flow through the respiratory chain complex I. J Biol Chem 1998 273:12662–12668

Korvald C, Elvenes OP, Myrmel T 2000 Myocardial substrate metabolism influences left ventricular energetics *in vivo*. Am J Physiol Heart Circ Physiol 278:H1345–1351

Levy B, Gibot S, Franck P, Cravoisy A, Bollaert PE 2005 Relation between muscle Na+K+ ATPase activity and raised lactate concentrations in septic shock: a prospective study. Lancet 365:871–875 Erratum in Lancet 366:122

Novel-Chate V, Rey V, Chiolero R et al 2001 Role of Na+-K+-ATPase in insulin-induced lactate release by skeletal muscle. Am J Physiol Endocrinol Metab 280:E296–300

Piquet MA, Fontaine E, Sibille B, Filippi C, Keriel C, Leverve XM 1996 Uncoupling effect of polyunsaturated fatty acid deficiency in isolated rat hepatocytes: effect on glycerol metabolism. Biochem J 317:667–674

Inhibiting glycogen synthase kinase 3β in sepsis

Laura Dugo*, Marika Collin*, David A. Allen*, Nimesh S.A. Patel*, Inge Bauer†, Eero M.A. Mervaala‡, Marjut Louhelainen‡, Simon J. Foster§, Muhammad M. Yaqoob* and Christoph Thiemermann*

*Centre for Experimental Medicine, Nephrology and Critical Care Medicine, The William Harvey Research Institute, St. Bartholomew's and The Royal London School of Medicine and Dentistry, Charterhouse Square, London EC1M 6BQ, UK, † Department of Anesthesiology and Critical Care Medicine, University of the Saarland, Homburg, Germany, ‡ Institute of Biomedicine, Pharmacology, Biomedicum Helsinki, FIN-00014, University of Helsinki, Finland and § Department of Molecular Biology and Biotechnology, University of Sheffield, Western Bank, Sheffield S10 2TN, UK

Abstract. The serine-threonine protein kinase glycogen synthase kinase (GSK)-3 is involved in the regulation of many cell functions, but its role in the regulation of the inflammatory response is unknown. Here we investigate the effects of GSK-3β inhibition on organ injury/dysfunction caused by endotoxaemia or severe inflammation in the rat. Rats received either intravenous *Escherichia coli* lipopolysaccharide (LPS) (6 mg/kg) or LPS (1 mg/kg) plus *Staphylococcus aureus* peptidoglycan (PepG) (0.3 mg/kg) or their vehicle (saline). The GSK-3β inhibitors TDZD-8, SB415286 (both 1 mg/kg, i.v.), and SB216763 (0.6 mg/kg i.v.), or vehicle (10% dimethyl sulfoxide) were administered 30 min before LPS or LPS/PepG. Both endotoxaemia and co-administration of LPS/PepG resulted in multiple organ injury and dysfunction. The GSK-3β inhibitors attenuated the organ injury/dysfunction caused by LPS or LPS/PepG. GSK-3β inhibition reduced the Ser536 phosphorylation of nuclear factor (NF)-κB subunit p65 and the mRNA expression of NF-κB-dependent pro-inflammatory mediators, but had no effect on the NF-κB/DNA binding activity in the lung. GSK-3β inhibition reduced the increase in NF-κB p65 activity caused by interleukin (IL)1 in human embryonic kidney cells *in vitro*. We propose that GSK-3β inhibition may be useful in the therapy of sepsis, shock and other diseases associated with local or systemic inflammation.

2007 Sepsis—new insights, new therapies. Wiley, Chichester (Novartis Foundation Symposium 280) p 128–146

Glycogen synthase kinase (GSK)-3 is a ubiquitous serine-threonine protein kinase that participates in a multitude of cellular processes, ranging from cell membrane–nucleus signalling, gene transcription, translation and cytoskeletal organization to cell cycle progression and survival (Cohen & Abraham 1999, Embi et al 1980, Woodgett 2001). Two closely related isoforms have been found in mammals, GSK-3α and GSK-3β. Unlike most kinases, GSK-3 is constitutively active in cells and a wide range of extracellular stimuli, including insulin, epidermal growth factor (EGF) and fibroblast growth factor (FGF) exert their effects by inhibiting GSK-3 activity (Cross et al 1995). Phosphorylation in a specific serine residue (Ser21 in GSK-3α and Ser9 in GSK-3β) located in its N-terminal domain inhibits GSK-3 activity and, hence, reduces its activity to alter cell function (Woodgett 2001).

Recently, GSK-3β knockout mice showed a similar phenotype to mice in which the gene for p65 or I-κB kinase 2 (and hence, the activation of NF-κB) had been deleted (Hoeflich et al 2000). Similar to the disruption of the p65 gene, disruption of the murine GSK-3β gene resulted in embryonic lethality caused by severe liver degeneration (Beg et al 1995, Hoeflich et al 2000, Li et al 1999). This finding is the basis for the hypothesis that GSK-3β may play a pivotal role in the regulation of the inflammatory response.

Hence, this study was designed to elucidate the effects of GSK-3β inhibition on the renal dysfunction, hepatocellular injury, pancreatic injury and neuromuscular injury caused by systemic inflammation in the rat. Systemic inflammation was induced by (i) administration of lipopolysaccharide (LPS) (endotoxaemia, model of systemic inflammation with hypotension) or (ii) co-administration of LPS and peptidoglycan (model of systemic inflammation without hypotension) (Dugo et al 2004). To investigate the mechanisms by which GSK-3β inhibition may alleviate the organ injury/dysfunction associated with systemic inflammation, we measured the effects of various chemically distinct GSK-3β inhibitors (TDZD-8, SB216763 and SB415286) on the NF-κB/DNA binding, the phosphorylation of serine residue 536 (Ser536) on NF-κB subunit p65, and the mRNA expression of NF-κB-dependent pro-inflammatory cytokines (interleukin [IL]1β and IL6), adhesion molecules (ICAM1 and VCAM1) and monocyte chemoattractant protein (MCP1) in tissues from rats subjected to systemic inflammation and treated with GSK-3β inhibitors. To obtain a more mechanistic insight in to the effects of these compounds, we evaluated the effects of GSK-3β inhibitors on the phosphorylation of the residue Ser9 of GSK-3β and on the p65 activity *in vitro*.

Materials and methods

Surgical procedure and quantification of organ injury/dysfunction

This study was carried out on 99 male Wistar rats (Charles River, UK) weighing 230–300 g, receiving a standard diet and water *ad libitum*. The investigation was performed in accordance with the Home Office *Guidance on the Operation of the Animals (Scientific Procedures) Act 1986*, published by HMSO, London.

TABLE 1   Experimental design: study I

Group	Group ID	Treatment	Dose	n
1	Sham Control	Vehicle-10% DMSO	1 ml/kg	12
2	LPS Control	LPS + Vehicle-10%DMSO	6 mg/kg + 1 ml/kg	12
3	LPS + TDZD-8	LPS + TDZD-8	1 mg/kg i.v.	8
4	LPS + SB216763	LPS + SB216763	1 mg/kg i.v.	8

n is the number of animals used in the study.

All animals were anaesthetised with thiopentone sodium (Intraval®, 120 mg/kg, i.p.), and anaesthesia was maintained by supplementary injections of thiopentone sodium (approximately 1–2 mg/kg/h i.v.) as required. The general surgical procedures and collection of the samples were performed as previously described (Thiemermann et al 1995).

Experimental design

Study I. Animals were assigned to four experimental groups. Rats were subjected to either (i) the surgical procedure alone, without inducing endotoxaemia, or (ii) induction of endotoxaemia by administration of *Escherichia coli* LPS (serotype 0127:B8), which was given slowly over 10 min, for a period of 6 h and pre-treated with either the vehicle (10%DMSO, 1 ml/kg), TDZD-8 (1 mg/kg i.v.) or SB216763 (1 mg/kg i.v.) 30 min prior to the administration of LPS (Table 1).

Study II. Animals were assigned to four experimental groups. Rats were subjected to either (i) the surgical procedure alone, without inducing systemic inflammation, or (ii) induction of systemic inflammation by administration of *E. coli* LPS (serotype 0127:B8) and *Staphylococcus aureus* peptidoglycan, which was given slowly over 10 min, for a period of 6 h and pre-treated with either the vehicle (10%DMSO, 1 ml/kg), TDZD-8 (1 mg/kg i.v.) or SB415286 (1 mg/kg i.v.) 30 min prior to the administration of LPS (Table 2).

The effects of the selective GSK-3β inhibitors TDZD-8, SB216763 and SB415286 on renal dysfunction, hepatocellular injury, pancreatic injury and neuromuscular injury were also investigated in sham-operated animals (not subjected to administration of any bacterial cell wall components). The doses of SB216763 and SB415286 were chosen based on a previous report demonstrating GSK-3β inhibition *in vivo* (Gross et al 2004). The dose of TDZD-8 used was chosen based on the IC_{50} values for the inhibition of GSK-3β (published by the supplier) as well as preliminary experiments.

TABLE 2   Experimental design: study II

Group	Group ID	Treatment	Dose	n
1	Sham Control	Vehicle-10% DMSO	1 ml/kg	10
2	LPS + PepG Control	LPS + PepG + Vehicle 10%DMSO	1 mg/kg + 0.3 mg/kg + 1 ml/kg	10
3	LPS + PepG + TDZD-8	LPS + TDZD-8	1 mg/kg + 0.3 mg/kg + 1 mg/kg	10
4	LPS + PepG + SB415286	LPS + SB415286	1 mg/kg + 0.3 mg/kg + 1 mg/kg	10

n is the number of animals used in the study.

Nuclear extracts and electrophoretic mobility shift assay (EMSA)

Nuclear extracts were prepared from frozen lung sections using a modification of a method by Dignam et al (1983) as described in detail previously (Rensing et al 2001). Double-stranded NF-κB consensus oligonucleotide probe (NF-κB: AGTTGAGGGGACTTTCCCAGGC) was end-labelled with $\gamma[^{32}P]$ (Amersham, Freiburg, FRG) (Essani et al 1996).

Western blot analyses

Six hours after co-administration of LPS and peptidoglycan, lung samples were collected, immediately frozen in liquid nitrogen, and stored at −80 °C. Tissue homogenates were obtained by 20 strokes of a sintered glass homogenizer in two volumes of ice-cold lysis buffer (phosphate buffered saline pH 7.4 containing 0.5% sodium deoxycholate, 1 mM EDTA, 1% SDS and 1% NP40 and protease inhibitor cocktail (1:50, Sigma-Aldrich, UK). Homogenates were centrifuged at 16000 g for 15 min at 4 °C. The supernatant was removed and total protein measured using the bicinchoninic acid assay (BCA, Pierce). Lysates (50 μg) were resolved on a 4–12% NuPage gel and transferred to PVDF membrane (Immobilon-P, Millipore). Membranes were blocked for 2 h at room temperature and incubated overnight at 4 °C with anti-NF-κB p65 (serine 536) monoclonal antibody (1:1000, Cell Signaling Technology). Membranes were incubated with HRP-conjugated anti-mouse antibody followed by detection using chemiluminescence. Densitometric analysis was performed using Gelblot Pro software (UVP Ltd, Cambridge, UK) and results expressed as relative peak area (fold of control). For *in vitro* experiments, 50 μg of whole-cell (human embryonic kidney 293 cells; HEK293) lysate was analysed by SDS-PAGE as above. Membranes were probed with anti-phospho-GSK-3β antibody (Ser21/9, 1:1000, Cell Signaling Technology) overnight at 4 °C followed by anti-rabbit IgG-HRP.

Real time (RT)-PCR analysis

Six hours after co-administration of LPS and peptidoglycan, lung tissues were collected and immediately frozen in liquid nitrogen. Samples were stored at −80 °C. Total RNA from the rat lungs were collected with Trizol (Gibco), treated with DNAse 1 (deoxyribonuclease 1, Sigma Chemicals Co., St Louis, MO, USA) and reverse transcribed (Enhanced avian HS RT-PCR kit, Sigma Chemicals Co.). 2 μl of cDNA was subjected to a quantitative real time polymerase chain reaction by Lightcycler instrument (Roche diagnostics, Neuilly sur Seine, France) for detection of IL1β, IL6, VCAM1, ICAM1, MCP1 and GAPDH mRNAs. GAPDH served as housekeeping gene. The samples were amplified by using FastStart DNA Master SYBR Green 1 (Roche diagnostics) in presence of 0.5 μM of the following primers: MCP (Heyen et al 2002) forward GCAGGTCTCTGTCACGCTTCT, reverse GGCTGAGACAGCACGTGGAT; ICAM1 (Heyen et al 2002) forward ACCTGCAGCCGGAAAGC, reverse CCCGTTTGACAGACTTCACCAT; VCAM1 (Heyen et al 2002) forward GAAGCCGGTCATGGTCAAGT, reverse GGTCACCCTTGAACAGTTCTATCTC; IL1β (Heyen et al 2002) for-ward AGGAAGGCAGTGTCACTCATTGT, reverse CTTGGGTCCTCATCCT GGAA; IL6 (Heyen et al 2002) forward ATATGTTCTCAGGGAGATCTTG GAA, reverse GTGCATCATCGCTGTTCATACA; GAPDH (Farjah et al 2003) forward GGATGCAGGGATGATGTTCT, reverse GAAGGGCTCATGACCA CAGT. The quantities of IL1β, IL6, VCAM1, ICAM1, MCP1 and GAPDH PCR products were quantified with an external standard curve amplified from purified PCR product.

NF-κB p65 activity

HEK293 cells were obtained from the American Type Culture Collection (LGC Promochem Ltd, UK) and maintained in Dulbecco's modified Eagles medium containing 10% v/v FCS, 100 U/mL penicillin, 100 μg/mL streptomycin and 0.25 μg/mL amphotericin B. Cells were incubated in serum free media for 2 h prior to stimulation with IL1β (25 ng/mL) for 30 min. Where indicated, inhibitors of GSK-3β were incubated with HEK293 cells 30 min prior to stimulation with IL1β. NF-κB activity was detected in whole cell lysates of HEK293 cells. Briefly, following stimulation the cells were harvested by pipetting and lysed in modified RIPA buffer as before. 10 μg of lysate was used to detect NF-κB p65 activity in a microplate assay (TransAM p65, Active Motif, Belgium).

Purification of peptidoglycan

Peptidoglycan was isolated from *S. aureus* as previously described (Foster 1992).

Materials

TDZD-8 was purchased from Alexis Corporation (UK) (Bingham, Nottingham, UK). SB216763 and SB415286 were purchased from Tocris Cookson Ltd. (Avonmouth, Bristol, UK). *E. coli* LPS (serotype 0127:B8) was obtained from Sigma-Aldrich Company Ltd. (Poole, Dorset, UK). Thiopentone sodium (Intraval Sodium®) was obtained from Rhône Mérieux Ltd. (Harlow, Essex, UK). All stock solutions were prepared in non-pyrogenic saline (0.9% NaCl; Baxter Healthcare Ltd., Thetford, Norfolk, UK) or 10% DMSO (Sigma).

Statistical analysis

All data are presented as means ± SEM of n observations, where n represents the number of animals or blood samples studied. For repeated measurements (haemodynamics) a two-way analysis of variance (ANOVA) was performed, followed by Bonferroni post test. Data without repeated measurements (organ injury/dysfunction) were analysed by one-way ANOVA, followed by a Dunnett's test for multiple comparison.

Results and discussion

Here we investigated the effects of GSK-3β inhibition on the systemic inflammatory response caused by acute severe endotoxaemia in the rat. We demonstrate that endotoxaemia caused a substantial increase in the serum level of creatinine, AST and ALT indicating the development of acute renal dysfunction and hepatocellular injury (Fig. 1A, Fig. 2A,B). In addition, endotoxaemia was associated with an increase in the serum lipase and CK, indicative of pancreatic and neuromuscular (skeletal or cardiac) injury. A favourable haemodynamic response was also observed in animals treated with TDZD-8, as the hypotension associated with the progression of endotoxaemia was attenuated in these animals. This may explain some of the protection afforded by this GSK-3β inhibitor against the organ injury and dysfunction caused by endotoxaemia. However, prevention of hypotension is not likely to be of pivotal importance in the mechanism(s) underlying the beneficial effects of this non-ATP-competitive GSK-3β inhibitor, as another potent, ATP-competitive inhibitor of this enzyme, SB216763, elicited no significant favourable haemodynamic effect, but was nevertheless able to protect the organs against the injury and dysfunction caused by severe endotoxaemia. To investigate whether prevention of hypotension does indeed contribute to the observed beneficial effects of the GSK-3β inhibitors, we repeated the experiment in another model of systemic inflammation, which is not associated with significant hypotension (Dugo et al 2004).

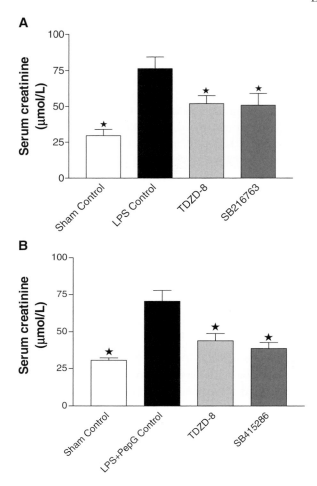

FIG. 1. Alterations in the serum levels of creatinine in endotoxaemia and systemic inflammation. (A) Serum levels of creatinine in rats subjected to the surgical procedure and pre-treated
with 10% DMSO (Sham Control, $n = 12$). Rats subjected to endotoxaemia (LPS 6 mg/kg i.v.)
were pre-treated with either 10% DMSO (LPS Control, $n = 12$), TDZD-8 (1 mg/kg, i.v.,
$n = 8$), or SB216763 (0.6 mg/kg, i.v., $n = 8$) 30 min prior to administration of LPS. (B) Serum
levels of creatinine in rats subjected to the surgical procedure and pre-treated with 10% DMSO
(Sham Control, $n = 10$). Rats subjected to co-administration of LPS (1 mg/kg i.v.) and
peptidoglycan (0.3 mg/kg i.v.) were pre-treated with either 10% DMSO (LPS+PepG Control,
$n = 10$), TDZD-8 (1 mg/kg, i.v., $n = 10$), or SB415286 (1 mg/kg, i.v., $n = 10$) 30 min prior to the
co-administration of LPS and peptidoglycan. *$P < 0.05$ when compared with LPS Control by
ANOVA followed by Dunnett's *post hoc* test.

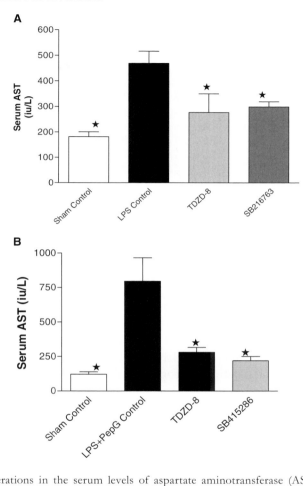

FIG. 2. Alterations in the serum levels of aspartate aminotransferase (AST) and alanine aminotransferase (ALT) in endotoxaemia and systemic inflammation. Serum levels of (A) AST and (B) ALT in rats subjected to the surgical procedure and pre-treated with 10% DMSO (Sham Control, $n = 12$). Rats subjected to endotoxemia (LPS 6 mg/kg i.v.) were pre-treated with either 10% DMSO (LPS Control, $n = 12$), TDZD-8 (1 mg/kg, i.v., $n = 8$), or SB216763 (0.6 mg/kg, i.v., $n = 8$) 30 min prior to administration of LPS. Serum levels of (C) AST and (D) ALT in rats subjected to the surgical procedure and pre-treated with 10% DMSO (Sham Control, $n = 10$). Rats subjected to co-administration of LPS (1 mg/kg i.v.) and peptidoglycan (0.3 mg/kg i.v.) were pre-treated with either 10% DMSO (LPS+PepG Control, $n = 10$), TDZD-8 (1 mg/kg, i.v., $n = 10$), or SB415286 (1 mg/kg, i.v., $n = 10$) 30 min prior to the co-administration of LPS and peptidoglycan. *$P < 0.05$ when compared with LPS Control by ANOVA followed by Dunnett's *post hoc* test.

TABLE 3   Serum parameters of organ injury/dysfunction in Sham-operated animals and sham-operated animals treated with the GSK-3β inhibitors TDZD-8, SB216763 and SB415286

		Serum parameters of organ injury/dysfunction				
Group	*n*	*Creatinine* *(μmol/L)*	*AST* *(iu/L)*	*ALT* *(iu/L)*	*Lipase* *(iu/L)*	*CK* *(iu/L)*
Sham Control	12	30 ± 4	182 ± 19	66 ± 5	18 ± 3	318 ± 80
Sham + TDZD-8	7	30 ± 2	215 ± 22	73 ± 11	13 ± 4	323 ± 21
Sham + SB216763	6	30 ± 3	131 ± 10	57 ± 3	19 ± 1	212 ± 33
Sham + SB415286	6	27 ± 3	143 ± 28	57 ± 11	10 ± 1	272 ± 50

n, number of animals per group; AST, aspartate transaminase; ALT, alanine transaminase; CK, creatine kinase.

Here we demonstrate that co-administration of LPS and peptidoglycan caused substantial increases in the serum levels of creatinine and the transaminases AST and ALT and, hence, renal dysfunction and liver injury, but did not cause hypotension (Fig. 1B, Fig. 2C,D). We also demonstrate that pre-treatment of rats with the GSK-3β inhibitors TDZD-8 and SB415286 markedly reduced the renal dysfunction and hepatocellular injury caused by co-administration of LPS and peptidoglycan in the rat, but these compounds have no effect in normal rats (Table 3).

Many reports have recently demonstrated a link between GSK-3β and NF-κB activity *in vitro* (Demarchi et al 2003, Hoeflich et al 2000, Schwabe & Brenner 2002, Takada et al 2004). For instance, deletion of GSK-3β had no effect on the tumour necrosis factor (TNF)α-induced I-κBα degradation or on the nuclear translocation of the subunit p65, but prevented the activation of NF-κB by an unknown mechanism (Hoeflich et al 2000). Our finding that the GSK-3β inhibitor TDZD-8 had no effect on the DNA binding activity of NF-κB *in vivo* is consistent with this hypothesis. However, GSK-3β has also been suggested to be needed for IKK activation, I-κBα phosphorylation and degradation, and NF-κB/DNA binding using fibroblasts derived from GSK-3β knock-out mice (Takada et al 2004). Very recently, it was reported that activation of NF-κB by phosphorylation of Ser536 on subunit p65 leads to basal and IL1-induced transcription of IL8 *in vitro* (Buss et al 2004). Therefore, in an attempt to clarify the mechanism for the protection afforded by GSK-3β inhibitors, we investigated whether these compounds would have any effect on the phosphorylation of this particular p65 residue, using lung biopsies obtained from rats subjected to co-administration of LPS and peptidoglycan. We report here, in concert with the previous report, that co-administration of LPS and peptidoglycan caused a significant increase in the phosphorylation of Ser536 on p65 in the lung at 6 h, whereas pre-treatment with

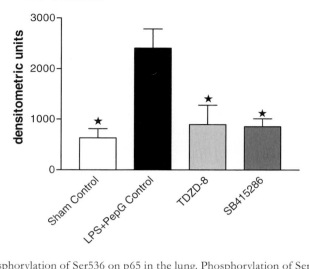

FIG. 3.   Phosphorylation of Ser536 on p65 in the lung. Phosphorylation of Ser536 on NF-κB subunit p65 measured by Western blot analysis in the lung of rats subjected to the surgical procedure and pre-treated with 10% DMSO (Sham, *n* = 3). Rats subjected to co-administration of LPS (1 mg/kg i.v.) and peptidoglycan (0.3 mg/kg i.v.) were pre-treated with either 10% DMSO (Control, *n* = 3), TDZD-8 (*n* = 3, 13 mg/kg i.v.) or SB415286 (*n* = 3, 13 mg/kg i.v.) 30 min prior to the co-administration of LPS and peptidoglycan. *$P < 0.05$ when compared with LPS+PepG Control by ANOVA followed by Dunnett's *post hoc* test.

the GSK-3β inhibitor TDZD-8 significantly reduced this phosphorylation (Fig. 3). However, it has been recently reported that GSK-3β-dependent phosphorylation of another serine residue, Ser468, of p65 blocks the activation of NF-κB and that inhibition of GSK-3β was associated with increased p65 activity (Buss et al 2004). This may contribute to the constitutive NF-κB activity seen in some inflammatory states. Taken together, the balance between pro-inflammatory and pro-survival roles of NF-κB may depend on the phosphorylation status of p65, and GSK-3β may play a central role in this process. The exact molecular mechanism(s) by which GSK-3β amplifies the inflammatory response and, ultimately, the associated organ injury and dysfunction warrants further investigation. As there is good evidence that the activation of NF-κB plays a fundamental role in the development of the multiple organ injury and dysfunction syndrome in systemic inflammation caused by endotoxaemia or co-administration of LPS and peptidoglycan *in vivo* (Wang et al 2004, Wray et al 2001), we also investigated whether the inhibition of GSK-3β would have an effect on the expression of NF-κB–dependent genes such as the pro-inflammatory cytokines IL1β and IL6, adhesion molecules ICAM1 and VCAM1, and the chemokine MCP1. We found that co-administration of LPS and peptidoglycan resulted in significant increases in the expression of the mRNA of these pro-inflammatory mediators in the lung. Most notably, pre-treatment with the GSK-3β inhibitor TDZD-8 abolished the up-regulated expression of the mRNA of these NF-κB-dependent genes (Fig. 4).

To obtain a more mechanistic insight into the effects of the GSK-3β inhibitors, we carried out *in vitro* experiments using HEK293 cells. Using this *in vitro* system, we investigated whether TDZD-8, SB216763 or SB415286 are able to phosphorylate the Ser9 residue on GSK-3β, the key site determining the activity of this kinase (Eldar-Finkelman 2002). We demonstrate that all three compounds phosphorylate residue Ser9 on GSK-3β, and, hence, are likely to inhibit the activity of the kinase (Fig. 5A) (Woodgett 2001). In addition, we investigated the effects of the GSK-3β inhibitors on NF-κB activation *in vitro*. There is good evidence that the p65 activity is increased in HEK293 cells by IL1β (Kirschning et al 1998). We show here that the IL1β - induced increase in the p65 activity in these cells was significantly decreased by the GSK-3β inhibitors (Fig. 5B). These findings support our *in vivo* data, and lend support to the concept of the inhibitory effect of GSK-3β inhibition on NF-κB activity.

It should be noted that other mechanisms and signalling pathways may also be involved in the protective effects of GSK-3β inhibitors observed in this study. In intact cells different protein kinases, such as protein kinase B (PKB), PKC and PKA, are able to phosphorylate GSK-3β on Ser9 (Eldar-Finkelman 2002). Activation of these protein kinases is dependent on the external stimuli. However, although the signalling pathways converge at GSK-3, phosphorylation of the enzyme by a certain signal will not lead to activation of all targets, but to a selected target determined by the type of signal (Eldar-Finkelman 2002). The precise molecular mechanisms of GSK-3β in the regulation of the inflammatory response will be a subject for future studies.

Hence, we propose that the activation of GSK-3β plays a pivotal role in the pathophysiology of organ injury/dysfunction associated with systemic inflammation (caused by severe endotoxaemia or co-administration of LPS and peptidoglycan). This implies that potent and selective inhibitors of the activity of GSK-3β may be useful for the prevention of the organ injury/dysfunction associated with systemic inflammation (and potentially septic shock). In the present study, however, a pre-treatment regime was employed. To accurately evaluate whether GSK-3β inhibitors are indeed effective in preventing the development of multiple organ failure, further studies employing a therapeutic (post-treatment) administration of these compounds are warranted.

In conclusion, our results demonstrate that activation of GSK-3β contributes to the organ injury/dysfunction caused by excessive, systemic inflammation (caused by severe endotoxaemia or co-administration of LPS and peptidoglycan). The mechanism(s) of the observed beneficial effects of the inhibitors of GSK-3β may involve the inhibition of the phosphorylation of the Ser536 residue on p65, prevention of the activation of NF-κB, and/or reduction of the expression of NF-κB-

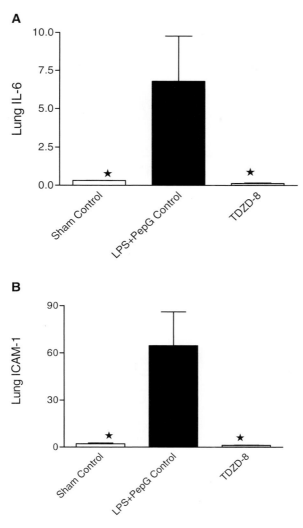

FIG. 4.   IL1β, IL6, ICAM1, VCAM1 and MCP1 mRNA expression in the lung. Expression of (A) IL1β, (B) IL6, (C) ICAM1, (D) VCAM1 and (E) MCP1 measured by RT-PCR in the lung of rats subjected to the surgical procedure and pre-treated with 10% DMSO (Sham, *n* = 4). Rats subjected to co-administration of LPS (1 mg/kg i.v.) and peptidoglycan (0.3 mg/kg i.v.) were pre-treated with either 10% DMSO (Control, *n* = 4) or TDZD-8 (1 mg/kg i.v., *n* = 4) 30 min prior to the co-administration of LPS and peptidoglycan. *$P < 0.05$ when compared with LPS+PepG·Control by ANOVA followed by Dunnett's *post hoc* test.

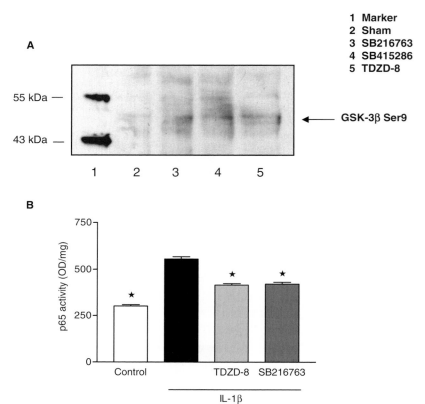

FIG. 5.   Effect of GSK-3β inhibitors on the phosphorylation of Ser9 on GSK-3β and p65 activity. (A) HEK293 cells were incubated in serum free media for 2 h and stimulated with 30 μM SB216763, 10 μM SB415286 or 10 μM TDZD-8 for 30 min. Whole cell lysates were analysed by SDS-PAGE and phosphorylation of GSK-3 detected with anti-phospho GSK-3α/β (Ser21/9). (B) The effect of GSK-3β inhibitors on NF-κB p65 activity was measured in IL1β-stimulated HEK293 cells ($n = 3$/group). *$P < 0.05$ when compared with IL1β-stimulated untreated cells by ANOVA followed by Dunnett's *post hoc* test. OD, optical density.

dependent pro-inflammatory genes. We propose the novel concept that GSK-3β inhibition may be a new strategy for the prevention or therapy of the organ injury/dysfunction associated with sepsis, shock, and other conditions associated with local or systemic inflammation.

Acknowledgements

This study was supported by grants provided by the William Harvey Research Foundation, UK, and Emil Aaltonen Foundation and Helsingin Sanomat Centennial Foundation, Finland.

References

Beg AA, Sha WC, Bronson RT, Ghosh S, Baltimore D 1995 Embryonic lethality and liver degeneration in mice lacking the RelA component of NF-κB. Nature 376:167–170

Buss H, Dorrie A, Schmitz ML, Hoffmann E, Resch K, Kracht M 2004 Constitutive and interleukin-1-inducible phosphorylation of p65 NF-κ B at serine 536 is mediated by multiple protein kinases including Iκ B kinase (IKK)-α, IKKβ, IKKε, TRAF family member-associated (TANK)-binding kinase 1 (TBK1), and an unknown kinase and couples p65 to TATA-binding protein-associated factor II31-mediated interleukin-8 transcription. J Biol Chem 279:55633–55643

Cohen J, Abraham E 1999 Microbiologic findings and correlations with serum tumor necrosis factor-alpha in patients with severe sepsis and septic shock. J Infect Dis 180:116–121

Cross DA, Alessi DR, Cohen P, Andjelkovich M, Hemmings BA 1995 Inhibition of glycogen synthase kinase-3 by insulin mediated by protein kinase B. Nature 378:785–789

Demarchi F, Bertoli C, Sandy P, Schneider C 2003 Glycogen synthase kinase-3 beta regulates NF-kappa B1/p105 stability. J Biol Chem 278:39583–39590

Dignam JD, Lebovitz RM, Roeder RG 1983 Accurate transcription initiation by RNA polymerase II in a soluble extract from isolated mammalian nuclei. Nucleic Acids Res 11:1475–1489

Dugo L, Collin M, Cuzzocrea S, Thiemermann C 2004 15d-prostaglandin J(2) reduces multiple organ failure caused by wall-fragment of Gram-positive and Gram-negative bacteria. Eur J Pharmacol 498:295–301

Eldar-Finkelman H 2002 Glycogen synthase kinase 3: an emerging therapeutic target. Trends Mol Med 8:126–132

Embi N, Rylatt DB, Cohen P 1980 Glycogen synthase kinase-3 from rabbit skeletal muscle. Separation from cyclic-AMP-dependent protein kinase and phosphorylase kinase. Eur J Biochem 107:519–527

Essani NA, McGuire GM, Manning AM, Jaeschke H 1996 Endotoxin-induced activation of the nuclear transcription factor kappa B and expression of E-selectin messenger RNA in hepatocytes, Kupffer cells, and endothelial cells in vivo. J Immunol 156:2956–2963

Farjah M, Roxas BP, Geenen DL, Danziger RS 2003 Dietary salt regulates renal SGK1 abundance: relevance to salt sensitivity in the Dahl rat. Hypertension 41:874–878

Foster SJ 1992 Analysis of the autolysins of Bacillus subtilis 168 during vegetative growth and differentiation by using renaturing polyacrylamide gel electrophoresis. J Bacteriol 174:464–470

Gross ER, Hsu AK, Gross GJ 2004 Opioid-induced cardioprotection occurs via glycogen synthase kinase beta inhibition during reperfusion in intact rat hearts. Circ Res 94:960–966

Heyen JR, Blasi ER, Nikula K et al 2002 Structural, functional, and molecular characterization of the SHHF model of heart failure. Am J Physiol Heart Circ Physiol 283:H1775–1784

Hoeflich KP, Luo J, Rubie EA, Tsao MS, Jin O, Woodgett JR 2000 Requirement for glycogen synthase kinase-3beta in cell survival and NF-κB activation. Nature 406:86–90

Kirschning CJ, Wesche H, Merrill AT, Rothe M 1998 Human toll-like receptor 2 confers responsiveness to bacterial lipopolysaccharide. J Exp Med 188:2091–2097

Li Q, Van Antwerp D, Mercurio F, Lee KF, Verma IM 1999 Severe liver degeneration in mice lacking the IkappaB kinase 2 gene. Science 284:321–325

Rensing H, Jaeschke H, Bauer I et al 2001 Differential activation pattern of redox-sensitive transcription factors and stress-inducible dilator systems heme oxygenase-1 and inducible nitric oxide synthase in hemorrhagic and endotoxic shock. Crit Care Med 29:1962–1971

Schwabe RF, Brenner DA 2002 Role of glycogen synthase kinase-3 in TNF-alpha-induced NF-kappaB activation and apoptosis in hepatocytes. Am J Physiol Gastrointest Liver Physiol 283:G204–211

Takada Y, Fang X, Jamaluddin MS, Boyd DD, Aggarwal BB 2004 Genetic deletion of glycogen synthase kinase-3beta abrogates activation of IκBα kinase, JNK, Akt, and p44/p42 MAPK but potentiates apoptosis induced by tumor necrosis factor. J Biol Chem 279:39541–39554

Thiemermann C, Ruetten H, Wu CC, Vane JR 1995 The multiple organ dysfunction syndrome caused by endotoxin in the rat: attenuation of liver dysfunction by inhibitors of nitric oxide synthase. Br J Pharmacol 116:2845–2851

Wang X, Li W, Lu J, Li N, Li J 2004 Lipopolysaccharide suppresses albumin expression by activating NF-κB in rat hepatocytes. J Surg Res 122:274–279

Woodgett JR 2001 Judging a protein by more than its name: GSK-3. Sci STKE 2001: RE12–22

Wray GM, Foster SJ, Hinds CJ, Thiemermann C 2001 A cell wall component from pathogenic and non-pathogenic gram-positive bacteria (peptidoglycan) synergises with endotoxin to cause the release of tumour necrosis factor-α, nitric oxide production, shock, and multiple organ injury/dysfunction in the rat. Shock 15:135142

DISCUSSION

Marshall: An obvious candidate as a target is I-κB. You may be increasing the inhibitory activity for binding or transcription. Has this been looked at? What is the effect on neutrophil accumulation?

Thiemermann: I-κB phosphorylation has been looked at in a number of *in vitro* studies. This was not affected. What you are asking about has not been looked at. This might be an easier way to look at it than looking at p65 phosphorylation. With regard to neutrophil recruitment, we usually look at the lung because activated neutrophils adhere to the endothelium and stick in the pulmonary circulation. This was also reduced in animals treated with inhibitors of GSK-3, and in the colitis study (DNBS-induced colitis) neutrophil recruitment into the colon was reduced in animals treated with inhibitors of GSK-3. We are now collaborating with Dr Jacob Wang in Oslo (Norway) using his rat model of cecal ligation and puncture (CLP). We find an increase in AST and ALT, but when we give appropriate fluid resuscitation, we do not see an increase in creatinine. We did detect a significant neutrophil recruitment into the lung, which was missing in Mervyn Singer's study. Thus, accumulation of neutrophils in the pulmonary circulation with acute lung injury was seen in the CLP model and our acute LPS model.

Gilroy: Some time ago we showed that there is a shift of NF-κB subunits from onset when p50/p65 drove the response to predominantly p50/p50 suppressor homodimer during resolution (Lawrence et al 2001). This is almost reminiscent of an attempt at restoration to normal physiology. Specifically, an active attempt to restore the injured tissue to it's prior physiological functioning. As part of that we have evidence showing that there is a p65 present in the form of a cleavage product that may be important for apoptosis (work in progress). Have you taken your studies out to later time points to see what the consequences of inhibiting GSK are on recovery or resolution?

Thiemermann: We have limited our work to acute experiments in anaesthetized animals, so we have not done the suggested studies.

Gilroy: If you came into the pathways through the disease process with your inhibitors, what would happen to the resolution?

Thiemermann: We haven't tried this. In our collagen-induced arthritis studies, we gave the GSK-3 inhibitors between day 10 and 25, but did not look at resolution of inflammation.

Radermacher: I have a question about the role of NF-κB in the resumption of inflammation. Do you think there is a time window for the GSK inhibition? In other words, would a type of ischaemia–reperfusion injury be a more appropriate way of using it as a therapeutic? Under these conditions you know the time when the challenge was set, and you can use your joker as a pre-treatment or a very early post-challenge treatment.

Thiemermann: That is a good question. It is likely that there is a specific time window for the administration of inhibitors of GSK-3. We carried out preliminary studies using a model of ischaemia–reperfusion injury in the kidney, and pre-treatment with one of these inhibitors was beneficial. This was again a relatively acute study in which we looked at bilateral renal ischaemia for 45 min followed by reperfusion for six hours. We looked at renal and tubular dysfunction, as well as secondary lung injury. We found a reduction in the renal injury and are now looking at the secondary lung injury. There is a recent study indicating that inhibition of GSK-3β may play a role in protecting the heart against ischaemia–reperfusion injury (Park et al 2006). We tried these inhibitors, but did not see a significant effect in ischaemia–reperfusion injury of the heart. This indicates to me that inhibitors of GSK-3 are useful in conditions associated with excessive inflammation. In our heart model, inflammation is not the major cause of necrosis or apoptosis, as the injury is driven by ROS-mediated activation of PARP.

Szabó: The story that NF-κB plays a role in shock and inflammation has been out for a long time. This concept that NF-κB inhibition could be of some use has been argued for colitis. But no one is really going after NF-κB as a target. Why do you think this is, and how would your approach be different?

Thiemermann: I don't know, but in colitis, for example, people used to say that molecules which inhibit the effects of TNF are not an effective strategy. But now anti-TNF drugs represent a very effective strategy in colitis. Whether inhibitors of GSK-3 may be as effective (or better) that anti-TNF strategies in colitis is unknown.

Fink: NF-κB is being developed as a drug target. Approaches using proteasome inhibitors are being tried for both acute and chronic indications. Part of the story is that the original Baltimore and colleagues patent on NF-κB as a drug target has made it difficult for people. I think this is one of the reasons why the proteasome inhibitor approach is being taken.

Thiemermann: We looked at the patent situation around GSK-3β inhibitors. Many drug companies appear to have patented GSK-3 inhibitors for a number of disease targets including neurodegenerative disorders, Alzheimer's disease and inflammation.

Van den Berghe: What you hinted at is that part of the insulin effects are mediated via this pathway. I don't think you should extrapolate from your model, because it is a hypoglycaemic model, meaning that these animals are insulin-sensitive, whereas our patients are not.

Thiemermann: That's true, but the first time I came across insulin was in the late 1970s, when a number of people tried to use infusions of insulin, glucose and K^+ as a cardioprotective solution. Insulin can be used in many models of acute tissue injury as a very effective survival strategy.

Radermacher: You mentioned that it was also active on hypotension. Was it really anti-hypotensive? Is that mainly through the cardiac function *per se* or an improved or restored vasomotor response?

Thiemermann: When I say it was effective, I mean that the effect of the GSK-3 inhibitor on the hypotension was statistically significant, but the observed effect was not very dramatic. We don't know whether any of the observed effects of these compounds are on cardiac (dys)function or on systemic vascular resistance (hypotension).

Singer: My question is also dealing with the hypoglycaemic issue. We noticed that in our shock model, so we give them a lot of glucose to try to keep them normo-glycaemic. Why, despite the acute phase response, do they become hypoglycaemic? Do they become hyperinsulaemic or is it an increased sensitivity? Or is it a problem of substrate? Why does it happen?

Van den Berghe: In the human the insulin signal varies dramatically within a few hours, and varies for days after. We don't really know what happens.

Thiemermann: It is certainly not a question of the substrate support. In our rodent models, we have infused glucose, but the animals still became hypoglycaemic. They have a markedly reduced gluconeogenesis. It seems to be a problem with the gluconeogenesis in the liver itself, independent of perfusion or substrate delivery.

Griffiths: The trouble with a lot of rodent experiments is the timing of eating. They eat at night. Their glycogen stores are relatively limited because they are continuous eaters.

Thiemermann: There is always a debate, as to whether any given animal model is clinically relevant. Clearly with respect to plasma glucose levels, the CLP model is hypoglycaemic, the pig model is hypoglycaemic, so we all seem to be dealing with acute models of hypoglycaemia, while critically ill patients are hyperglycaemic.

Annane: Have you tried to set up your models at different levels of blood glucose giving them various doses of exogenous glucose, to see whether this changes the activity of GSK? Or did you look at insulin-sensitive versus insulin-insensitive tissues? Or insulin receptor knockout mice?

Thiemermann: We have used as much glucose as it takes to bring the glucose level back to normal, to see whether this has any effect on outcome.

Hellewell: Do you know anything about the pharmacokinetics of these compounds? You are giving them with a 40 min pre-treatment and then you are looking six hours later. How long is the kinase inhibited for?

Thiemermann: We don't know. We know that TDZD-8 is a non-competitive inhibitor of GSK-3 which has been reported to have relatively long-lasting effects. The activation of NF-κB occurs within 30 min of the administration of lipoteichoic acid and peptidoglycan. This is why we used this pre-treatment paradigm. We don't have to be effective for six hours, just for the first two or three, during which the NF-κB activation occurs, which then drives all the other disease processes.

Hellewell: What is the cellular target? Is it the neutrophil?

Thiemermann: Macrophages would be a target. Kupffer cells would also be a target, because the cytokine formation in the rat can come from both the peripheral blood mononuclear cells as well as from the Kupffer cells. It could be many other cells. In the lung we look at recruitment of neutrophils, and in this case the endothelial cells or the neutrophils themselves would be a target.

Cavaillon: Because of the effects of the GSK-3β inhibitor and its consequences for p65, have you had a chance to check for the presence of the homodimer p50/p50, which is by itself an inactive form and an inhibitor of NF-κB?

Thiemermann: We haven't done this, but it's a good question.

Evans: The fact that these reagents are acting quite a long way downstream from the activation, makes them potentially attractive drug targets because they are more likely to have a delayed effect. Is there any more mechanistic insight into how they work downstream?

Thiemermann: Not in the last six months since the papers came out. You are right that because they act further downstream, maybe you can give these compounds later. Many years ago we worked with calpain inhibitor 1, when we realised that the activation of NF-κB activation was important in inducible nitric oxide synthase (iNOS) induction. When given as a pre-treatment these compounds were very effective, but as a post-treatment they did not work.

Fink: Valproic acid is also a good GSK-3β inhibitor. It has a great safety profile. Please try it!

Thiemermann: I agree, and another one is lithium.

References

Lawrence T, Gilroy DW, Colville-Nash PR, Willoughby DA 2001 Possible new role for NF-kappaB in the resolution of inflammation. Nat Med 7:1291–1297

Park SS, Zhao H, Jang Y, Mueller RA, Xu Z 2006 *N*6-(3-iodobenzyl)-adenosine-5'-*N*-methylcarboxamide confers cardioprotection at reperfusion by inhibiting mitochondrial permeability transition pore opening via glycogen synthase kinase 3 beta. J Pharmacol Exp Ther 318:124–131

Ethyl pyruvate: a novel treatment for sepsis

Mitchell P. Fink

Departments of Critical Care Medicine and Surgery, University of Pittsburgh Medical School, 616 Scaife Hall, 3550 Terrace Street, Pittsburgh PA 15261, USA

Abstract. Ethyl pyruvate (EP), a simple aliphatic ester derived from pyruvic acid, improves survival and ameliorates organ system dysfunction in mice with peritonitis induced by caecal ligation and perforation, even when treatment is started as late as 12–24 hours after the onset of sepsis. In studies using lipopolysaccharide-stimulated RAW 264.7 murine macrophage-like cells, EP inhibits activation of the pro-inflammatory transcription factor, NF-κB, and down-regulates secretion of a number of pro-inflammatory cytokines, such as tumour necrosis factor (TNF). In this reductionist *in vitro* system, EP also blocks secretion of the late-appearing pro-inflammatory cytokine-like molecule, high mobility group box 1 (HMGB1). In murine models of endotoxaemia or sepsis, treatment with EP decreases circulating levels of TNF and HMGB1. While the molecular events responsible for the salutary effects of EP remain to be elucidated, one mechanism may involve covalent modification of a critical thiol residue in the p65 component of NF-κB. EP warrants evaluation as a therapeutic agent for the treatment of sepsis in humans.

2007 Sepsis—new insights, new therapies. Wiley, Chichester (Novartis Foundation Symposium 280) p 147–159

The anti-inflammatory effects of ethyl pyruvate

At physiological pH values, pyruvic acid, which is a relatively strong carboxylic acid, is almost completely ionized. Pyruvate (CH_3COCOO^-), the anionic form of pyruvic acid, is a three-carbon intermediate in the metabolism of glucose and numerous amino acids. Under anaerobic conditions, much of the pyruvate generated by glycolysis is reduced to form lactate. In contrast, under aerobic conditions, most of the pyruvate formed in the cytosol is transported into mitochondria where it is oxidized to form acetyl coenzyme A. This reaction is the first and rate-limiting step in the tricarboxylic acid (TCA) cycle, the predominant source of ATP in cells.

Although pyruvate plays a central role in intermediary metabolism, this simple organic anion also functions in cells as an endogenous antioxidant and free radical scavenger. The capacity of pyruvate to function as an antioxidant was first reported by Holleman, who showed that α-keto carboxylates with the general structure, RCOCOO⁻, reduce hydrogen peroxide (H_2O_2) nonenzymatically (Holleman 1904). In the case of pyruvate, this oxidative decarboxylation reaction yields acetate, water and carbon dioxide. This reaction is both rapid and stoichiometric. In addition to H_2O_2, pyruvate is also capable of scavenging another highly reactive oxygen species (ROS), the hydroxyl radical (OH·) (Dobsak et al 1999).

Prompted by the recognition that pyruvate is an effective ROS scavenger, many laboratories have tested the hypothesis that this compound might be a useful therapeutic agent for the treatment of various pathological conditions that are thought to be mediated by the formation of H_2O_2 and related partially reduced forms of oxygen. For example, Salahudeen et al (1991) showed that infusing a solution of sodium pyruvate preserves kidney function in rat models of ROS-mediated acute renal failure. Other investigators reported that treatment with pyruvate ameliorates organ injury or dysfunction in animal models of redox stress, such as transient myocardial (Bunger et al 1989), intestinal (Cicalese et al 1999), or hepatic (Sileri et al 2001) ischaemia followed by reperfusion.

Despite these promising findings, the usefulness of pyruvate as a therapeutic agent is probably limited by its poor stability in solution. Aqueous solutions of pyruvate rapidly undergo a spontaneous condensation reaction to form parapyruvate (2-hydroxy-2-methyl-4-ketoglutarate), a compound that inhibits a key step in the TCA cycle (Montgomery & Webb 1956).

In order to circumvent this issue, our laboratory carried out experiments using the ethyl ester of pyruvic acid, i.e. ethyl pyruvate (EP). In an initial study, Sims et al (2001) found that treatment with EP ameliorates much of the structural and functional damage to the intestinal mucosa that normally occurs when rats are subjected to mesenteric ischaemia and reperfusion (Sims et al 2001). Interestingly, in this study, treatment with EP seemed to be more effective than treatment with an equimolar dose of sodium pyruvate. Similar findings indicating that EP is more effective than pyruvate were reported by Varma et al (1998), who compared the two compounds in an *in vitro* study of redox-mediated cellular injury.

In a subsequent study, Yang et al (2002) compared the effects of resuscitation with a solution of EP instead of Ringer's lactate solution (RLS) on several parameters in a murine model of hemorrhagic shock. This study provided the first evidence that EP has anti-inflammatory properties, since treatment with the compound decreased activation of the pro-inflammatory transcription factor, NF-κB, in liver and colonic mucosa following resuscitation from haemorrhagic shock and also decreased the expression of transcripts for several pro-inflammatory genes, including inducible nitric oxide synthase (iNOS), tumour necrosis factor (TNF), cyclooxygenase 2 (COX-2), and interleukin (IL)6 in liver, ileal mucosa and colonic mucosa.

Effect of treatment with ethyl pyruvate on outcome in animal models of sepsis

Venkataraman and colleagues evaluated the effects of EP in a rat model of profound arterial hypotension induced by the intravenous injection of a large dose of *Escherichia coli* lipopolysaccharide (LPS) (Venkataraman et al 2002). When mean arterial pressure (MAP) decreased to 60 mmHg, the endotoxaemic rats were randomized to resuscitation with either EP solution or RLS, the volume of fluid being titrated to maintain MAP greater than 60 mmHg until a total volume of 7 ml/kg was infused. Resuscitation with REPS as compared to RLS significantly prolonged survival time. Resuscitation with EP solution was also associated with significantly lower circulating concentrations of nitrite/nitrate (markers of nitric oxide synthesis) and IL6 and higher plasma levels of IL10. Thus, delayed treatment with an EP-containing resuscitation fluid shifted the response to LPS challenge toward increased production of an anti-inflammatory cytokine (IL10) and away from production of the pro-inflammatory cytokine (IL6).

Pursuing this line of investigation still further, Ulloa and colleagues investigated the effects of EP on LPS-induced inflammatory responses *in vitro* and *in vivo* (Ulloa et al 2002). In these studies, incubation of LPS-stimulated RAW 264.7 murine macrophage-like cells with EP inhibited release of TNF and decreased steady-state levels of TNF mRNA. In this same system, EP blocked NF-κB DNA binding and down-regulated phosphorylation of p38 mitogen activated protein kinase. When mice were pretreated with EP prior to being challenged with a lethal dose of LPS, survival was significantly improved and circulating concentrations of TNF were decreased. Remarkably, treatment with EP four hours after the injection of LPS (i.e. well after the monophasic spike in circulating TNF levels) also improved survival in this murine model of systemic inflammation.

For many reasons, acute endotoxaemia models in rodents are not ideal for carrying out preclinical studies of novel agents for the treatment of human sepsis (Fink & Heard 1990). Compared to humans, rats and mice are far less sensitive to the pro-inflammatory and lethal effects of LPS. Furthermore, in acute endotoxaemia, the inflammatory response is exclusively deleterious; therefore most effective anti-inflammatory agents tend to improve organ function and/or survival. However, in sepsis (defined as systemic inflammation secondary to acute infection), the inflammatory response has both salutary and deleterious effects. On the positive side of the ledger, the inflammatory response in septic animals or patients is essential for eradicating the microbes responsible for causing the underlying infection. On the negative side, the inflammatory response is also the cause for organ system dysfunction and mortality. Thus, in animal models of sepsis, anti-inflammatory strategies can sometimes be beneficial and in other cases actually worsen outcome.

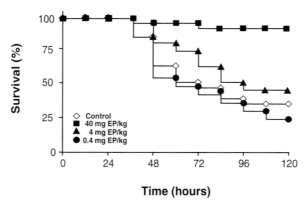

Time (hours)

FIG. 1.   Effect of treatment with EP on the survival of mice with severe sepsis induced by caecal ligation and puncture (CLP). Beginning 24 h after the induction of sepsis, surviving mice were treated with five intraperitoneal doses of vehicle or EP (0.4, 4 or 40 mg/kg per dose). Doses of vehicle or drug were administered at these times after CLP: 24, 30, 36, 42 and 48 h. Adapted with permission from Ulloa et al (2002).

In view of these considerations, Ulloa et al (2002) evaluated the therapeutic effects of EP using a well-studied animal model of severe sepsis: caecal ligation and perforation (CLP) in mice. Polymicrobial peritonitis was induced in all of the rodents and 12 hours later the animals were treated with a single dose of a broad-spectrum antibiotic (Imipenem). After another 12 hours (i.e. 24 hours after the induction of sepsis), the animals were randomized to receive treatment with either vehicle alone or vehicle containing graded dosed of EP (0.4, 4 or 40 mg/kg per dose for five doses). Treatment with the highest dose of EP significantly improved survival (Fig. 1).

Some of the beneficial effects of EP in murine endotoxaemia and sepsis may be because this compound inhibits secretion by immunostimulated macrophages of a cytokine-like protein, high mobility group box 1 (HMGB1). First described as a non-histone nuclear protein with high electrophoretic mobility, HMGB1 has been identified as a late-acting mediator of LPS- (Wang et al 1999) or sepsis-induced (Yang et al 2004) lethality. Ulloa et al (2002) showed that incubating LPS-stimulated RAW 264.7 cells with EP blocks the release of HMGB1 *in vitro*. Furthermore, these investigators documented that treatment of mice with EP decreases circulating levels of HMGB1 following administration of LPS or induction of sepsis (Ulloa et al 2002).

Acute renal failure (ARF) is one of the most common complications of sepsis (Klenzak & Himmelfarb 2005). Until recently, however, progress toward the development of new therapeutic agents to prevent or treat sepsis-related ARF was hampered by the lack of a good animal model for this condition. In 2003, however, a group of investigators at the National Institutes of Health in the USA reported that aged mice with CLP-induced sepsis develop clinical and pathological findings that are remarkably similar to those observed in humans with ARF (Miyaji et al 2003). In view of the apparent clinical relevance of this model, it is noteworthy that Miyaji et al (2003) showed that treatment with a single intraperitoneal dose of EP immediately after surgery significantly inhibits development of ARF. Importantly, these investigators documented that the therapeutic benefit of EP is still apparent, even if treatment is delayed until 12 hours after the onset of sepsis. Furthermore, treatment with EP decreases expression in the kidney of several proteins (TNF, tissue factor, and plasminogen activator inhibitor 1) that have been implicated in the pathogenesis of organ dysfunction due to sepsis (Miyaji et al 2003). In a more recent study from the same laboratory, treatment with EP was shown to ameliorate sepsis-induced renal dysfunction, as detected by dendrimer-enhanced magnetic resonance imaging (Dear et al 2005).

As noted above, rodents are far less sensitive to LPS than are humans. Pigs, however, are not only exquisitely sensitive to the pro-inflammatory effects of LPS, but also respond to the infusion of endotoxin by developing a hyperdynamic hypotensive cardiovascular profile that is very reminiscent of the high cardiac output state commonly observed in adequately resuscitated septic patients. A German group, under the direction of Peter Radermacher, has perfected a porcine subacute endotoxaemia model that recapitulates many aspects of severe sepsis in humans. In this paradigm, anaesthetized and mechanically ventilated pigs are continuously infused with LPS for 24 hours. Using this model, Hauser et al (2005) randomized animals to treatment with vehicle or a continuous infusion of EP, beginning at 12 hours after the onset of endotoxaemia. Treatment with EP significantly reduced intrapulmonary venous admixture and resulted in significantly greater PaO_2/FIO_2 ratio at 24 hours after induction of 'sepsis.' Despite comparable urine production in the two groups during the first 18 hours of endotoxaemia, treatment with EP significantly increased diuresis during the last six hours of the study. LPS-induced systemic and post-hepatic venous metabolic acidosis were significantly ameliorated by EP treatment. Endotoxaemia increased both blood nitrate + nitrite and isoprostane concentrations, and therapy with EP had salutary effects on these markers of nitric oxide production and lipid peroxidation, respectively. Collectively, these data obtained in a large animal model of severe sepsis support the view that delayed treatment with EP ameliorates many of the deleterious consequences of systemic inflammation.

The biochemical basis for the anti-inflammatory effects of EP

Sen & Baltimore (1986) originally identified NF-κB as a transcription factor involved in the activation of κ light chain genes in B lymphocytes. Subsequently,

NF-κB has been shown to regulate the transcription of approximately 200 genes. Many of these genes, such as TNF, IL6, IL8, COX-2 and iNOS, are involved in the inflammatory response.

The term NF-κB describes a family of transcription factors formed by the hetero- or homodimerization of proteins from the Rel family. There are five Rel proteins: p50, p65 (RelA), c-Rel, p52 and RelB. In resting cells, the homo- or heterodimeric forms of NF-κB exist in the cytoplasm in an inactive form due to binding by a third inhibitory protein, called I-κB. In mammalian cells, several I-κB-like proteins have been identified: I-κBα, I-κBβ, I-κBε, and Bcl-3. Upon stimulation of the cell by a proinflammatory trigger—for example, cytokines like TNF or IL1β or the bacterial product, LPS—Iκ-B is phosphorylated on two key serine residues (Ser32 and Ser36 in I-κBα). Phosphorylation of I-κB targets the molecule for ubiquitination and subsequent proteasomal degradation. Phosphorylation of I-κB is mediated by an enzyme complex called I-κB kinase (IKK) that contains two catalytic subunits, IKKα and IKKβ. Phosphorylation, release and degradation of I-κB permits translocation of the transcriptionally competent form of NF-κB into the nucleus, where it can bind to *cis*-acting elements in the promoter regions of various NF-κB-responsive genes. The upstream events that lead to IKK activation depend upon the nature of the initiating stimulus. In the canonical NF-κB activation scheme, IKK activation is mediated by NF-κB-inducing kinase, although other kinases, notably MEKK1, also can activate IKK.

Our laboratory has employed the electrophoretic mobility shift assay to show that EP inhibits activation of NF-κB in a variety of *in vitro* and *in vivo* systems. Since an oxidizing environment, particularly in the cytosol, favours activation of NF-κB, and EP, like pyruvate, is an antioxidant (Varma et al 1998, Tawadrous et al 2002, Tsung et al 2005), it is possible that EP inhibits activation of NF-κB by scavenging ROS. Several observations, however, suggest that EP-mediated inhibition of NF-κB activation may entail more than an antioxidant effect.

First, oxidant stress (1–10 mM H_2O_2) fails to activate NF-κB in Caco-2 (Parikh et al 2000) or DLD-1 (Salzman et al 1996) enterocyte-like cells, yet EP blocks activation of NF-κB in cytomix-stimulated Caco-2 cells (Sappington et al 2003b).

Second, other well known ROS scavengers fail to block IL1β-induced NF-κB activation in Caco-2 cells (Parikh et al 2000), yet EP effectively inhibits cytomix-induced NF-κB activation in this same cell line (Sappington et al 2003b).

Third, *N*-acetylcysteine (NAC), an effective ROS scavenger, fails to inhibit activation of NF-κB induced by TNF or IL1β in ECV304 endothelial cells (Bowie et al 1997). NAC also fails to block LPS-induced NF-κB activation in J774.1 murine macrophage-like cells (Chandel et al 2000). In contrast, EP inhibits activation of NF-κB induced by cytomix (TNF, IL1β, plus IFNγ) in Caco-2 cells (Sappington et al 2003b) or by LPS in RAW 264.7 cells (Ulloa et al 2002). Indeed, when we carried out a head-to-head comparison of EP and NAC in experiments using LPS-stimulated RAW 264.7 cells, EP was clearly a more potent inhibitor of NF-κB DNA binding (Song et al 2004).

Fourth, if the anti-inflammatory effects of EP are due mainly to its actions as an ROS scavenger, then one would predict that the parent compound, pyruvate, would be equally effective in this regard. However, just the contrary has been observed in multiple studies. Whereas, EP effectively down-regulates the expression of pro-inflammatory mediators in a variety of systems, pyruvate exhibits little or no anti-inflammatory activity (Yu et al 2005, Kim et al 2005, Sappington et al 2003b).

Fifth, effective scavenging of H_2O_2 or other reactive species requires that the scavenger be present in the location (cell or extracellular milieu) where the reactive species are being produced. But, after transient exposure to EP, its anti-inflammatory effects are durable both *in vitro* and *in vivo*. For example, when Caco-2 cells are incubated with EP and then the compound is removed by extensive washing of the cells, anti-inflammatory effects remain apparent for at least 6 hours (Sappington et al 2003a). Similarly, when mice are injected with a single dose of EP, anti-inflammatory effects are demonstrable for at least 6 hours (Sappington et al 2003a).

Sixth, if the anti-inflammatory effects of EP were related to its ability to scavenge H_2O_2 or other oxidants, then one would predict that co-incubation of LPS-stimulated RAW 264.7 cells with a second ROS scavenger, such as glutathione ethyl ester, would either have no effect or would further augment the anti-inflammatory effects of EP. But, just the contrary result has been observed; the anti-inflammatory effects of EP are partially *reversed* when RAW 264.7 cells are also treated with glutathione ethyl ester (Song et al 2004).

Since EP is such a simple molecule, what possible mechanism other than ROS scavenging could explain its ability to inhibit NF-κB activation? One hypothesis is suggested by recent observations regarding the mechanism of action of parthenolide and other sesquiterpene lactones that inhibit NF-κB activation. These agents alkylate a critical cysteine residue (Cys38) in the p65 subunit, and thereby interfere with DNA binding by activated NF-κB heterodimers (Lyss et al 1998, Schmidt et al 1999, Garcia-Pineres et al 2001). The key functionality in this class of NF-κB inhibitors is an exocyclic methylene group conjugated to a carbonyl group. This highly reactive pharmacophore reacts with nucleophiles, especially cysteine sulfhydryl groups, in a Michael-type addition (Dupuis et al 1974, Hay et al 1994, Schmidt 1999). Although its structure does not precisely recapitulate the sesquiterpene lactone pharmacophore, EP in solution exists in tautomeric equilibrium with another compound, ethyl-2-hydroxyacrylate, which does. It is noteworthy, therefore, that 2-acetamidoacrylate, a compound that is closely related to the ethyl-2-hydroxyacrylate tautomeric form of EP, has been shown to have anti-inflammatory properties both *in vitro* and *in vivo* (Sappington et al 2005). Interestingly, the ester, methyl-2-acetamidoacrylate, which is known to be a much more potent Michael acceptor than is the parent compound (Snow et al 1976), is also a much more potent anti-inflammatory agent than is 2-acetamidoacrylate (Sappington et al 2005).

In order to obtain further evidence for the idea that EP targets a critical sulf-hydryl group in the NF-κB complex, we carried out series of experiments using cells transfected with plasmids encoding wild-type (wt) and mutant (Cys38→Ser and Cys120→Ala) forms of p65 (Han et al 2005). Treatment with EP inhibited binding by wild-type p65 homodimers and also inhibited DNA binding by p65 homodimers when an alanine residue was substituted for Cys120. EP, however, failed to inhibit binding by p65 homodimers with a Cys38→Ser mutation. In addition, EP failed to inhibit degradation of I-κBα or I-κBβ induced by LPS in RAW 264.7 cells; thus, the effect of EP appears to be downstream of the step in the activation pathway that permits transcriptionally active Rel protein dimers to translocate into the nucleus. Collectively, these data support the view that EP covalently modifies Cys38 in p65 and thereby inhibits NF-κB-dependent signalling by interfering with binding of the transcription factor to *cis*-acting response elements in the promoter regions of target genes.

References

Bowie AG, Moynagh PN, O'Neill LAJ 1997 Lipid peroxidation is involved in the activation of NF-kB by tumor necrosis factor but not interleukin-1 in the human endothelial cell line ECV304. J Biol Chem 272:25941–25950

Bunger R, Mallet RT, Hartman DA 1989 Pyruvate-enhanced phosphorylation potential and inotropism in normoxic and postischemic isolated working heart. Near-complete prevention of reperfusion contractile failure. Eur J Biochem 180:221–233

Chandel NS, Trzyna WC, McClintock DS, Schumacker PT 2000 Role of oxidants in NF-kappa B activation and TNF-alpha gene transcription induced by hypoxia and endotoxin. J Immunol 165:1013–1021

Cicalese L, Lee K, Schraut W, Watkins S, Borle A, Stanko R 1999 Pyruvate prevents ischemia-reperfusion mucosal injury of rat small intestine. Am J Surg 171:97–100

Dear JW, Kobayashi H, Jo SK et al 2005 Dendrimer-enhanced MRI as a diagnostic and prognostic biomarker of sepsis-induced acute renal failure in aged mice. Kidney Int 67: 2159–2167

Dobsak P, Courdertot-Masuyer C, Zeller M et al 1999 Antioxidative properties of pyruvate and protection of the ischemic rat heart during cardioplegia. J Cardiovasc Pharmacol 34: 651–659

Dupuis G, Mitchell JC, Towers GH 1974 Reaction of alantolactone, an allergenic sesquiterpene lactone, with some amino acids. Resultant loss of immunologic reactivity. Can J Biochem 52:575–581

Fink MP, Heard SO 1990 Research review: laboratory models of sepsis and septic shock. J Surg Res 49:186–196

Garcia-Pineres AJ, Castro V, Mora G et al 2001 Cysteine 38 in p65/NF-kappaB plays a crucial role in DNA binding inhibition by sesquiterpene lactones. J Biol Chem 276:39713–39720

Han Y, Englert JA, Yang R, Delude RL, Fink MP 2005 Ethyl pyruvate inhibits NF-{kappa}B-dependent signaling by directly targeting p65. J Pharmacol Exp Ther 312:1097–1115

Hauser B, Kick J, Asfar P et al 2005 Ethyl pyruvate improves systemic and hepato-splanchnic hemodynamics and prevents lipid peroxidation in a porcine model of resuscitated hyperdynamic endotoxemia. Crit Care Med 33:2034–2042

Hay AJB, Hamburger M, Hostettmann K, Hoult JRS 1994 Toxic inhibition of smooth muscle contractility by plant-derived sesquiterpenes caused by their chemically reactive alpha-methylenebutyrolactone functions. Br J Pharmacol 112:9–12

Holleman MAF 1904 Notice sur l'action de l'eau oxygénée sur les acétoniques et sur le dicétones 1.2. Recl Trav Chim Pays-bas Belg 23:169–171

Kim JB, Yu YM, Kim SW, Lee JK 2005 Anti-inflammatory mechanism is involved in ethyl pyruvate-mediated efficacious neuroprotection in the postischemic brain. Brain Res 1060:188–192

Klenzak J, Himmelfarb J 2005 Sepsis and the kidney. Crit Care Clin 21:211–222

Lyss G, Knorre A, Schmidt TJ, Pahl HL, Merfort I 1998 The anti-inflammatory sesquiterpene lactone helenalin inhibits the transcription factor NF-kappaB by directly targeting p65. J Biol Chem 273:33508–33516

Miyaji T, Hu X, Yuen PST et al 2003 Ethyl pyruvate decreases sepsis-induced acute renal failure and multiple organ damage in aged mice. Kidney Int 64:1620–1631

Montgomery CM, Webb JL 1956 Metabolic studies on heart mitochondria. II. The inhibitory action of parapyruvate on the tricarboxylic acid cycle. J Biol Chem 221:359–368

Parikh AA, Moon MR, Pritts TA et al 2000 IL-1beta induction of NF-kappaB activation in human intestinal epithelial cells is independent of oxyradical signaling. Shock 13:8–13

Salahudeen AK, Clark EC, Nath KA 1991 Hydrogen peroxide-induced renal injury. A protective role for pyruvate in vitro and in vivo. J Clin Invest 88:1886–1893

Salzman AL, Denenberg AG, Ueta I, O'Connor M, Linn SC, Szabo C 1996 Induction and activity of nitric oxide synthase in cultured human intestinal epithelial monolayers. Am J Physiol 270:G565–573

Sappington PL, Fink ME, Yang R, Delude RL, Fink MP 2003a Ethyl pyruvate provides durable protection against inflammation-induced intestinal epithelial barrier dysfunction. Shock 20:521–528

Sappington PL, Han X, Yang R, Delude RL, Fink MP 2003b Ethyl pyruvate ameliorates intestinal epithelial barrier dysfunction in endotoxemic mice and immunostimulated Caco-2 enterocytic monolayers. J Pharmacol Exp Ther 304:464–476

Sappington PL, Cruz RJ Jr, Harada T et al 2005 The ethyl pyruvate analogues, diethyl oxaloproprionate, 2-acetamidoacrylate, and methyl-2-acetamidoacrylate, exhibit anti-inflammatory properties in vivo and/or in vitro. Biochem Pharmacol 70:1579–1592

Schmidt TJ 1999 Toxic activities of sesquiterpene lactones: structural and biochemical aspects. Curr Org Chem 3:577–608

Schmidt TJ, Lyss G, Pahl HL, Merfort I 1999 Helenanolide type sesquiterpene lactones. Part 5: the role of glutathione addition under physiological conditions. Bioorg Med Chem 7: 2849–2855

Sen R, Baltimore D 1986 Inducibility of kappa immunoglobulin enhancer-binding protein NF-kappaB by a posttranslational mechanism. Cell 47:921–928

Sileri P, Schena S, Morini S et al 2001 Pyruvate inhibits hepatic ischemia-reperfusion injury in rats. Transplantation 72:27–30

Sims CA, Wattanasirichaigoon S, Menconi MJ, Ajami AM, Fink MP 2001 Ringer's ethyl pyruvate solution ameliorates ischemia/reperfusion-induced intestinal mucosal injury in rats. Crit Care Med 29:1513–1518

Snow JT, Finley JW, Friedman M 1976 Relative reactivities of sulfhydryl groups with N-acetyl dehydroalanine and N-acetyl dehydroalanine methyl ester. Int J Peptide Protein Res 8:57–64

Song M, Kellum JA, Kaldas H, Fink MP 2004 Evidence that glutathione depletion is a mechanism responsible for the anti-inflammatory effects of ethyl pyruvate in cultured LPS-stimulated RAW 264.7 cells. J Pharmacol Exp Ther 308:307–316

Tawadrous ZS, Delude RL, Fink MP 2002 Resuscitation from hemorrhagic shock with Ringer's ethyl pyruvate solution improves survival and ameliorates intestinal mucosal hyperpermeability in rats. Shock 17:473–477

Tsung A, Kaizu T, Nakao A et al 2005 Ethyl pyruvate ameliorates liver ischemia-reperfusion injury by decreasing hepatic necrosis and apoptosis. Transplantation 27:196–204

Ulloa L, Ochani M, Yang H et al 2002 Ethyl pyruvate prevents lethality in mice with established lethal sepsis and systemic inflammation. Proc Natl Acad Sci USA 99:12351–12356

Varma SD, Devamanoharan PS, Ali AH 1998 Prevention of intracellular oxidative stress to lens by pyruvate and its ester. Free Rad Res 28:131–135

Venkataraman R, Kellum JA, Song M, Fink MP 2002 Resuscitation with Ringer's ethyl pyruvate solution prolongs survival and modulates plasma cytokine and nitrite/nitrate concentrations in a rat model of lipopolysaccharide-induced shock. Shock 18:507–512

Wang H, Bloom O, Zhang M et al 1999 HMG-1 as a late mediator of endotoxin lethality in mice. Science 285:248–251

Yang R, Gallo DJ, Baust JJ et al 2002 Ethyl pyruvate modulates inflammatory gene expression in mice subjected to hemorrhagic shock. Am J Physiol Gastrointest Liver Physiol 283:G212–222

Yang H, Wang H, Li J et al 2004 Reversing established sepsis with antagonists of endogenous HMGB1. Proc Natl Acad Sci USA 101:296–301

Yu YM, Kim JB, Lee KW, Kim SY, Han PL, Lee JK 2005 Inhibition of the cerebral ischemic injury by ethyl pyruvate with a wide therapeutic window. Stroke 36:2238–2243

DISCUSSION

Marshall: What is the effect of these compounds on antimicrobial defences, bacterial growth and cell killing?

Fink: Before we gave ethyl pyruvate (EP) to Louis Ulloa, New York, we looked at its effects on caecal ligation and puncture (CLP). We got negative results with a pre-treatment paradigm. If anything, the animals died faster. Louis post-treated the animals after treating them with antibiotics. Our suspicion is that if you give a potent anti-inflammatory agent to an animal that has an adequately treated infection, this is good. But, if the infection hasn't been adequately treated, then administering an anti-inflammatory agent might not be good. *In vitro*, EP is not antibacterial, so its effects on animal models of sepsis cannot be explained this way.

Marshall: Do they have any activity on histone deacetylases (HDACs)?

Fink: This is on our 'to do' list of experiments. HDAC inhibitors are anti-inflammatory and are beneficial in a number of model systems. It is possible this compound works that way. Valproic acid is not only a GSK-3β inhibitor, but also an HDAC inhibitor.

Gilroy: Your data are heartening. We work on prostaglandin D2, which breaks down to cyclopentenone prostaglandins. Like your compounds, they are very electrophilic and form Michael addition reactions with proteins. We are getting criticised by certain groups who argue that these compounds aren't formed naturally *in vivo* (we now have LC/MS/MS data to prove they do exist in inflammation) and when you put them back into inflammatory models to exert an anti-inflammatory effect people say that they are non-specific and will bind onto every protein with an SH group that is available. How would you address this issue with your compounds? How specific are they?

Fink: The people who review our papers have been kind enough to make the same points! Any molecule that is as simple as EP cannot be specific. There is not enough geometry to impose much specificity on the molecule. It is also not a very potent electrophile. I think this is exactly where the selectivity comes from. The sulfhydryl (SH) group on Cys38 in p65 sits in a pocket surrounded by arginine residues. It is a basic environment and this environment favours the formation of S^-. It is a wonderful target for even a weak electrophile. The key SH groups in Keap1 also are easily oxidized. Their job in the cell is to detect weak electrophiles. Really potent electrophiles are alkylating agents that will alkylate DNA and kill the cell. I think the beauty of EP is that it is a weak electrophile and it only targets these very sensitive electrophilic targets. I suspect the cyclopentanones are in the same category.

Evans: Can it target SH groups in caspases? Is there a displacement of nitrosylated SH groups?

Fink: We don't know this yet.

Cohen: It affects both HMG and NF-κB. But those two are apparently separate or independent. Do you think its effect is because it affects both, or have you been able to do experiments that dissect whether it is effective due to one or the other?

Fink: No, we haven't done these experiments. I would presume that the effects Louis observed in the CLP model, where the drug is started 24 h after the onset of inflammation, have to be related largely to the inhibition of HMGB1 or some other late-acting mediator. NF-κB signalling in that model is largely all over by 24 h. You are coming in so late I can't imagine that the inhibition of NF-κB is important. In an endotoxin model where you are pretreating, you can knock down the whole cytokine storm, and the HMGB1 part of the story is probably unimportant. It is mostly about inhibiting NF-κB.

Thiemermann: Earlier I asked Dr Wang whether HMGB1 signals by activation of NF-κB. There is a lot of evidence that HMGB1 can activate NF-κB. When I was asking this I was wondering whether there is a biphasic activation of NF-κB: an early one, and then a late release of mediators such as HMGB1 which then drive a secondary inflammatory event.

Fink: I think that's a good question. With respect to EP, it not only blocks HMGB1 release, it also blocks the pro-inflammatory effects of HMGB1. If you add HMGB1 to macrophages or epithelial cells and coincubate with EP, you inhibit activation of those cells. You are right: there are probably waves of inflammation. There are alarm phase and late phase mediators which are released and interact with one another.

Annane: Does EP influence the anti-inflammatory cytokines?

Fink: That's a good question. We haven't measured the effects of EP on IL10 *in vitro*. Ethacrinic acid *in vitro* down-regulates IL10 secretion at least as much as it down-regulates IL6 secretion.

Griffiths: Clearly it is a concern when you have an increased problem with the pre-treatment. Do you think these compounds are having any effects on cellular protective mechanisms, such as glutathione or heat shock proteins?

Fink: Potentially. We haven't seen problems with pre-treatment in ischaemia/reperfusion models. The only place we have had a problem with pre-treatment is in infection models. I'm not surprised about this. You'd see the same if you gave any effective anti-inflammatory agent as a pre-treatment in a CLP model.

Ulloa: We don't believe that EP is doing everything through inhibition of NF-κB. I am wondering about alternative mechanisms. Can EP work as an antioxidant?

Fink: It is a good peroxide scavenger, so it is an antioxidant. But the fact that it works in the reactive oxygen species (ROS) cell system after washing it out suggests that this isn't all that important to the pharmacology of the compound. We haven't done any experiments to see whether PARP activation is inhibited, but I would suspect it is. If you pacify the cell and make it quiescent, I don't think there will be oxidants that are produced that will damage DNA and activate PARP. But we haven't done the experiments.

Szabó: If it is an antioxidant, it would probably inhibit PARP (indirectly, by preventing DNA breakage). It is just a matter of concentration. I am trying to reconcile the *in vitro* concentrations with the *in vivo* dose. If you use 10 mM *in vitro* and then give 40 mg/kilogram, because the molecular weight is about 100, it is hard for me to imagine that you would find millimolar concentrations in blood or extracellular fluids. Have you measured plasma levels of EP?

Fink: That's a great question. EP has been licensed to a biotechnology company called Critical Therapeutics that is trying to develop it as a drug. The company needed to get pharmacokinetic information for an FDA submission document, and they have attempted to measure EP levels in the circulation. It is impossible to measure. After administration, it disappears from the plasma almost instantaneously. There is a drug called CNI1493, which is another macrophage-pacifying drug. This works in cell culture at millimolar concentrations but works *in vivo* at much lower concentrations. The initial presumption was that CNI1493 worked by shutting down macrophages. The way it really works is by telling the brain to increase vagal outflow, which is what causes the anti-inflammatory effects. I have a feeling that EP works centrally *in vivo*. Kevin Tracey and his group have done some preliminary experiments showing that i.p. injection of EP causes increased vagal nerve firing in mice. I think that it crosses the blood–brain barrier (it is lipophilic) and tells the vagus to increase traffic.

Radermacher: I assume it cleaves almost immediately when it is injected. Has anyone tried the equimolar combination of ethanol and pyruvic acid? Or lactate and ethanol?

Fink: A number of people have suggested that experiment, but we haven't tried it yet. The fact that we can't find it in the circulation doesn't necessarily mean that it is cleaved instantaneously. It is very lipophilic, and I think it dissolved into cells rapidly.

Herndon: What dose was it given in Vincent's sheep model?

Fink: I am not certain of the dose.

Radermacher: Our dose was 30 mg/kg as a bolus over 10 minutes, and thereafter a continuous i.v. infusion at 30 mg/kg/h over 12 hours. We didn't find any pyruvate increase. We didn't look at ethanol.

Cavaillon: Because of the properties of EP and analogues, could they also induce some negative regulators of the signalling cascade within the cell. Have you checked some of them such as, for example, SOCS1, IRAK-M, MyD88short, ST2, etc?

Fink: That is a great suggestion. We haven't done this experiment. We need an explanation for why a host of these phase II enzyme inducers have anti-inflammatory effects.

Pugin: Does it have an influence on the balance of survival and cell death *in vitro*? Is there a shift from necrosis or apoptosis to survival?

Fink: I am not aware of anyone who has looked at this in cell culture.

Wang: For *in vitro* studies, such as macrophages stimulated with lipopolysaccharide (LPS), do any of your compounds block cytokine release if they are added after LPS?

Fink: We haven't looked at this.

Ulloa: Since tumour necrosis factor (TNF) is induced after LPS stimulation, we studied whether EP was able to inhibit TNF-induced HMGB1 release. Our experiments indicated that EP was able to inhibit both LPS- and TNF-induced extracellular release of HMGB1 in culture of macrophages. These results were in agreement with our previous studies *in vivo*, indicating that EP can control serum levels of cytokines even when administered after the onset of sepsis.

GENERAL DISCUSSION I

Thiemermann: In animal models of disease, such as models of endotoxaemia, we often assume that what we see in response to endotoxin is the acute cytokine storm, with a rapid formation of both pro- and anti-inflammatory cytokines including tumour necrosis factor (TNF), interleukin (IL)1 and IL6 and IL10. When people say this is an acute model and is therefore not relevant, this may be true, but by the same token there is an implication that hyper-inflammation is not as important. In contrast, many anti-inflammatory therapeutic strategies are effective in models of caecal ligation and perforation (CLP). There must be a case for a significant degree of inflammation in the first 24–72 h in these models during which multiple organ failure and injury occurs.

Gilroy: You are injecting lipopolysaccharide (LPS), which is a chemical, versus bugs. If you dampen down the immune response then bugs will run riot. The two can't be compared.

Thiemermann: But the patients will be treated with antibiotics. Assuming that you remove the focus in the CLP model, or give antibiotics, they can be compared.

Singer: There are now a few registries and retrospective databases showing that, on average, the clinician gets the choice of antibiotic right less than 50% of the time. Interestingly, the literature is split as to how much impact this has on outcome.

Cohen: That's rubbish! There are papers showing that selection of the correct antibiotic does have a profound and measurable effect on outcome (Ibrahim et al 2000, Leroy et al 2003, Garnacho-Montero et al 2003).

Singer: Certainly, if I was ill I would want an appropriate antibiotic. However, it doesn't make as much difference as we would like to believe.

Radermacher: Let's go back to animals, where we know the bug in question and where antibiotics do make a difference. In Steve Hollenberg's mouse CLP model he has shown that by adding antibiotics and fluid resuscitation, he markedly improved the outcome and morbidity of his animals (Hollenberg et al 2000, 2001). Still, an anti-inflammatory approach had an additional marked improvement.

Gilroy: How efficient would it be in the absence of the antibiotics?

Radermacher: We haven't tried this because the idea was to use the appropriate antibiotic to get rid of the criticism that a model not treated with antibiotics would be less clinically relevant.

Singer: With an abscess, antibiotics aren't that effective.

Radermacher: I take that point. We didn't remove the abscess.

Fink: I don't even take that point. Antibiotics are quite effective in an abscess. You can treat hepatic abscesses with antibiotics. We used to operate on them.

Cohen: That's a different discussion, although you would normally prefer to drain an abscess. There is an interesting issue to do with animal models. They ask different questions. Providing one recognizes this, they are fine for providing mechanisms. The danger is if we extrapolate from animal models to patients with sepsis.

Marshall: There is another fundamental issue in trial design that is often overlooked. You want to evaluate a compound with this additional activity in a patient who has been adequately resuscitated, who has had source control and has had antibiotics, but has not responded as one anticipates. This is not the way we have traditionally identified patients.

Singer: In PROWESS, over 90% were community-acquired sepsis.

Marshall: I'm thinking more of the temporal aspect. Most patients will respond appropriately to fluid resuscitation, antibiotics and source control. Patients with severe sepsis who would be optimal candidates for adjuvant therapies represent a small subgroup who don't respond appropriately and die. This is the group we need to be targeting for trials.

Fink: Natanson and colleagues did a famous experiment many years ago where they randomized dogs with clot-induced peritonitis to nothing, fluids, antibiotics or fluids and antibiotics. The animals treated with fluids and antibiotics survived. The survival in the other three treatment groups was relatively poor (Natanson et al 1990).

Radermacher: The same is true for Steve Hollenberg's work. Mice without any resuscitation had a 48h mortality of 100% (sham-operation: 0%), while approximately 50% of the animals survived when fluid resuscitation were administered together with antibiotics. Antibiotics and fluids alone were associated with a 20–30% survival. (Hollenberg et al 2001).

Singer: There is a healthy animal literature showing the opposite: antibiotics increase mortality. It just depends.

Radermacher: The essential point is adding fluid resuscitation to the antibiotics. The antibiotics alone only resulted in 20–30% mortality. The combination was important.

Fink: I think the literature you are referring to, Mervyn Singer, is with i.v. bugs followed by a cell wall active antibiotic. This turns the i.v. bug model into an acute endotoxaemia model.

Piantadosi: You can do something similar with CLP and a static antibiotic, where the animals fare better than with a bacteriocidal antibiotic. I want to reiterate the point about animal models. To drug companies, sepsis has been hands-off because it is a huge money drain, and many clinical trials have been negative. Now the views have changed about preclinical models: we don't want to know about pre-treatment or whether it works in the absence of antibiotics. We want established sepsis with fluids and antibiotics on board. Then, if you can show an additional effect, someone might consider funding a trial.

Szabó: How much can you tell us about the clinical development plans for ethyl pyruvate?

Fink: I can tell you everything that is public knowledge. The company we were talking about was founded by H. Shaw Warren, Kevin Tracey and me about five years ago. I am an advisor to the company but also a shareholder, so I am hugely conflicted here. The company is in the midst of a 150 patient cardiopulmonary bypass trial, and about 100 patients have been enrolled so far. It is a pre- and post-treatment study with a read-out of total complications. The patients are pre-screened so that they have a predicted mortality of greater than 15%. There have also been two phase I studies in humans. The first used peripheral administration of ethyl pyruvate at graded concentrations. It caused thrombophlebitis in several of the subjects when administered through a peripheral vein. In the second phase I study, the drug was infused through a central vein. At the highest dose, some of the normal subjects complained of blurred vision and CNS effects. As soon as the drug was stopped, these side-effects went away.

Wang: Is it advantageous to develop therapeutic agents with multiple protective effects? For instance, one such compound is ethyl pyruvate, which not only has anti-inflammatory activities, but it also works well in animal models for ischaemia/reperfusion.

Fink: I'll comment on that not with respect to ethyl pyruvate, but with respect to compounds in general. The Holy Grail for the pharmaceutical industry has been to find compounds that are exquisitely specific and target a single enzyme. The rationale is that these will have a better side-effect profile because of their specificity. But it is turning out that the compounds that are the most useful actually lack specificity. The kinase inhibitors that are showing great efficacy in cancer were originally developed to target a specific RTK, but they actually target a bunch of RTKs. The same is true in the psychiatry literature. The most effective drugs for the treatment of depression affect multiple signalling pathways. In a disease as complicated as sepsis, the notion that you want to target a single node in this massively complex signalling cascade is hopelessly simplistic.

Marshall: Isn't Gleevec very specific?

Fink: No, there was a recent paper showing how Gleevec needs to target more than one kinase to be effective (Wong et al 2004).

Szabó: In the literature there are more and more papers on what people call 'selectively non-selective' compounds. They are looking for things that globally modulate cellular functions, as opposed to homing in on one narrow particular molecular pathway. Really successful drugs, such as aspirin or steroids, affect dozens of pathways. The concepts in drug development are changing. For example, there is this new concept that what we are supposed to be doing is cell-based screens based around cell functions. You don't always need to know the mechanisms of action to find an active compound.

Piantadosi: That doesn't make it conceptually correct. Take for example a genetic disease: sickle cell anaemia. We understand the molecular cause of the disease. We don't understand the molecular cause of sepsis. Given our level of sophistication your approach may be appropriate. But there is the hope that we will be able to sort the mechanisms out and that molecular specificity will be important.

Szabó: There are very few single-gene diseases that can be compared to sickle-cell disease. Most diseases affect complex pathways and therapies should also deal with them simultaneously.

Piantadosi: The new molecular medicine work being done to identify single nucleotide polymorphisms (SNPs) I think will identify important mutations but just yet, we cannot do anything about them.

Annane: What we are talking about is translational research, moving from animal models to humans. One major gap that remains to be filled is integrating all these pieces of the puzzle. As we saw earlier, we have PARP, GSK and other pieces for which we are getting more information, but we don't know how to put them together.

Griffiths: With regard to the specificity, I would still prefer to have an antibiotic that hits an invading meningococcus specifically.

Szabó: Do you care about the mode of action?

Griffiths: Not really. The issue regarding the animal models is that they are not reflecting what our real clinical population is: that of an ageing population. More of our model systems used in sepsis research need to reflect this, in particular what goes wrong with the complex signalling and defence mechanisms with ageing. Most of my work is on muscle damage and we are interested in the elderly. There, many of the cellular systems are impaired with age for instance protection against damage and the ability to repair.

Fink: The model of renal failure by Star and colleagues is a huge advance because it is a realistic model. The only way he could get the mice to respond appropriately was by making them old.

Thiemermann: Many drug targets start as a specific target (i.e. angiotensin-converting enzyme [ACE] inhibitors) and then over time, as we learn more about pathophysiology and the pharmacology of these drugs, these compounds turn out to be less specific. Here's another example, peroxisome proliferator-activated receptor (PPAR)γ agonists are very specific for PPARγ, but the more we learn about PPARγ, the more non-specific effects of these compound may be discovered. The same is true for erythropoietin, which is in clinical use for the treatment of anaemia in patients with chronic renal failure, but is has become recently apparent that this drug has a number of pleiotropic effects.

Fink: ACE inhibitors are an interesting example. They inhibit ACE, but they also promote bradykinin production. And they have an active sulfhydryl group so they are antioxidants. The notion of specificity is largely illusory.

References

Garnacho-Montero J, Garcia-Garmendia JL, Barrero-Almodovar A, Jimenez-Jimenez FJ, Perez-Paredes C, Ortiz-Leyba C 2003 Impact of adequate empirical antibiotic therapy on the outcome of patients admitted to the intensive care unit with sepsis. Crit Care Med 31: 2742–2751

Hollenberg SM, Broussard M, Osman J et al 2000 Increased microvascular reactivity and improved mortality in septic mice lacking inducible nitric oxide synthase. Circ Res 86: 774–778

Hollenberg SM, Dumasius A, Easington C et al 2001 Charactarization of a hyperdynamic murine model of resuscitated sepsis using echocardiography. Am J Respir Crit Care Med 164:891–895

Ibrahim EH, Sherman G, Ward S, Fraser VJ, Kollef MH 2000 The influence of inadequate antimicrobial treatment of bloodstream infections on patient outcomes in the ICU setting. Chest 118:146–155

Leroy O, Meybeck A, d'Escrivan T, Devos P, Kipnis E, Georges H 2003 Impact of adequacy of initial antimicrobial therapy on the prognosis of patients with ventilator-associated pneumonia. Intensive Care Med 29:2170–2173

Natanson C, Danner RL, Reilly JM et al 1990 Antibiotics versus cardiovascular support in a canine model of human septic shock. Am J Physiol 259:H1440–1447

Wong S, McLaughlin J, Cheng D, Zhang C, Shokat KM, Witte ON 2004 Sole BCR-ABL inhibition is insufficient to eliminate all myeloproliferative disorder cell populations. Proc Natl Acad Sci USA 101:17456–174561

Cytoprotective and anti-inflammatory actions of carbon monoxide in organ injury and sepsis models

Stefan W. Ryter and Augustine M.K. Choi[1]

Department of Medicine, Division of Pulmonary, Allergy and Critical Care Medicine, The University of Pittsburgh School of Medicine, MUH 628 NW, 3459 Fifth Ave, Pittsburgh, PA 15213, USA

Abstract. Carbon monoxide (CO) can exert potent anti-inflammatory effects in animal and cell culture models of sepsis, despite well-known lethal effects at high concentration. Endogenous biological CO arises from the enzymatic degradation of haem, mainly from haemoglobin turnover, catalysed by haem oxygenases (HO). The inducible form of HO, haem oxygenase 1 (HO-1) participates in endogenous cellular defence against oxidative stress. HO-1 confers cytoprotection in many models of organ and tissue injury where inflammatory processes are implicated, including sepsis. When applied exogenously at low concentration, CO mimics the cytoprotective potential of HO-1 induction in these models. CO confers protection against endotoxin shock *in vitro* and *in vivo* by inhibiting the production of pro-inflammatory cytokines, in a mechanism involving the modulation of p38 mitogen activated protein kinase. CO protection against vascular injury may involve both anti-inflammatory and antiproliferative effects. The protection afforded by CO against liver failure and inflammatory lung injury was associated with the modulation of inducible nitric oxide synthase. Recent *in vitro* studies indicate that CO inhibits proinflammatory signalling by differentially inhibiting the trafficking of toll-like receptors (TLRs) to lipid rafts. Additional candidate mechanisms in anti-inflammatory effects of CO include the increased expression of heat shock proteins and the tumour suppressor protein caveolin 1.

2007 Sepsis—new insights, new therapies. Wiley, Chichester (Novartis Foundation Symposium 280) p 165–181

The identification of endogenously produced nitric oxide (NO) gas as a potent vasodilating substance formerly known as endothelium-derived relaxing factor (EDRF) led to a revolution in life sciences research, ultimately recognized by the Nobel Prize in Physiology (1998) awarded to its discoverers Drs Murad, Furchgott and Ignarro. This discovery led to the widespread recognition that endogenously-

---

[1]This paper was presented at the symposium by Augustine M.K. Choi, to whom correspondence should be addressed.

derived gases, such as NO, could participate in the regulation of vital physiological processes. Biological NO arises during the metabolic conversion of L-arginine to L-citrulline by constitutive and inducible nitric oxide synthases (NOS; E.C 1:14:13:39). NO produces its vasodilatory effect by binding to and activating soluble guanylyl cyclase (sGC), leading to the enhanced production of guanosine 3′,5′-monophosphate (cGMP), which in turn activates G kinase-dependent protein phosphorylation cascades. By this mechanism, NO can act as an autocrine or paracrine factor to stimulate intracellular signal transduction pathways, leading to a host of physiological effects, including smooth muscle relaxation. By the same mechanism, it has been recently recognized that carbon monoxide (CO), another small gas molecule may also potentially exert physiological effector functions despite its well-known toxicity at high concentrations (Ryter et al 2004). Unlike NO, which is a free radical gas capable of undergoing complex redox chemistry, CO is relatively inert in biological systems with its reactivity restricted to forming complexes with haem moieties (Ryter & Otterbein 2004). Elevated concentrations of CO produce hypoxaemia, eventually leading to death, by competition for oxygen binding sites in haemoglobin (Von Berg 1999). Endogenous CO arises principally during haem degradation catalysed by the haem oxygenase (HO) enzymes (EC 1:14.99.3) (Tenhunen et al 1969). The HO enzymes occur as two genetically-distinct isozymes, a constitutive form (HO-2) and an inducible form (HO-1), both of which catalyse the degradation of haem to biliverdin, CO and iron (Ryter et al 2006). The haem degradative pathway culminates in the reduction of biliverdin to the lipophillic bile pigment bilirubin by NADPH biliverdin reductase (Tenhunen et al 1969). HO-1 responds to transcriptional induction by a broad spectrum of environmental agents (such as heavy metals and other xenobiotics) as well as endogenous factors associated with pro-inflammatory stress, such as cytokines (Ryter et al 2006). This general inducible response to stress belongs to a larger family of stress protein responses, associated with cellular adaptation to environmental stimuli, among which include the well-known heat shock protein (HSP) response. HO-1, as an inducible stress protein, confers protection against oxidative stress conditions *in vitro* and *in vivo*, by exerting antioxidative, anti-apoptotic and anti-inflammatory actions. The underlying mechanisms of HO-dependent cytoprotection remain incompletely understood (Ryter et al 2006, Ryter & Tyrrell 2000). HO exerts antioxidative functions by converting haem, a potential pro-oxidant molecule, into the bile pigments, biliverdin-IXα, and bilirubin-IXα, which have demonstrated antioxidant properties (Fig. 1). HO-derived iron may stimulate the synthesis of ferritin, which can confer cytoprotection related to the sequestration of potentially reactive iron (Ryter et al 2006, Ryter & Tyrrell 2000, Vile & Tyrrell 1993). Since these and other cytoprotective mechanisms associated with HO-derived iron and/or biliverdin/

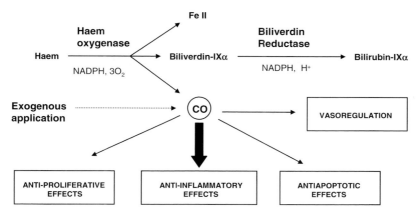

FIG. 1.   Exogenous application of carbon monoxide mimics endogenous cytoprotective pathways. Induction of haem oxygenase 1 (HO-1) is associated with tissue protection in multiple organ injury models. HO-1 activity generates carbon monoxide, biliverdin-IXα, and ferrous iron from the oxidative degradation of haem. BV is converted to bilirubin-IXα by NADPH biliverdin reductase. The exogenous application of CO gas can mimic many of the cytoprotective effects of endogenous HO-1 activation. These include general cytoprotective effects involving antiapoptotic, anti-inflammatory, and anti-proliferative mechanisms. Vascular effects of CO include modulation of vessel tone, the inhibition of platelet aggregation, and the inhibition of vascular smooth muscle proliferation, leading to prevention of tissue remodelling.

bilirubin have been extensively reviewed elsewhere, the current paper will focus on mechanisms involving the endogenous production of HO-derived CO (see previous reviews Ryter et al 2006, Ryter & Tyrrell 2000).

CO affects vascular function by influencing the regulation of vessel tone, platelet aggregation, and smooth muscle proliferation (Ryter et al 2006, Furchgott & Jothianandan 1991, Morita et al 1995, 1997, Kim et al 2006). Our previous studies have identified a potent anti-inflammatory effect of CO involving the inhibition of pro-inflammatory cytokine production following inducing stimuli, dependent on the modulation of mitogen activated protein kinase (MAPK)-signalling cascades (Otterbein et al 2000). More recent studies imply multiple mechanisms in the anti-inflammatory potential of CO, involving the potential participation of secondary factors such as heat shock proteins (Kim et al 2005a), inducible nitric oxide synthases (Sarady et al 2004), caveolin 1 (Wang et al unpublished studies), and peroxisome proliferator-activated receptor (PPAR)γ (Bilban et al 2006). Recent studies also identify effects of CO on early events in pro-inflammatory signalling involving the regulation of Toll-like receptor trafficking (Nakahira et al 2006). This brief monograph will summarize the current state of the CO field with emphasis on anti-inflammatory mechanisms.

Carbon monoxide inhibits pro-inflammatory cytokine production in a macrophage model of sepsis

CO has been shown in a number of models to exert a potent anti-inflammatory effect at low concentration (Otterbein et al 1999, 2000, 2003, Sarady et al 2004, Morse et al 2003). *In vitro*, CO prevented the lipopolysaccharide (LPS)-induced production of pro-inflammatory cytokines such as tumor necrosis factor (TNF)α, interleukin (IL)1β and macrophage inflammatory protein 1β (MIP1β) in cultured macrophages (Otterbein et al 2000). This protection mimicked that which could be achieved by the artificial overexpresion of HO-1 in this model, suggesting a link between CO and the cytoprotective effect of HO-1 induction. CO treatment also promoted the increased production of the anti-inflammatory cytokine interleukin-10 (IL-10) during LPS challenge. Inhibitor studies determined that the anti-inflammatory effects of CO in this model were independent of sGC activation or endogenous NO production (Otterbein et al 2000). Recent studies also suggest an anti-inflammatory mechanism involving increased ROS production and expression of PPARγ (Bilban et al 2006). The LPS-dependent stimulation of pro-inflammatory cytokines in macrophages involved the activation of MAPK signalling pathways, including the p38 MAPK, extracellular regulated kinase 1/2 (ERK1/2) and c-Jun N-terminal kinase (JNK) pathways. In the presence of LPS, CO increased p38 MAPK activation, and its upstream kinases MKK3 and MKK6 in macrophages (Otterbein et al 2000).

In murine models of endotoxaemia, CO preconditioning reduced the production of serum TNFα, interleukin (IL)1β, interleukin 6 (IL6) and prolonged survival following LPS challenge (Otterbein et al 2000, Morse 2003). Mice received injections of LPS (1 mg/kg) with or without CO pretreatment (250 ppm). CO dose-dependently inhibited LPS-inducible serum TNFα levels and increased LPS-inducible IL10 production. The responsiveness of TNFα to LPS treatment was decreased in $Mkk3^{-/-}$ mice compared to wild-type mice. CO failed to further down-regulate TNFα levels or up-regulate IL10 levels in LPS-treated $Mkk3^{-/-}$ mice. In $Il10^{-/-}$ mice, CO inhibited TNFα levels within the first hour of LPS treatment to a similar extent as in wild-type mice, excluding a role for IL10 in the early anti-inflammatory effects of CO (Otterbein et al 2000).

Carbon monoxide protects in ischaemia–reperfusion (I/R) injury and vascular injury models

CO confers tissue protection in several preclinical animal models of disease, including oxidative and inflammatory lung injury, I/R injury, and cardiovascular injury/disease (reviewed in Ryter et al 2006, Slebos et al 2003). The protection afforded by CO against I/R injury has been demonstrated in multiple organ models including lung, liver, kidney, intestine and heart (Zhang et al 2003, Fujita et al 2001, Amersi et al 2002, Nakao et al 2003, 2005). In the lung I/R model CO diminished proapoptotic markers induced by I/R including caspase 3 activation (Zhang et al 2003). The protective effects of CO in I/R injury are related to anti-apoptotic and anti-inflammatory effects with a possible contribution from vascular effects (Zhang et al 2003, Fujita et al 2001, Amersi et al 2002, Nakao et al 2003, 2005). CO also protected against hyperoxic lung injury by reducing the expression of proinflammatory mediators (Otterbein et al 1999, 2003a). In a model of intimal hyperplasia, where smooth muscle cells proliferate uncontrollably following balloon angioplasty of the carotid artery, exposure to CO also completely prevented vascular stenosis (Otterbein et al 2003b). Pre-treatment with CO (250 ppm) for just 1 h significantly reduced the neointimal proliferation seen at 14 days post-balloon angioplasty relative to control rats that did not receive CO treatment. This effect was attributed to the inhibition of smooth muscle cell proliferation by CO in mechanisms dependent on activation of soluble guanylate cyclase and p38 MAPK, resulting in the up-regulation of $p21^{Waf1/Cip1}$ (Otterbein et al 2003b).

Role of inducible nitric oxide synthase (iNOS) in anti-inflammatory properties of CO

In a model of acute liver failure induced by TNFα, low dose CO conferred organ protection associated with the transcriptional up-regulation of iNOS. The authors proposed a complementary adaptive response whereby the up-regulation of iNOS by CO treatment promoted the subsequent NO-dependent induction of HO-1. The protection afforded by CO was diminished in *Inos*-deleted hepatocytes, but could be compensated for in this case by HO-1 expression. On the other hand, *Ho1* was essential for the cytoprotective potential of CO in this model (Zucker-braun et al 2003). In a model of LPS-induced multiorgan failure, CO protected against the lethal effects of LPS (Sarady et al 2004). CO had reciprocal effects on iNOS expression in an organ-specific fashion. CO inhibited the induction of iNOS and NO production in the lung whereas it increased the expression of iNOS and NO in the liver. This specificity was also observed *in vitro* such that CO inhibited LPS-induced cytokine production while reducing LPS-induced iNOS expression in lung macrophages. On the other hand, CO protected hepatocytes from LPS-induced apoptosis but increased iNOS expression in hepatocytes (Sarady et al 2004). Furthermore, the cytoprotection afforded by CO during kidney and intestinal transplant-associated I/R injury was associated with the inhibition, rather than up-regulation of iNOS expression (Nakao et al 2003, 2005). In conclusion, the up-regulation of iNOS by CO appears to be specific to the liver, with down-regulation of iNOS observed in other organs. The relationship between iNOS activity and CO-mediated cytoprotection remains unclear.

Role of heat shock factor and heat shock protein in anti-inflammatory properties of CO

Low dose CO was shown to up-regulate the expression of Hsp70 in mouse lung endothelial cells, which can confer cross-resistance to a number of agents in addition to thermal stress. In mouse lung endothelial cells this expression of Hsp70 contributed to the apparent cytoprotection conferred by CO against pro-apoptotic stimuli, such as TNFα/actinomycin D (Kim et al 2005a). The cytoprotective effect of CO against TNFα/ActD was diminished in fibroblasts derived from heat shock factor deficient mice $(Hsf^{-/-})$ as well as in fibroblasts derived from p38 MAPK deficient mice. Anti-inflammatory effects of CO, with respect to modulation of pro- or anti-inflammatory cytokines were diminished in heat shock factor knockout mice, indicating a potential role for the heat shock response in CO-dependent cytoprotection (Kim et al 2005a). To assess the protective role of CO *in vivo*, $Hsf1^{-/-}$ and heterozygous mice were administered LPS and survival rates were monitored for 192 h. Exposure with CO (250 ppm) in heterozygote mice lengthened the survival after LPS challenge to 192 h which correlated with high levels of Hsp70 in lung tissue. In the absence of HSF1, the effect of CO on survival rate in HSF knockout mice was significantly reduced (Kim et al 2005a).

CO differentially inhibits TLR receptor trafficking and downstream signalling in macrophages

Our recent studies have identified a novel mechanism by which CO may exert anti-inflammatory effects involving the down-regulation of Toll-like receptor (TLR) trafficking. The trafficking of TLRs to specialized membrane lipid raft domains represents an early upstream event in the activation of TLR-dependent signalling pathways associated with pro-inflammatory stimuli. We investigated the effect of CO on cytokine production in RAW 264.7 cells induced with various TLR ligands (TLR ligands: TLR2, peptidoglycan [PGN] or Pam₃CSK4 [Pam]; TLR3, double-stranded RNA poly(I:C); TLR4, LPS; TLR5, flagellin (Fla); and TLR9, CpG) (Nakahira et al 2006). CO exposure inhibited TLR2, 4, 5 and 9 ligand-induced TNFα production, but did not affect poly(I:C)-induced TNFα production. The effect of CO on LPS-induced cytokine production was dose-dependent over a range of 50–500 ppm. The effect of CO on TNFα production in mouse peritoneal macrophages was consistent with that observed in RAW 264.7 macrophages. Activation of both TLR3 and TLR4 signalling cascades induces interferon (IFN)β through the activation of IRF3, leading to the production of IFN-inducible gene products, such as IFNγ inducible protein 10 (IP10) and RANTES. Although CO significantly inhibited LPS-induced

IFNβ gene expression and the production of IP10 and RANTES, the induction of these cytokines by poly(I:C) was not inhibited by CO. Since NF-κB and IRF3 are key transcription factors activated in TLR3 and TLR4 signalling pathways, we examined the effect of CO on the ligand-induced activation of NF-κB and IRF3. CO inhibited NF-κB activation, induced by LPS, Pam, Fla and CpG. Nuclear translocation of IRF3 increased after LPS treatment, and CO significantly suppressed this translocation. CO had no effect on poly(I:C)-induced NF-κB activation and translocation of IRF3. With the exception of TLR3, all the TLRs interact with an adaptor protein, MyD88. TLR3 uses only the adaptor molecule TRIF to activate IRF3, and TLR4 also activates IRF3 through TRIF. We observed increased interaction not only between TLR4 and MyD88 but also that of TLR4 and TRIF at 5 min after LPS treatment; however, CO markedly attenuated both interactions. Although poly(I:C) treatment also increased the interaction of TLR3 and TRIF, CO did not suppress the TLR3 and TRIF interaction.

To address the involvement of lipid rafts on TLR signalling pathways and the potential role of CO on the membrane rafts, cells were stimulated with LPS or poly(I:C) in the presence or absence of CO and incubated with FITC-CTx. CTx specifically binds to the glycosphingolipid 1 (GM1), which is enriched in lipid rafts. In the resting RAW 264.7 cells, TLR4 localized, both in the membrane and intracellular compartment. After LPS treatment, a large fraction of TLR4 translocated to the plasma membrane and co-localized with GM1. In CO-treated cells, the LPS-induced translocation of TLR4 to the membrane rafts was significantly inhibited. In contrast, TLR3 localized in the intracellular compartment in the resting cells, and remained unchanged after poly(I:C) stimulation, even when CO was added. To investigate whether CO modulates the translocation of TLR4 and its adaptor molecules to lipid rafts, we isolated raft fractions and examined the translocation of the proteins involved in TLR signalling by immunoblotting. TLR4 and its adaptor molecules (MyD88 and TRIF), as well as MD2, IRAK1, TRAF6, p65 and I-κBα rapidly translocated to lipid rafts after LPS stimulation, whereas TRAF2 was not translocated. In contrast, CO significantly inhibited the LPS-induced recruitment of TLR4 and other signalling molecules to lipid rafts. The distribution of TLR4 was not affected by CO treatment alone. CD14 was constitutively expressed mainly in lipid rafts of resting cells and its expression was unaffected by LPS or CO treatment. To confirm the differential localization and translocation patterns of TLRs, TLR3, 4 and 9 were immunoprecipitated with each antibody and immunoblotted with the same antibody using Triton X-100-soluble and -insoluble raft fractions. After the ligand stimulation, TLR4 and 9 translocated to the rafts fraction while TLR3 did not. In addition, the adaptor protein TRIF interacted with TLR4 in the rafts fraction by LPS stimulation, but not with TLR3 by poly(I:C) (Nakahira et al 2006).

Reactive oxygen species (ROS) exert critical roles in intracellular signalling including the TLR signalling pathway. Scavenging of ROS or inhibition of NADPH oxidase suppresses LPS-induced cytokine production. To examine if ROS are involved with the TLR signalling pathway and trafficking of TLR to lipid rafts, RAW 264.7 cells were pretreated with the antioxidant N-acetyl-L-cysteine (NAC) or a NADPH oxidase inhibitor, diphenylene iodonium (DPI) for 30 min, followed by incubation with TLR ligands. NAC dose-dependently suppressed LPS-induced TNFα production. DPI significantly suppressed TNFα production induced by LPS, Pam and CpG, but not by poly(I:C) treatment. DPI also inhibited LPS-induced interaction of TRIF and TLR4. Furthermore, the LPS-induced transloca-tion of TLR4 to lipid rafts was inhibited by DPI treatment. These results indicate that inhibition of NADPH oxidase suppresses the TLR signalling pathway by modulating events upstream of the pathway. Furthermore, cellular stimulation with H_2O_2 and PMA also recruits TLR4 to lipid rafts. We investigated the involve-ment of CO on TLR ligands-induced ROS generation. CO significantly suppressed LPS and Pam-induced ROS production. CO failed to inhibit poly(I:C)-induced ROS production in macrophages. Upon stimulation, ROS are generated by NADPH oxidase, which forms a membrane-bound complex, including p22^{phox} and gp91^{phox} and cytosolic proteins such as p47^{phox}. The complex of gp91^{phox} and p47^{phox} increased 5 min after LPS treatment while complex formation was inhibited by CO as well as DPI treatment. Furthermore, superoxide anion production, detected in isolated membrane fractions from LPS-treated macrophages, was inhibited when the cells were exposed to CO. Peritoneal macrophages from gp91^{phox} deficient (gp91$^{phox-/-}$) mice significantly produced less TNFα in response to LPS than the cells from the wild-type control. The effect of CO on LPS-induced TNFα production was impaired in gp91^{phox}-deficient cells. TLR4 interacted with gp91^{phox} in response to LPS treatment, while DPI treatment inhibited the interaction. CO inhibited the LPS-induced complex formation of TLR4 and gp91^{phox}. To confirm if NADPH oxidase is involved in the LPS-induced translocation of TLR4 to lipid rafts, we isolated lipid rafts from peritoneal macrophages from gp91$^{phox-/-}$ mice. TLR4 translocated to lipid rafts 5 min after LPS treatment in the wild type cells, however, the translocation of TLR4 by LPS was suppressed in gp91^{phox}-deficient cells. These results suggest that gp91^{phox} is involved with LPS-induced translocation of TLR4 to lipid rafts and that the effect of CO on trafficking to lipid rafts is potentially mediated by modulation of gp91^{phox} and suppression of NADPH oxidase activity. In summary, these data suggest that the involvement of lipid rafts in TLR signal-ling is dependent on the specificity of the TLRs. Furthermore, the negative regula-tion of CO on TLR signalling pathways is likely to be dependent not on adaptor proteins, but on the specificity of TLRs. These observations add CO to the list of natural inhibitors of TLR signalling pathways, and furthermore identify ROS as an important mediator of TLR4 trafficking (Nakahira et al 2006) (Fig. 2).

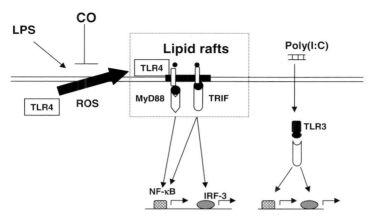

FIG. 2.   The anti-inflammatory effect of carbon monoxide involves differential regulation of Toll-like receptor (TLR) trafficking. The trafficking of TLRs to specialized membrane lipid raft domains represents an early upstream event in the activation of TLR-dependent signalling pathways associated with pro-inflammatory stimuli. The activated receptors associate with multiple adaptor molecules (i.e. MyD88, TRIF). Proinflammatory signalling culminates in the activation of transcription factors (i.e. NF-κB, IRF3) which regulate multiple cytokine genes. We found that TLR4 trafficking to lipid rafts in response to lipopolysaccharide (LPS) stimulation is dependent on the endogenous production of reactive oxygen species (ROS). On the other hand stimulation of TLR3-dependent signalling pathways by the TLR3 ligand poly (I-C) did not involve TLR3 trafficking to the lipid raft. Carbon monoxide, which has known anti-inflammatory effects with respect to macrophage production of cytokines, specifically inhibited TLR4 trafficking to the lipid raft during LPS stimulation, through a mechanism involving the down-regulation of NADPH oxidase-dependent ROS production. On the other hand, CO did not inhibit poly (I-C)-induced activation of TLR3 signalling pathways.

Other mechanisms

Previously we have shown that the tumour suppressor protein caveolin 1 mediates the antiproliferative effects of CO in vascular smooth muscle cells. CO treatment induces the expression of caveolin 1 in smooth muscle cells. The anti-proliferative potential of CO was lost in smooth muscle cells deficient in caveolin 1 expression (Kim et al 2005b). We hypothesized that caveolin 1 may mediate the anti-inflammatory properties of CO as well. In recent unpublished studies from our laboratory, we have found that the anti-inflammatory effect of CO in macrophages also depended on functional caveolin 1 expression. In macrophages isolated from caveolin 1 deficient mice (*Cav*$^{-/-}$) the anti-inflammatory effect of CO against LPS stimulation was abolished (Wang et al, unpublished studies). Furthermore caveolin 1 was shown to associate with and down-regulate the activity of HO-1 in endothelial cells and macrophages (Kim et al 2004, Wang et al unpublished studies).

Conclusions

Despite inherent toxicity at high concentration, the application of CO at low concentration provides protection in multiple models of organ injury. CO provides potent anti-inflammatory protection in models of endotoxinaemia, oxidative lung injury and transplant-associated I/R injury. Much previous research has examined downstream signalling pathways associated with this protection, including the participation of p38 MAPK. The recent identification of CO effects on TLR trafficking provides an additional novel mechanism for the anti-inflammatory effect of CO, and this study is the first to examine upstream events in this pathway. Further work in progress aims to elucidate complex interactions between the HO/CO system and caveolin 1, and their relevance to inflammation. A complete understanding of the underlying mechanisms of CO-mediated tissue protection may lead to the rational design of anti-inflammatory therapies for clinical application.

References

Amersi F, Shen XD, Anselmo D et al 2002 *Ex vivo* exposure to carbon monoxide prevents hepatic ischemia/reperfusion injury through p38 MAP kinase pathway. Hepatology 35: 815–823

Bilban M, Bach FH, Otterbein SL et al 2006 Carbon monoxide orchestrates a protective response through PPARgamma. Immunity 24:601–610

Fujita T, Toda K, Karimova A et al 2001 Paradoxical rescue from ischemic lung injury by inhaled carbon monoxide driven by derepression of fibrinolysis. Nat Med 7:598–604

Furchgott RF, Jothianandan D 1991 Endothelium-dependent and independent vasodilation involving cyclic GMP: relaxation induced by nitric oxide, carbon monoxide and light. Blood Vessels 28:52–61

Kim HP, Wang X, Galbiati F, Ryter SW, Choi AMK 2004 Caveolae compartmentalization of heme oxygenase-1 in endothelial cells. FASEB J 18:1080–1089

Kim HP, Wang X, Zhang J et al 2005a Heat shock protein 70 mediates the cytoprotective effect of carbon monoxide: involvement of p38B MAPK and heat shock factor-1. J Immunol 175:2622–2629

Kim HP, Wang X, Nakao A et al 2005b Caveolin-1 expression by means of p38β mitogen activated protein kinase mediates the antiproliferative effect of carbon monoxide. Proc Natl Acad Sci 102:11319–11324

Kim HP, Ryter SW, Choi AM 2006 CO as a cellular signaling molecule. Ann Rev Pharm Tox 46:411–449

Morita T, Perrella MA, Lee ME, Kourembanas S 1995 Smooth muscle cell-derived carbon monoxide is a regulator of vascular cGMP. Proc Natl Acad Sci USA 92:1475–1479

Morita T, Mitsialis SA, Koike H, Liu Y, Kourembanas S 1997 Carbon monoxide controls the proliferation of hypoxic vascular smooth muscle cells. J Biol Chem 272:32804–323809

Morse D, Pischke SE, Zhou Z et al 2003 Suppression of inflammatory cytokine production by carbon monoxide involves the JNK pathway and AP-1. J Biol Chem 278:36993–36998

Nakahira K, Kim HP, Geng XH et al 2006 Carbon monoxide differentially inhibits TLRs signaling pathways by regulating ROS-induced trafficking of TLRs to lipid rafts. J Exp Med 203:2377–2389

Nakao A, Kimizuka K, Stolz DB et al 2003 Protective effect of carbon monoxide inhalation for cold-preserved small intestinal grafts. Surgery 134:285–292

Nakao A, Neto JS, Kanno S et al 2005 Protection against ischemia/reperfusion injury in cardiac and renal transplantation with carbon monoxide, biliverdin and both. Am J Transplant 5:282–291

Otterbein LE, Mantell LL, Choi AM 1999 Carbon monoxide provides protection against hyperoxic lung injury. Am J Physiol 276:L688–L694

Otterbein LE, Bach FH, Alam J et al 2000 Carbon monoxide has anti-inflammatory effects involving the mitogen-activated protein kinase pathway. Nat Med 6:422–428

Otterbein LE, Otterbein SL, Ifedigbo E et al 2003a MKK3 mitogen activated protein kinase pathway mediates carbon monoxide-induced protection against oxidant induced lung injury. Am J Pathol 163:2555–2563

Otterbein LE, Zuckerbraun BS, Haga M et al 2003b Carbon monoxide suppresses arteriosclerotic lesions associated with chronic graft rejection and with balloon injury. Nat Med 9:183–190

Ryter SW, Tyrrell RM 2000 The heme synthesis and degradation pathways: role in oxidant sensitivity. Heme oxygenase has both pro- and antioxidant properties. Free Radic Biol Med 28:289–309

Ryter SW, Otterbein L 2004 Carbon monoxide in biology and medicine. Bioessays 26:270–280

Ryter SW, Morse D, Choi AMK 2004 Carbon monoxide: to boldly go where NO has gone before. Sci STKE 230:re6

Ryter SW, Alam J, Choi AM 2006 Heme oxygenase-1/carbon monoxide: from basic science to therapeutic applications. Physiol Rev 86:583–650

Sarady JK, Zuckerbraun BS, Bilban M et al 2004 Carbon monoxide protection against endotoxic shock involves reciprocal effects on iNOS in the lung and liver. FASEB J 18:854–856

Slebos DJ, Ryter S, Choi AM 2003 Heme oxygenase-1 and carbon monoxide in pulmonary medicine. Respir Res 4:7

Tenhunen R, Marver HS, Schmid R 1969 Microsomal heme oxygenase. Characterization of the enzyme. J Biol Chem 244:6388–6394

Vile GF, Tyrrell RM 1993 Oxidative stress resulting from ultraviolet A irradiation of human skin fibroblasts leads to a heme oxygenase-dependent increase in ferritin. J Biol Chem 268:14678–14681

Von Berg R 1999 Toxicology update. Carbon monoxide. J Appl Toxicol 19:379–386

Zhang X, Shan P, Otterbein LE et al 2003 Carbon monoxide inhibition of apoptosis during ischemia-reperfusion lung injury is dependent on the p38 mitogen-activated protein kinase and involves caspase-3. J Biol Chem 278:1248–1258

Zuckerbraun BS, Billiar TR, Otterbein SL et al 2003 Carbon monoxide protects against liver failure through nitric oxide-induced heme oxygenase-1. J Exp Med 198:1–11

DISCUSSION

Marshall: There is an evolving literature on the anti-inflammatory effects of carbon dioxide (CO_2). Is there any interaction between oxygen intermediates that might result in carbon monoxide (CO) being converted to CO_2?

Choi: I have talked to other biochemists such as Claude Piantadosi and there is an interaction. It is an interesting question.

Piantadosi: Mitochondria oxygenate CO to CO_2, which is a disposal mechanism for CO. This goes back to L. Young and W. Caughey in the 1980s, whose work clearly showed that when cytochrome oxidase binds CO (and would inhibit respiration) the mitochondria respond by oxygenating it to CO_2.

Choi: We don't know how much of that is happening *in vivo*.

Marshall: The issue here would be that in inflammation you might get increased conversion of CO to CO_2.

Piantadosi: It is a small amount. Roughly 98% of all CO is excreted by the lungs, and 2% is converted this way.

Choi: We have measured CO and CO_2 in blood gases. In the injury models we don't get a bump of CO_2, so it is a small effect.

Fink: Haemoglobin binds CO with high avidity, so all the *in vitro* stuff is straightforward, because there is no haemoglobin. But *in vivo* the CO will be bound to haemoglobin. Is haemoglobin a transport protein for CO?

Choi: Absolutely. There are some studies that suggest that these effects may be independent of CO being delivered with haemoglobin to the sites. When I see data on MAPK *in vivo*, kinases don't have a haem moeity, but still can do their thing.

Fink: One approach to address this question *in vivo* would be to do experiments in animals that are very anaemic, so that presumably the plasma fraction of the haemoglobin would be higher and you ought to be able to show that lower concentrations of CO produce the same biological effect.

Choi: I don't know of anyone who has done that. There is now a Japanese company that can measure CO in tissues and in blood independent of haem. We have shown that if you expose the animals to 250 ppm CO, there is about a tenfold increase of tissue, cellular and plasma CO.

Fink: In the elegant *in vitro* work you have described, can you recapitulate what you see with 8-bromo-cGMP?

Choi: That's a good question; we haven't done the experiment. In macrophages we know that CO antiinflammatory effects are independent of the cGMP pathway. In the proliferation effects, however, cGMP is critically important. Without this CO will not work.

Radermacher: I love the ideas you presented, and in particular the analogy you made to nitric oxide (NO). Michael Pinsky found out that when he changed the air supply from environmentally contaminated air to medical gas, the inherent contamination of the environment with NO had a therapeutic effect. Is the same true for CO?

Choi: You are right. I think NO contamination is a real story. At NIH there is an NO contamination in the order of 3–5 ppm. So we had to buy medical air, which is a lot more expensive. I don't know whether this would hold true for CO.

Radermacher: At the end of the day you are looking for a therapeutic application. Do you think that there is a species-specific dose–response for CO? I raise this because there was a paper last year from Florian Mayr in Vienna. He injected endotoxin into volunteers, and exposed them to the same concentrations of CO you used. He couldn't produce any of the anti-inflammatory effects (Mayr et al 2005).

Choi: I know that study well. There are also other studies in preclinical models of CO where it doesn't have much effect. Is it a kinetics problem? Or is it possible that CO will not work in higher animals? Experimentally, the only large mammals that have been looked at are pigs, and it does a similar thing. In the humans, I like to think that this negative study is because of kinetics and not because of a species problem. The study was done very carefully. There is now a study from iNO therapeutics who have all the rights to CO and NO. They are now doing a 6 months study giving people 250 ppm CO five days a week.

Radermacher: There are already large animal data. The pig is not all that far from humans. We lack primate data, but still we do have some data that are relevant, not only with exogenous CO supplementation but also with haem oxygenase inhibition (Nalos et al 2003, Lavitrano et al 2004, Mazzola et al 2005, Moore et al 2005).

Choi: There are several papers in the pig. They show that if you give CO at the same concentration we used in smaller animals, it has pretty good effects. We are probably about two years away from a first use in transplantation.

Ayala: You made an elegant case for MAP kinase and p38, but then you went to the NF-κB and the TLR story. Do you not see those pathways as comparative?

Choi: Toll is upstream to MAP kinase. NF-κB is downstream. I was trying to show a model in which we start off with the MAP kinase pathway, going upstream to the TLR signalling. We think it is a continuum.

Hellewell: Has haem oxygenase been knocked out *in vivo*?

Choi: Yes. It's lethal, but few do survive with lots of problems. It is one of the few delayed genes which is lethal if it is knocked out. In most knockout mice you have to knock out upstream molecules for it to be lethal. In 1999 Yachie published the first human case report of an *HO1*-deficient patient (Yachie et al 1999). The problems were anaemia, mental and somatic retardation, and pronounced proinflammatory indices. This patient died aged 9. The feeling is that this is one of the rare *HO1* knockout babies that survived a natural abortion.

Hellewell: What about the heterozygous knockouts?

Choi: They behave like controls. They have enough HO-1 protein.

Hellewell: If you were to knock it down with siRNA, what would happen?

Choi: There is one paper on this. Zhang et al (2004) gave intranasal siRNA and knocked down *HO1* nicely. She has an ischaemia–reperfusion model in the lung, and it did what it is supposed to do.

Fink: HO-1 does two things. It makes CO, but it also makes bilirubin, which is nature's version of a very effective ROS scavenger.

Choi: I do not want to down play ferritin and bilirubin. When we got into this field and did a PubMed search, we picked up a couple of dozen papers on ferritin being a very cytoprotective agent, especially in the vascular endothelium. It has been known for a long time that bilirubin is as potent as vitamins C and E in scavenging superoxide. If you give bilrubin or biliverdin it mimics CO effects in the selective models.

Thiemermann: In your lipopolysaccharide (LPS) model, many of the animals in the survival studies died within two hours. Often, rats will die if you give them a lot of LPS by pulmonary vasoconstriction and a secondary fall in cardiac output. Pigs will do the same if they get anywhere near LPS. When we did pig studies in 1985, we did a comparison between NO inhalation and iNOS inhibitors. We found, to our surprise, NO inhalation is therapeutic in this pig model, because opening of the pulmonary circulation brought the cardiac output and blood pressure back to normal. In your model, if you inhale CO, are these dramatic effects on survival caused by opening up the pulmonary circulation?

Choi: The NO people tell me that in the vasculature we should get out of the field, because NO has 200 times more affinity for cGMP. This is true, but I challenge them by saying that there may be a cGMP independent pathway. If you take pulmonary vasculature and hit it with NO and CO, there is no comparison. The protective mechanism could be anti-proliferation of smooth muscle cells, endothelium protection and all the other things that go on in vascular injury.

Thiemermann: It was 2 h to the death of the animals, so presumably this is something very acute.

Cavaillon: Because IL10 is inducing HO-1, how much is CO contributing to the anti-inflammatory properties of IL10?

Choi: Good question. There is a Taiwanese group that reported that not only does it induce HO-1, but also it requires HO-1 to be an anti-inflammatory molecule.

Griffiths: HO-1 is so incredibly induced: does your giving CO impact on that inducibility?

Choi: We have data that CO induces HO-1. There may be a positive feedback. We also have data showing that in some cells CO down-regulates HO-1, so it depends on the cell type and the model.

Griffiths: What's the relationship between NO and HO-1?

Choi: Many people have shown that CO induces iNOS and NO induces HO-1. It depends on the system.

Griffiths: But perhaps this is occurring in a different time frame.

Choi: That's another area that needs to be dealt with. There is definitely cross-talk between CO and NO and there is also cross-regulation of each process.

Griffiths: Isn't the iNOS induction quicker than the HO induction?

Choi: It depends on your stimulus. With LPS the kinetics are similar.

Fink: Is there a proteomic way of finding out what the target is?

Choi: People are doing this now. There might be a proteomic way of finding non-haem moiety proteins. We are doing this too.

Piantadosi: CO is relatively inert: it does a limited number of things in the cell. The main thing it does is to bind to reduced transition metals. There may be other minor effects, but nothing like the effect on iron, which has huge implications for ROS and NO signalling. CO will displace NO from iron, for example. This means the entire NO handling system of the cell is changed by the presence of CO. Another thing that CO does is to re-route electrons. We look for electron transport effects of CO, for example in the mitochondrion, where it increases the H_2O_2 leak rate by binding to cytochrome a,a3. I have been a proponent for a long time of the idea that these effects of CO are double-edged both in terms of the effects on iron-dependent redox systems and on NO-metal chemistry.

Fink: In the cell based system, in a highly reducing environment created by adding dithiothreitol, for example can you abrogate the CO effects?

Piantadosi: This would facilitate them by increasing iron (II).

Fink: But you might scavenge the ROS that are leaking from mitochondria.

Choi: Sol Snyder published several years ago that HO-1 is a critical regulator of iron efflux from the cell.

Piantadosi: There is a clear link between CO and iron, and between CO and NO. This is what gives CO its pleiotropic effects. It accounts for some good things and some bad things. What happens in the body when we give CO? My issue there is always do a hypoxia control, because CO lowers the tissue PO_2. That said, CO is also carried out of the body by haemoglobin. If you tie up the normal CO binding sites in the haemoglobin, the back pressure of endogenous CO in the cell rises. We can demonstrate this now that we can measure cellular CO. If you have 10 or 15% carboxyhaemoglobin in the blood, CO made by haem oxygenase is retained in the cell. You have retarded the CO egress from the cell, and this raises the partial pressure of CO in the cell. The positive effect of breathing CO may be because HO, being stimulated by mild hypoxia, is making CO in the cell. Also, this may cause haem release from the mitochondria like it does iron release.

Choi: It may be that CO is having its beneficial effects through hypoxic conditions. There's evidence from preclinical human data in the cardiovascular literature that hypoxic conditions are a big deal.

Fink: You ought to be able to block this by giving adenosine deaminase.

Choi: Yes, is it just a conditioning response, and then when they are hit with stress they are protected?

Cohen: How does it know that it is supposed to decrease transcription for pro-inflammatory cytokines, but increase it for anti-inflammatory cytokines?

Choi: That's a great question. It happens in the same animal. It goes back to my bias about homeostasis. I think there is a homeostatic balance: if the cell is stressed it needs to get back to its homeostasis. The macrophage is bringing down bad TNF and augmenting IL10 to dampen that.

Cohen: There must be a separation of pathways.

Choi: TNF is early and IL10 comes on a few hours later, so kinetics might be involved.

Singer: What sorts of pathophysiological levels of CO can you get from HO-1 induction?

Choi: In sepsis patients you can measure up to about 3–5, depending on whether this is in the trauma unit or with a surgical patient. In exhaled breath, non-smokers exhale about 1–2 ppm, and this can rise to 3 or 4. This is given the limitations of the technology (carboxyhaemoglobin).

Piantadosi: Perhaps 5% is enough to raise the PCO in tissue if you have haem oxygenase cranked up.

Singer: We have shown that the tissue PO_2 goes up with septic insults, presumably because the mitochondria aren't using the oxygen. Therefore it will be competing with the same binding sites. What about the hyperoxia story?

Choi: It may be displacing the O_2. I like to think that CO is not just displacing the O_2, but that it has inherent anti-inflammatory effects in hyperoxic models.

Piantadosi: It's the ratio of the CO to O_2. Unless PO_2 is really high, there will be some binding of CO to haem proteins.

Singer: How do you quantitate that?

Piantadosi: That's a difficult question, especially *in vivo*.

References

Lavitrano M, Smolenski RT, Musumeci A et al 2004 Carbon monoxide improves cardiac energetics and safeguards the heart during reperfusion after cardiopulmonary bypass in pigs. FASEB J 18:1093–1095

Mayr FB, Spiel A, Leitner J et al 2005 Effects of carbon monoxide inhalation during experimental endotoxemia in humans. Am J Respir Crit Care Med 171:354–360

Mazzola S, Forni M, Albertini M, Bacci ML et al 2005 Carbon monoxide pretreatment prevents respiratory derangement and ameliorates hyperacute endotoxic shock in pigs. FASEB J 19:2045–2047

Moore BA, Overhaus M, Whitcomb J et al 2005 Brief inhalation of low-dose carbon monoxide protects rodents and swine from postoperative ileus. Crit Care Med. 33:1317–1326

Nalos M, Vassilev D, Pittner A et al 2003 Sn-mesoporphyrin to inhibit heme oxygenase during long-term hyperdynamic porcine endotoxemia. Shock 19:526–532

Yachie A, Niida Y, Wada T et al 1999 Oxidative stress causes enhanced endothelial cell injury in human heme oxygenase-1 deficiency. J Clin Invest 103:129–135

Zhang X, Shan P, Jiang D, Noble PW, Abraham NG, Kappas A, Lee PJ 2004 Small interfering RNA targeting heme oxygenase-1 enhances ischemia-reperfusion-induced lung apoptosis. J Biol Chem 279:10677–10684

The hypothalamic pituitary adrenal axis in sepsis

Andrea Polito, Jérôme Aboab and Djillali Annane[1]

Hospital Raymond Poincaré (AP-HP), University of Versailles SQY, 104 Boulevard Raymond Poincaré, Garches 92380

Abstract. At the beginning of the 20th century, observations of apoplectic adrenal glands in fatal meningococcemia underlined their key role in host defence against infection. Thirty years later, cortisone was discovered and rapidly proven to have numerous and diversified physiological functions in the host response to stress. Corticosteroids were introduced in the treatment of severe infection as early as in the 1940s. Several 'negative' randomized controlled trials of high-dose of glucocorticoids given for a short period of time in the early course of severe sepsis or acute respiratory distress syndrome raised serious doubts as to the benefit of this treatment. Recently, a link between septic shock and adrenal insufficiency, or systemic inflammation-induced glucocorticoid receptor resistance has been established. This finding prompted renewed interest in a replacement therapy with low doses of corticosteroids during longer periods. We will review the key role of the hypothalamic–pituitary–adrenal axis in the host response to stress.

2007 Sepsis—new insights, new therapies. Wiley, Chichester (Novartis Foundation Symposium 280) p 182–203

Regulation of the hypothalamic–pituitary–adrenal axis

At rest

The adrenal gland is made up of two functional units, the medulla which produces cathecolamines and cortex composed of three zones: zona glomerulosa, superficially located, producing mineralocorticoids (aldosterone and corticosterone), zona reticularis deeper sited producing weak androgens and zona fasciculata producing corticosteroids (cortisol and corticosterone) (Fig. 1).

Cortisol, the main corticosteroid, is a steroid hormone of 19 carbon atoms derived from cholesterol by an enzyme of the P450 cytochrome complex. Cortisol circulates in plasma either in its free and active form (which accounts only for

---

[1]This paper was presented at the symposium by Djillali Annane, to whom correspondence should be addressed.

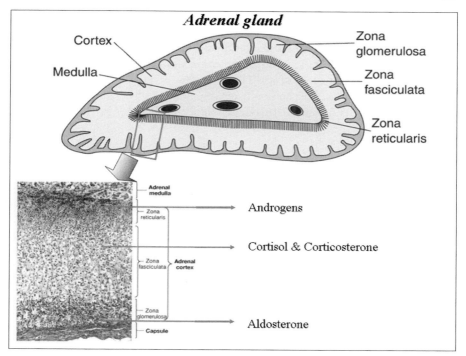

FIG. 1.   Main hormones secreted by the cortex of the adrenal gland.

5–10% of total cortisol) or in its inactive form, reversibly bound to proteins. The two main binding proteins are the cortisol-binding globulin (CBG) and albumin (Orth et al 1992).

Production of corticosteroids is regulated by the hypothalamic–pituitary–adrenal (HPA) axis. Cortisol production and secretion is stimulated mainly by the adrenocorticotrophic hormone (ACTH). This is a 39 amino acid peptide produced in the anterior pituitary. It is obtained after the cleavage of a large precursor, the pro-opiomelanocortin, which also liberates other peptides (β-endorphin, lipotropin, melanocyte-stimulating hormone). In the short term, ACTH stimulates cortisol production and secretion even if cortisol storage in adrenal glands is low; in the longer term, ACTH also stimulates the synthesis of enzymes that are involved in cortisol production, as well as their cofactors and adrenal receptors for low-density lipoprotein cholesterol. ACTH also stimulates the production of adrenal androgens and, to a lesser extent, mineralocorticoids (Orth et al 1992).

The half-life of ACTH is short and cortisol concentration in adrenal veins rises only a few minutes after ACTH secretion (Chrousos 1995). Secretion of ACTH is regulated by several factors, among which are the corticotrophin-releasing hormone (CRH) and arginine vasopressin (AVP), which are both secreted by the hypothalamus. AVP stimulates ACTH secretion only weakly but it strongly promotes CRH action. Catecholamines, angiotensin II, serotonin and vasoactive intestinal peptide are also known stimulators of ACTH secretion. Finally, some inflammatory cytokines influence ACTH secretion, exerting either a stimulatory action (interleukin [IL]1, IL2, IL6, tumour necrosis factor [TNF]α) or an inhibitory one (transforming growth factor β) (Chrousos 1995, Cavaillon 2000, Tsigos & Chrousos 2002).

CRH is a 41-amino-acid peptide secreted by the hypothalamus. Liberated in the hypothalamic–pituitary portal system, it stimulates the production and the secretion of pro-opiomelanocortin. Adrenergic agonists (noradrenaline) and serotonin stimulate its production whereas substance P, opioids and γ-aminobutyric acid inhibit it. Inflammatory cytokines (IL1, IL2, IL6, TNFα) also influence production of CRH (Chrousos 1995, Cavaillon 2000, Tsigos & Chrousos 2002, Marik & Zaloga 2002).

Finally, corticosteroids exert a negative feedback on the HPA axis, inhibiting ACTH production as well as pro-opiomelanocortin gene transcription, and CRH and AVP production. Secretion of the HPA axis hormones (ACTH, CRH and AVP) follows a pulsatile course with a circadian rhythm. The amplitude of the secretory pulses varies throughout the day and is greatest in the morning between 6 and 8 am, rapidly decreasing until noon and decreasing more slowly until midnight (Orth et al 1992).

However, the brain and the pituitary, which regulate the production of corticosteroid secretion through negative feedback by sensing time-integrated tissue exposure to corticosteroids, are also targets of corticosteroids. Thus, any generalized change in the corticosteroid signalling system will be followed by corrective, compensatory and generally protective changes in the activity of the HPA axis by adjusting target tissue effects to optimal levels (Chrousos 1995, Kino & Chrousos 2004). Absence of complete compensation—be it excessive or deficient—could result in chronically altered homeostasis or allostasis and target tissue pathology, as occurs in chronically stressed or depressed individuals who have mild but persistent hyper- or hyposecretion of cortisol (Chrousos 1995, Kino et al 2003a). The suprahypothalamic, hypothalamic, and pituitary corticosteroid-sensing network, however, differs from the networks of corticosteroid signalling systems in the arousal, associative, reward, metabolic, cardiovascular and immune systems. Any change in one or more molecules that participate in the corticosteroid signalling system could potentially produce a discrepancy in the sensitivity of target tissues to corticosteroids and result in pathology (Chrousos 1995, Chrousos et al 2004). For these reasons, any polymorphism or mutation of glucocorticosteriod receptor

(GR) gene may affect the corticosteroid signalling pathway and be responsible for different diseases according to corticosteroid tissue sensitivity that may be augmented (hypertension, diabetes mellitus II, visceral obesity-related insulin resistance) (Chrousos 1995, Kino & Chrousos 2004, Kino et al 2003) or decreased (asthma, ARDS) (Chrousos 1995, Kino et al 2003a). Moreover, tissue sensitivity to corticosteroids is affected by interactions of the host with viruses, such as human immunodeficiency viruses type 1, which increases corticosteroid sensitivity of host tissues, and the adenovirus, which decreases it (Kino et al 2003b, 2002).

During stress

Corticosteroids are the main mediators of the stress response. During a stressing event there is an immediate increment of ACTH secretion rapidly followed by increase in cortisol level (Lambers et al 1997). Moreover, the CBG level decreases and subsequently free cortisol rises (Beishuizen et al 2001a). Pro-inflammatory cytokines play a crucial role in the activation of the HPA axis (Franchimont et al 1999). These events are associated with a loss of the circadian rhythm of cortisol secretion secondary to an increase in CRH and ACTH production stimulated by inflammatory cytokines, vagal stimulation and reduction in cortisol-negative feedback (Lambers et al 1997, Chrousos 2000). All the changes during stress have the purpose to maintain homeostasis. Metabolic effects, especially hyperglycaemia, allow the redistribution of glucose toward insulin-dependent cells. The cardiovascular effects of corticosteroids aim to maintain normal vascular reactivity and almost all the components of the inflammatory cascade are prevented by cortisol. However, the ability of the HPA axis to respond to a sustained inflammatory insult like one resulting from severe infection, is likely to be a determinant of the progression from sepsis to septic shock and death.

It is unclear what the 'normal' concentration of circulating cortisol in critical illness is. It has been proposed that 15–20 μg/dL (Marik & Zalogo, McKee & Finlay 1983, Cooper & Stewart 2003, Annane et al 2002) is normal. Even if it is controversial, the higher the cortisol level at admission to the intensive care unit (ICU), the higher the mortality rate (Rothwell & Lawler 1995). Cortisol serum level seems to be an independent predictive factor for outcome, and likely also to be a marker of the severity of stress. However, it is more useful to determine the ability of the endocrine system to respond to sustained stress and thus dynamic testing of adrenal function is of paramount importance. The most convenient test in ICU is the standard ACTH stimulation test. Normally a rise of circulating cortisol concentration of 9 μg/dL or more is considered as a normal response (Rothwell et al 1991, Annane et al 2000).

Mechanism of altered HPA axis in sepsis

The recognition of various disorders that cause adrenal insufficiency (AI), either at a clinical or molecular level, often has implications for the management of the patient. Recent molecular genetic analysis for the disorder that causes AI gives valuable insights into adrenal organogenesis, regulation of steroid hormone biosynthesis, and developmental and reproductive endocrinology.

During sepsis numerous factors may interfere with HPA axis function, e.g. a pre-existing defect of the adrenal or pituitary gland, inflammation of the endocrine tissues, anatomical damage to the gland, or drugs inhibiting an enzymatic step of cortisol synthesis (e.g. etomidate, ketoconazole) or increasing cortisol metabolism (phenytoin, phenobarbital) (Lambers et al 1997, Soni et al 1995).

The various aetiologies of AI can be subgrouped into three categories: (1) impaired steroidogenesis, (2) adrenal dysgenesis/hypoplasia, and (3) adrenal destruction. AI develops only when a large part of the function of the adrenal gland is lost. Primary AI is caused by processes that damage the adrenal glands or by drugs that block cortisol synthesis. In contrast, secondary AI results from processes that reduce the secretion of ACTH by the pituitary gland due to a pituitary or hypothalamic pathology. More often in sepsis necrosis or haemorrhage of the hypothalamus or of the pituitary gland has been reported as a result of prolonged hypotension or severe coagulation disorders (Sharshar et al 2004). Sepsis may also exacerbate chronic known or latent secondary AI, which may be due to hypothalamic or pituitary tumours, chronic inflammation or congenital ACTH deficiency. Secondary AI may follow drug therapy. Previous treatment with corticosteroids reduces secretion of CRH and ACTH, resulting in slow onset of secondary AI. This suppression depends on duration of pre-treatment and on the type of corticosteroid used. Hydrocortisone is the least suppressive agent and dexamethasone the most (Melby 1974). The opioids reduce cortisol serum level probably by acting at the level of the hypothalamus (Hall et al 1990). Infectious diseases, especially viral and fungal, may cause chronic primary AI, particularly in immunosuppressed patients, like HIV patients (Marik & Zaloga 2002). Certain drugs may decrease steroidogenesis, such as etomidate. This effect persists as long as 24 hours after a single dose in critically ill patients (Absalomon et al 1999, Annane 2005). In addition cyclosporine (Abel & Back 1993) and clarithromycin (Ushiama et al 2002) accelerate cortisol metabolism.

Diagnosis of AI in sepsis

Usually, the adrenal crisis is characterized by fever, nausea, vomiting, abdominal pain, impaired consciousness, hypotension which is refractory to fluids and vasopressor therapy, hypoglycaemia, hyponatremia and hypereosinophilia. Unfortunately, these symptoms are very common during severe sepsis and thus they lack specificity to help in the decision making process. Thereafter, whenever AI is suspected endocrine tests are mandatory.

Non-stimulated serum cortisol

This test measures plasma ACTH and serum cortisol in the morning, when the latter peaks. The test requires that cortisol circadian rhythm is normal. A serum cortisol level of less than 3 μg/dL probably indicates AI (Oelker 1996). In the latter case, the plasma ACTH level will distinguish between primary and secondary AI. In primary AI, the ACTH level is almost invariably more than 100 pg/mL, while in secondary AI, plasma ACTH can be either low or inappropriately normal. In patients with severe stress, such as sepsis, serum cortisol level should be more than 18 μg/dL at any time. One exception may be the patient with severe hypoproteinaemia from whom total cortisol levels are no more accurate (Bernier et al 1998). However, in sepsis, high total cortisol levels may result from impaired cortisol clearance or tissue resistance and thus dynamic tests of adrenal function are essential to rule out AI.

Insulin-induced hypoglycaemia (insulin tolerance test, ITT)

This measures the patient's cortisol response to hypoglycaemia induced by the intravenous administration of insulin. This test is often considered as the gold standard because it assesses the ability of the entire HPA axis to respond to the stressful situation of hypoglycaemia. Following insulin (0.1 IU/kg) administration, blood is drawn during symptomatic hypoglycaemia (glucose should decrease to less than 40 mg/dl [<2.22 mmol/L]). In obese patients with insulin resistance, the usual dose of insulin should be increased to 0.15 IU/kg (Cordido et al 2003). A serum peak cortisol of more than 18 μg/dL is considered normal. ITT has some limitations in terms of reproducibility and clear cut-off levels (Pfeifer et al 2001, Nye et al 2001) and is contraindicated in patients with unstable haemodynamic status. In addition, peripheral insulin resistance that characterizes sepsis, made this test less accurate in this context.

Metyrapone test

The metyrapone test measures the ability of the HPA axis to respond to an acute reduction in serum cortisol levels. Metyrapone inhibits 11-hydroxylase, the enzyme involved in the last step of cortisol synthesis. This inhibition causes a decrease in cortisol that results in a compensatory increase in ACTH and in the cortisol precursor, 11-deoxycortisol. The administration of metyrapone (30 mg/kg;

maximal dose, 3000 mg) occurs at midnight, and blood is drawn the following morning at 8 am for cortisol and 11-deoxycortisol (Berneis et al 2002). In response to metyrapone, serum cortisol level should decrease to less than 5 µg/dL, and 11-deoxycortisol should increase to more than 7 µg/dL. This test can be done in healthy patients and it may be performed in ICU patients only when enteral nutrition is available. It should be administered very cautiously as it may cause adrenal crisis.

CRH stimulation test

The CRH stimulation test measures the ability of the pituitary gland to secrete ACTH in response to CRH. Ovine CRH (1 µg/dL) is injected intravenously, and cortisol is measured after 15, 30 and 60 minutes. The test has been proposed as a way to differentiate secondary (pituitary disease) from tertiary (hypothalamic disease) AI. However, the accuracy of this test remains very controversial (Schmidt et al 2003).

ACTH stimulation test

The ACTH stimulation test is based on the inability of a diseased adrenal gland to respond acutely to the injection of ACTH by secreting cortisol. ACTH is injected intravenously (or intramuscularly), and serum cortisol levels are measured at 30 or 60 minutes. In critical illness, cortisol levels less than 15 µg/dL or a cortisol increment of 9 µg/dL or less indicate AI and identify patients that require a replacement therapy (Cooper & Stewart 2003, Annane et al 2002, Doe et al 1964). Finally, an increase in cortisol level more than 9 µg/dL with the basal level above 34 µg/dL, suggests tissue resistance to corticosteroid.

As plasma ACTH levels following a bolus of 250 µg of ACTH exceed by several times the levels achieved during major surgery, it has been suggested that the 'high dose' test may miss 'mild' secondary AI (Graybeal & Fang 1985). Subsequently, the 1 µg ACTH test (LDST) was introduced as a more sensitive test (Dickstein et al 1991). However, 1 µg of ACTH induces supramaximal stimulation of the adrenals for only 30 min and may not appropriately evaluate the capacity of the adrenal glands to maintain maximal cortisol production in response to a major ongoing stress like sepsis. In addition, interpretation of the results of the 1 µg dose ACTH testing is highly dependent on determination of the lower limit of normality.

Given the uncertainty surrounding the reliability of the LDST in general, and the fact that in septic shock the benefit of cortisol replacement therapy has been shown only in non-responders to the 'High Dose' test, we strongly recommend use of the high dose ACTH test.

Molecular mechanism of action of corticosteroids

The human corticosteroid receptor gene (GR) is located on chromosome 5 and is responsible for the production of α and β subunits. The classic receptor has three major distinct functional domains—the N-terminal or immunogenic domain, the DNA binding domain (DBD), and the ligand-binding domain (LBD). In its unbound state, GRα is located primarily in the cytoplasm as part of a hetero-oligomeric complex that contains heat shock proteins (HSPs) 90, 70, 50 and 20 and, possibly, other proteins as well (Kino et al 2003a). After binding to an agonist ligand, GR undergoes conformational changes, dissociates from the HSPs and other chaperone proteins, and translocates into the nucleus through a nuclear pore as a monomer or dimer by means of an active ATP-dependent process mediated by its nuclear localization signals NL1 and NL2 (Kino et al 2003a). Once in the nucleus, ligand-activated GRα dimers interact directly with specific DNA sequences in the promoter regions of target genes (the corticosteroid response elements, GREs). Ligand-activated GRα monomers, interact with other transcription factors also, at the cytoplasm level (e.g. nuclear factor κB [NF-κB], activating protein 1 [AP-1], p53, CRE-binding protein [CREB], signal transducer and activator of transcription 5 [STAT5]) through protein–protein interactions, indirectly influencing the activity of the latter on their own target genes (Kino et al 2003a). GR contains two transactivation domains (activation function 1 [AF]-1 and AF-2) at its N-terminal and LBD, respectively. GR interacts through AF-1 and AF-2 with various protein complexes, including the nuclear receptor coactivator complexes (p160, p300/CREB-binding protein, CBP, and p300/CBP-associated factor, p/CAF) and other factors that can alter the transcription rates of corticosteroid-responsive genes (Kino et al 2003a) (Fig. 2). The GR isoform β does not itself bind corticosteroids, but rather exerts dominant negative effects on GRα through several mechanisms, such as heterodimerization and competition with GRα for GREs or transcriptional nuclear receptor coactivators (Kino & Chrousos 2004, Kino et al 2003a, Bamberger et al 1995, Charmandari et al 2005, Yudt et al 2003). GRα translational isoforms are differentially expressed in various cell lines (Lu & Cidlowski 2005). There are multiple mechanisms through which target cells alter the sensitivity and specificity of the response to corticosteroids. These take place at the levels of GR gene transcription, mRNA splicing, and mRNA translation, as well as through post-translational modifications and the inherent functional activity of the expressed isoform monomer(s) or dimer(s) on responsive genes. The N-terminal domain of GR substantially contributes to this regulatory diversity (Lu & Cidlowski 2005). The mineralocorticoid (MR), oestrogen (ER) and progesterone (Bernard et al 1987) receptors also contain potential alternative translation initiation sites in their N-terminal domains. Thus, like the GR gene, the genes encoding these receptors might

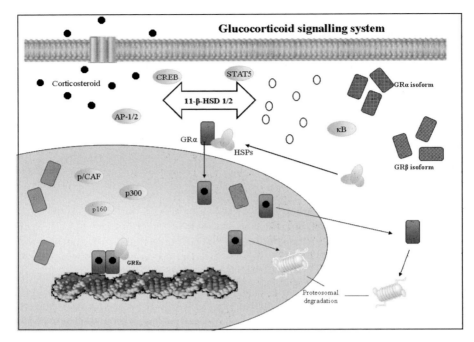

FIG. 2. Intracellular GR activation. 11β-hydroxysteroid dehydrogenase (HSD)1/2 regulates the conversion of inactive cortisone (white circle) to the active GR ligand cortisol (black circles). Cortisol binds to the cytoplasmic HSP-bound GR and translocates to the nucleus. There it interacts with DNA target sequences and glucocorticoid response elements (GREs). Alternatively, GR monomers interact with and alter the activity of a host of transcription factors such as NF-κB, AP-1 and STAT5.

produce N-terminal isoforms (Lu & Cidlowski 2005). Therefore, tissue-specific and regulated variable N-terminal isoform production may be a general mechanism that defines target tissue sensitivity to steroid hormones, further adding to the complexity of their own signal transduction systems.

It has been shown that corticosteroids up-regulate and down-regulate up to 2000 genes that are involved in regulation of the immune response (Galon et al 2002).

If cortisol is able to act in a genomic manner, it is also responsible for non-genomic interactions. Physiochemical interactions occur in-between the cell's membrane and corticosteriods inducing very rapid, non-specific, non-genomic effects (Almawi 2001). For example during acute stress the loss in interaction with hypothalamic synaptosomes may partly explain the loss in cortisol circadian rhythm (Edwardson & Bennett 1974). Moreover, corticosteroids act in this way in the immediate catecholamine release from sympathetic cells, restoration of sympathetic modulation on heart and vessel (Orlikowsky et al 2003), and sensitization to exogenous catecholamine in septic shock (Annane et al 1998, Bellisant & Annane 2000). In addition, through activation of endothelial nitric oxide synthase, they induce protective effects in ischaemic brain injury (Limbourg et al 2002), and in ischaemia/reperfusion injury (Hefezi-Moghadam et al 2002).

Main actions of corticosteroids in sepsis

Metabolic effects

With regard to carbohydrates, corticosteroids play a major role in glucose metabolism stimulating liver gluconeogenesis and glycogenolysis also promoting the secretion of glucagon and adrenaline. They inhibit cellular uptake of glucose by inducing peripheral insulin resistance. All these actions result in a rise in blood glucose concentration (Pikis & Granner 1992). In protein and fat metabolism, corticosteroids inhibit protein synthesis and activate proteinolysis in muscles, inhibit glucose uptake by adipocytes and activate lipolysis. Finally, they are involved in bone and mineral metabolism, activating osteoclasts, inhibiting osteoblasts, decreasing intestinal Ca^{2+} uptake and increasing Ca^{2+} urinary secretion by decreasing its renal reabsorption (Orth et al 1992).

Immune effects

The clinical relevance of corticosteroids in immune and inflammatory responses is controversial, although their affinity for immune cells is great. They can exert their influence through lymphocytes, natural killer (NK) cells, monocytes, macrophages, eosinophils, mast cells and basophils (Chrousos 2000). Corticosteroid administration is followed by a reduction of lymphocytes, which results in a passage of cells from blood to lymphoid organ. The opposite is true for granulocytes. They aid the reduction of inflammatory reactions by lowering chemokines and subsequently reducing neutrophil migration. Macrophage secretion is inhibited by the production of migration inhibitory factor (Beishuizen et al 2001b), while eosinophil apoptosis is stimulated (Beishuizen et al 1999).

Corticosteroids are involved in the immune response by inhibiting the production of IL12 by macrophages and monocytes, and influencing lymphocyte differentiation in favour of Th2 cells. This will result in a rise of IL4 and IL13 secretion (which is normally inhibited by IL12) and suppression of cellular immunity (Chrousos 2000). In patients with sepsis, hydrocortisone does not suppress IL12 secretion, an effect that resulted from hydrocortisone induced inhibition of the pro-inflammatory state (Keh et al 2003) (Fig. 3).

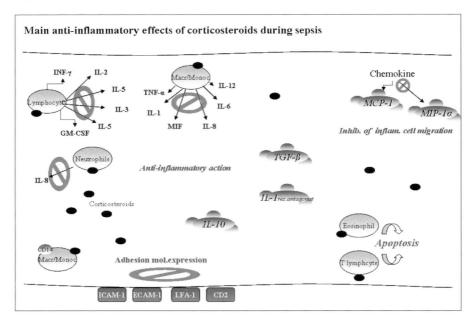

FIG. 3.   Major antinflammatory effects of corticosteroids during sepsis. The symbol of prohibition suggests inhibitory effects of corticosteroids on cytokine production.

Corticosteriods modulate the inflammatory response also acting on the cellular level by the inhibition of proinflammatory cytokines (IL1, IL2, IL3, IL6, interferon γ, TNFα), chemokines, eicosanoids, bradykinins and inhibitory factor (Cavillon 2000, Soni et al 1995, Beishuizen et al 2001b). This is possible by interaction of corticosteroid complex and DNA where it can activate and inhibit transcriptional factors (Almawi 2001).

In the last decade, corticosteroids have been shown to attenuate the inflammatory response in septic shock patients without causing immune suppression. Indeed, intravenous hydrocortisone decreased core temperature, heart rate and plasma levels of PLA_2 and C-reactive protein (Briegel et al 1994). It decreased circulating levels of IL6 and IL8, preventing endothelial activation and also decreased circulating levels of TNF soluble receptors I and II, and IL10. Hydrocortisone is also able to favour the expansion of peripheral blood-derived CD56[+] cells, allowing the differentiation of NK cells (Perez et al 2005).

Cardiovascular effects

Corticosteroids regulate vascular reactivity to vasoconstrictors. Physiological concentrations of corticosteroids play a key role in maintaining an appropriate vascular reactivity to vasoconstrictors, and hence normal blood pressure. Multiple mechanisms are involved in corticosteroid-mediated vascular responses. It is known that chronic excess of corticosteroids induces hypertension, whereas AI induces hypotension. Corticosteroids act on vascular endothelial cells and inhibit the release of endothelial vasodilators such as NO and PGI2 by down-regulating enzyme expression and activity. In vascular smooth muscle cells, corticosteroids enhance agonist-mediated pharmacomechanical coupling by increasing Ca^{2+} mobilization and Ca^{2+} sensitivity of myofilament. The corticosteroid-induced vascular changes occur within minutes and thus are unlikely to be dependent on genomic interactions. The precise mechanism of corticosteroid-induced changes in the endothelium and vascular smooth muscle cells is not clear.

Administration of hydrocortisone simultaneously with or just before infusion of lipopolysaccharide prevents vascular non-responsiveness to noradrenaline in healthy subjects, as well as hypotension and a rise in both heart rate and plasma adrenaline levels. In septic shock, AI was associated with a marked hyporesponsiveness to noradrenaline, which was fully reversed 1 h after 50 mg of intravenous hydrocortisone (Annane et al 1998). Corticosteroids regulate the response to noradrenaline and angiotensin II. The mechanism of action may be partially explained by iNOS pathway inhibition. Another study confirmed the ability of corticosteroids to reverse vessels' insensitivity within 1 h without using the renin–angiotensin system or the NO pathway (Bellisant & Annane 2000). Several placebo-controlled randomized studies have emphasized the cardiovascular effects of low dose corticosteroids (200–300 mg/day) for a prolonged period (Annane et al 2002, Keh et al 2003, Oppert et al 2005, Bollaert et al 1998, Briegel et al 1999, Chawla et al 1999). Hydrocortisone was associated with increased vascular resistance with little effect on cardiac index and pulmonary haemodynamics. It may be possible that the very early haemodynamic effects are nongenomic, whereas subsequent ones are partially due to iNOS inhibition (Keh et al 2003).

These trials also showed that use of corticosteroids reduces duration of shock and time of vasopressor weaning. The haemodynamic effect was confirmed by a phase III trial that also demonstrated survival benefit from a 7 day treatment with 50 mg of hydrocortisone every 6 h and 50 μg of fludrocortisone daily (Bernier et al 1998). The beneficial effect of corticosteroids is more pronounced in nonresponders to ACTH. In a more recent study, infusion of a 50 mg bolus of hydrocortisone followed by a continuous infusion of 0.18 mg/kg per h in 41 hyperdynamic septic shock patients, was associated with a dramatic reduction of vasopressor support (53 h vs. 120 h) and duration of shock and of proinflammatory cytokines. In this study the haemodynamic effects but not the immune effects of hydrocortisone were related to the adrenal status (Oppert et al 2005).

TABLE 1   Corticosteroid trials in severe sepsis and septic shock patients

Reference	Population (n)	Dose of cortisone vs. placebo	Results
Bollaert et al (1998)	Septic shock (41)	100 mg × 3 for 5 days of hydrocortisone	Reduction of mortality and shock reversal time
Briegel et al (1999)	Septic shock (40)	100 mg + 0.18 mg/kg/h of hydrocortisone	Reduction of time of vasopressor infusion
Chawla et al (1999)	Septic shock (44)	100 mg × 4 for 72 h of hydrocortisone	Reduction of shock reversal time and vasopressor infusion
Annane et al (2002)	Septic shock (300)	50 mg × 6 of hydrocortisone + fludrocortisone 50 μg for 7 days	Reduction of mortality and relative adrenal insufficiency
Yildiz et al (2002)	Severe sepsis (40)	Physiological dose of prednisolone for 10 days	Reduction of mortality
Confalonieri et al (2004)	Severe sepsis (46)	200 mg + 10 mg/h of hydrocortisone	Reduction of mortality and delayed of septic shock
Oppert et al (2005)	Septic shock (41)	50 mg + 0.18 mg/kg/h of hydrocortisone	Reduction of shock reversal time
Tandan et al (2005)	Septic shock (28)	Low doses of hydrocortisone	Reduction of mortality

Survival effects

Data extracted from the most important trials, show mortality rates in control groups and in treated groups were not significantly different. But subgroup analysis on trials with long timecourses (≥5 days) of low dose corticosteroids (≤300 mg hydrocortisone or equivalent) (Table 1) showed a significant reduction in mortality rate in favour of corticosteroids, at 28 days and at intensive care unit (ICU) and hospital discharge (Annane et al 2004).

Adverse events

In a recent meta-analysis of corticosteroid treatment during severe sepsis and septic shock there was no evidence for an increased risk of gastroduodenal bleeding (10 trials, $n = 1321$; 1.16, 0.82–1.65, $P = 0.40$), superinfection (12 trials, $n = 1705$; 0.93, 0.73–1.18, $P = 0.54$) or hyperglycaemia (6 trials, $n = 608$; 1.22, 0.84–1.78, $P = 0.30$) (Annane et al 2004). Only one trial reported a rise in serum sodium concentration (>155 mol/l) in 6/20 (30%) patients in the treated group and in 1/20 (5%) in the placebo group (Briegel et al 1999).

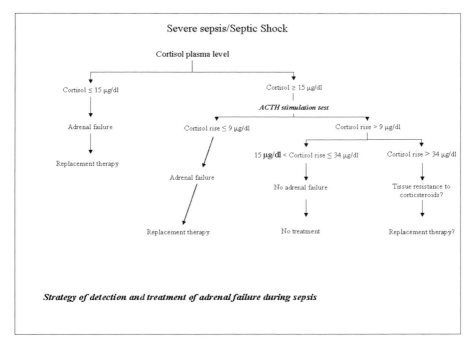

Severe sepsis/Septic Shock

Strategy of detection and treatment of adrenal failure during sepsis

FIG. 4.   Strategy of detection and treatment of adrenal failure during sepsis.

Conclusion and recommendations for clinical practice

During sepsis, haemodynamic instability and perpetuation of the inflammatory
state may result from AI. Thus, an ACTH test should be performed as soon as
possible to identify non overt AI (Fig. 4). It should be immediately followed by
a replacement therapy with i.v. bolus of 50 mg of hydrocortisone every 6 hours
combined with 50 µg of fludrocortisone once daily. When the results of the ACTH
test are available, treatment should be continued for 7 days in the non responders
to ACTH and withdrawn in the responders. Whether responders to ACTH with
high baseline cortisol levels (>34 µg/dl) have tissue resistance to cortisol and also
should receive exogenous hormones remains to be evaluated in clinical trials.

References

Abel SM, Back DJ 1993 Cortisol metabolism in vitro—III. Inhibition of microsomal 6 beta-
    hydroxylase and cytosolic 4-ene-reductase. J Steroid Biochem Mol Biol 46:827–832
Absalomon A, Pledger D, Kong A 1999 Adrenocortical function in critically ill patients 24 h
    after a single dose of etomidate. Anaesthesia 54:861–867

Almawi WY 2001 Molecular mechanisms of glucocorticoids effects. Mod Asp Immunobiol 2:78–82

Annane D 2005 ICU physicians should abandon the use of etomidate! Intensive Care Med 31:325–326

Annane D, Bellissant E, Sebille V et al 1998 Impaired pressor sensitivity to noradrenaline in septic shock patients with and without impaired adrenal function reserve. Br J Clin Pharmacol 46:589–597

Annane D, Sebille V, Troche G, Raphael JC, Gajdois P, Bellisant E 2000 A 3-level prognostic classification in septic shock based on cortisol levels and cortisol response to corticotropin. JAMA 283:1038–1045

Annane D, Sebille V, Carpentier C et al 2002 Effect of treatment with low doses of hydrocortisone and fludrocortisone on mortality in patients with septic shock. JAMA 288:862–871

Annane D, Bellissant E, Bollaert PE, Briegel J, Keh D, Kupfer Y 2004 Corticosteroids for treating severe sepsis and septic shock: a systematic review and meta-analysis. BMJ 329:480

Bamberger CM, Bamberger AM, de Castro M, Chrousos GP 1995 Glucocorticoid receptor beta, a potential endogenous inhibitor of glucocorticoid action in humans. J Clin Invest 95: 2435–2441

Beishuizen A, Vermes I, Hylkema BS, Haanen C 1999 Relative eosinophilia and functional adrenal insufficiency in critically ill patients. Lancet 353:1675–1676

Beishuizen A, Thijs LG, Vermes I 2001a Patterns of corticosteroid-binding globulin and the free cortisol index during septic shock and multitrauma. Intensive Care Med 27:1584–1591

Beishuizen A, Thijs LG, Haanen C, Vermes I 2001b Macrophage migration inhibitory factor and hypothalamo-pituitary-adrenal function during critical illness. J Clin Endocrinol Metab 86:2811–2816

Bellisant E, Annane D 2000 Effect of hydrocortisone on phenylephrine: mean arterial pressure dose-response relationship in septic shock. Clin Pharmacol Ther 68:293–303

Bernard GR, Luce JM, Sprung CL et al 1987 High-dose corticosteroids in patients with the adult respiratory distress syndrome. N Engl J Med 317:1565–1570

Berneis K, Staub JJ, Gessler A, Meier C, Girard J, Muller B 2002 Combined stimulation of adrenocorticotropin and compound-S by single dose metyrapone test as an outpatient procedure to assess hypothalamic-pituitary-adrenal function. J Clin Endocrinol Metab 87: 5470–5474

Bernier J, Jobin N, Emptoz-Bonneton A et al 1998 Decreased corticosteroid-binding globulin in burn patients: Relationship with interleukin-6 and fat in nutritional support. Crit Care Med 26:452–460

Bollaert PE, Charpentier C, Levy B et al 1998 Reversal of late septic shock with supraphysiologic doses of hydrocortisone. Crit Care Med 26:645–650

Briegel J, Kellermann W, Forst H et al 1994 Low-dose hydrocortisone infusion attenuates the systemic inflammatory response syndrome. The phospholipase A2 study group. Clin Investig 72:782–787

Briegel J, Forst H, Haller M et al 1999 Stress doses of hydrocortisone reverse hyperdynamic septic shock: a prospective, randomized, double-blind, single-center study. Crit Care Med 27:723–732

Cavaillon J 2000 Action of glucocorticoids in the inflammatory cascade. Réanim Urgences 9:605–612

Charmandari E, Chrousos GP, Ichijo T et al 2005 The human glucocorticoid receptor (hGR) beta-isoform suppresses the transcriptional activity of hGR-alpha by interfering with formation of active coactivator complexes. Mol Endocrinol 19:52–64

Chawla K, Kupfer Y, Tessler S 1999 Hydrocortisone reverses refractory septic shock. Crit Care Med 27:A33

Chrousos G 1995 The hypothalamic-pituitary-adrenal axis and immunomediated inflammation. N Engl J Med 332:1351–1362

Chrousos G 2000 The stress response and immune function: clinical implications. The 1999 Novera H. Spector lecture. In: Neuroimmunomodulation: perspectives at the new millennium p 38–67

Chrousos GP, Charmandari E, Kino T 2004 Glucocorticoid action networks-an introduction to systems biology. J Clin Endocrinol Metab 89:563–564

Confalonieri M, Urbino R, Potena A et al 2005 Hydrocortisone infusion for severe community-acquired pneumonia: a preliminary randomized study. Am J Respir Crit Care Med 171: 242–248

Cooper MS, Stewart P 2003 Corticosteroid insufficiency in acutely ill patients. N Engl J Med 348:727–734

Cordido F, Alvarez-Castro P, Isidro ML, Casanueva FF, Dieguez C 2003 Comparison between insulin tolerance test, growth hormone (GH)-releasing hormone (GHRH), GHRH plus acipimox and GHRH plus GH-releasing peptide-6 for the diagnosis of adult GH deficiency in normal subjects, obese and hypopituitary patients. Eur J Endocrinol 149: 117–122

Dickstein G, Shechner C, Nicholson WE et al 1991 Adrenocorticotropin stimulation test: effect of basal cortisol level, time of day and suggested new sensitive low dose test. J Clin Endocrinol Metab 72:773–778

Doe RP, Fernandez R, Seal US 1964 Measurement of corticosteroid-binding globulin in man. J Clin Endocrinol 24:1029–1039

Edwardson JA, Bennett GW 1974 Modulation of corticotropin-releasing factor release from hypothalamic synaptosome. Nature 251:425–427

Franchimont D, Martens H, Hagelstein MT et al 1999 Tumor necrosis factor alpha decreases, and interleukin-10 increases, the sensitivity of human monocytes to dexamethasone: potential regulation of the glucocorticoid receptor. J Clin Endocrinol Metab 84:2834–2839

Galon J, Franchimont D, Hiroi N et al 2002 Gene profiling reveals unknown enhancing and suppressive actions of glucocorticoids on immune cells. FASEB J 16:61–71

Graybeal ML, Fang V 1985 Physiological doses of exogenous ACTH. Acta Endocrinol 108: 401–406

Hall GM, Lacoumenta S, Hart GR, Burrin JM 1990 Site of action of fentanyl in inhibiting the pituitary-adrenal response to surgery in man. Br J Anaesth 65:251–253

Hefezi-Moghadam A, Simoncini T, Yang E et al 2002 Acute cardiovascular protective effects of corticosteroids are mediated by non-transcriptional activation of endothelial nitric oxide synthase. Nat Med 8:473–479

Keh D, BoehnkeT, Weber-Cartens S et al 2003 Immunologic and hemodynamic effects of 'low-dose' hydrocortisone in septic shock: a double-blind, randomized, placebo-controlled, crossover study. Am J Respir Crit Care Med 167:512–520

Kino T, Chrousos GP 2004 Glucocorticoid and mineralocorticoid receptors and associated diseases. Essays Biochem 40:137–155

Kino T, Gragerov A, Slobodskaya O, Tsopanomichalou M, Chrousos GP, Pavlakis GN 2002 Human immunodeficiency virus type 1 (HIV-1) accessory protein Vpr induces transcription of the HIV-1 and glucocorticoid-responsive promoters by binding directly to p300/CBP coactivators. J Virol 76:9724–9734

Kino T, De Martino MU, Charmandari E, Mirani M, Chrousos GP 2003a Tissue glucocorticoid resistance/hypersensitivity syndromes. J Steroid Biochem Mol Biol 85:457–467

Kino T, Mirani M, Alesci S, Chrousos GP 2003b AIDS-related lipodystrophy/insulin resistance syndrome. Horm Metab Res 35:129–136

Lambers SW, Bruining HA, de Jong FH 1997 Corticosteroid therapy in severe illness. N Engl J Med 337:1285–1292

Limbourg FP, Huang Z, Plumier JC et al 2002 Rapid nontranscriptional activation of endothelial nitric oxide synthase mediates increased cerebral blood flow and stroke protection by
corticosteroids. J Clin Invest 110:1729–1738

Lu NZ, Cidlowski JA 2005 Translational regulatory receptor gene, longevity, and the complex
disorders of Western societies. Mol Cell 18:331–342

Marik PE, Zaloga GP 2002 Adrenal insufficiency in the critically ill: a new look at an old
problem. Chest 122:1784–1796

McKee JI, Finlay WE 1983 Cortisol replacement in severely stressed patients [letter]. Lancet
1:484

Melby J 1974 Drug spotlight program: systemic corticosteroid therapy: pharmacology and
endocrinologic considerations. Ann Int Med 81:505–512

Nye EJ, Grice J, Hokgings GI et al 2001 The insulin hypoglycemia test: hypoglycemic criteria
and reproducibility. J Neuroendocrinol 13:524–530

Oelkers W 1996 Adrenal insufficiency. N Engl J Med 335:1206–1212

Oppert M, Schindler R, Husung C et al 2005 Low-dose hydrocortisone improves shock reversal
and reduces cytokine on early hyperdynamic septic shock. Crit Care Med 33:2457–
2464

Orlikowsky DST, Castel M, Annane D 2003 Acute effect of a single intravenous bolus of 50 mg
hydrocortisone on cardiovascular autonomic modulation in septic shock. Crit Care Med
31(suppl):A124

Orth DN, Kovacs WJ, DeBold CR 1992 In: Williams textbook of endocrinology. Wilson JD,
Foster DW (eds) W.B. Saunders Company, Philadelphia p 489–531

Perez SA, Mahaira LG, Demirtzoglou FJ et al 2005 A potential role for hydrocortisone in the
positive regulation of IL-15-activated NK cell proliferation and survival. Blood 106:
158–166

Pfeifer M, Kanc K, Verhovec R, Koijianic A 2001 Reproducibility of the ITT for assessment
of GH and cortisol secretion in normal and hypopituitary adult man. Clin Endocrinol
(Oxf)54:17–22

Pikis SJ, Granner D 1992 Molecular physiology of the regulation of the hepatic gluconeogenesis
and glycolysis. Annu Rev Physiol 54:885–909

Rothwell PM, Lawler PG 1995 Prediction of outcome in intensive care patients using endocrine
parameters. Crit Care Med 23:78–83

Rothwell PM, Udwadia ZF, Lawler PG 1991 Cortisol response to corticotropin and survival in
septic shock. Lancet 337:582–583

Schmidt IL, Lahner H, Mann K, Petersenn S 2003 Diagnosis of adrenal insufficiency: evaluation of the corticotropin-releasing hormone test and basal serum cortisol in comparison to
the insulin tolerance test in patients with hypothalamic-pituitary-adrenal disease. J Clin
Endocrinol Metab 88:4193–4198

Sharshar T, Annane D, de la Grandmaison GL, Brouland JP, Hopkinson NS, Francoise G 2004
The neuropathology of septic shock: a prospective case-control study. Brain Pathol 14:21–
33

Soni A, Pepper GM, Wyrwinski PM et al 1995 Adrenal insufficiency occurring during septic
shock: incidence, outcome, and relationship to peripheral cytokine levels. Am J Med
98:266–271

Tandan SM, Gupta N 2005 Low dose steroids and adrenocortical insufficiency in septic shock:
a double-blind randomised trial from India. Am J Respir Crit Care Med [A24]
[Poster:326]

Tsigos C, Chrousos GP 2002 Hypothalamic-pituitary-adrenal axis, neuroendocrine factors and
stress. J Psychosom Res 53:865–871

Ushiama H, Echizen H, Nachi S, Ohnishi A 2002 Dose-dependent inhibition of CYP3A activity by clarithromycin during Helicobacter pylori eradication therapy assessed by changes in

plasma lansoprazole levels and partial cortisol clearance to 6 beta-hydroxycortisol. Clin Pharmacol Ther 72:33–43

Yildiz O, Doganay M, Aygen B, Guven M, Keleutimur F, Tutuu A 2002 Physiological-dose steroid therapy in sepsis. Crit Care 6:251–259

Yudt MR, Jewell CM, Bienstock RJ, Cidlowski JA 2003 Molecular origins for the dominant negative function of human glucocorticoid receptor-beta. Mol Cell Biol 23:4319–4330

DISCUSSION

Choi: I was fascinated by the *Lancet* paper that showed sepsis induced haemorrhage and cell death (Sharshar et al 2003). Presumably these are not patients with meningitis. These are septic shock patients. Are there any data on cognitive function? Haemorrhage is regressible with repair, but what about apoptosis?

Annane: These data are from humans who died from septic shock so it is difficult to establish a causal relationship between apoptosis and septic encephalopathy. A few months later, our findings of sepsis induced neuronal apoptosis were confirmed in an animal model of sepsis (Messaris et al 2004).

Marshall: Just as you have shown loss of cells in the adrenal cortex, is it possible that necrosis in the adrenal medulla is responsible for the need for exogenous epinephrine and norepinephrine? Is there any evidence that a similar process might be behind septic shock? What is known about the regeneration of the adrenal gland, and the role of stem cells to restore those cortisol-producing cells that were lost?

Annane: In animals if you destroy the medulla but leave the cortex intact, they don't die, demonstrating that catecholamines released from adrenal cells are not essential to survive the septic insult. Moreover, vascular smooth muscles are more likely to be dependent on direct sympathetic discharges at terminal nerve endings rather than on circulating adrenal-derived catecholamines.

Marshall: Do they need pressors?

Annane: Animals in which the adrenal medulla is destroyed and the cortex is preserved don't develop shock after an endotoxin challenge. As far as the role of stem cells to restore adrenocortical cells is concerned, there are no data in an acute setting like sepsis. However, in chronic primary adrenal insufficiency, there are a growing number of experiments suggesting that in the near future, replacement of adrenocortical cells may be a valuable alternative for long term treatment of Addison disease.

Singer: A few weeks ago an endocrinologist told me he had a few patients who had survived sepsis but had chronic pituitary insufficiency. What is the natural recovery, both at the level of the adrenal gland, and looking at hypothalamic damage? In your *Lancet* paper the damage was limited to supraventricular and para-optic nuclei: it seemed to be a very specific apoptotic damage.

Annane: One reason why apoptosis was mainly confined to these areas was because these areas are highly vascularized. Indeed, the main trigger of apoptosis was iNOS-derived nitric oxide (NO), from smooth muscle cells of vessels neighbouring autonomic neurons. I am not aware of any data on how the adrenals or the hypothalamus are repaired following a septic insult. Of note, the reversibility of sepsis associated organ dysfunction is very common and not specific to the brain.

Singer: Jerome Pugin was telling me that the immune paresis continues for up to 24 months after sepsis. Has anyone done long-term stimulation tests on patients?

Annane: About 10 years ago, Joseph Briegel published a paper in which he repeated the ACTH tests after recovery from septic shock just before intensive care unit (ICU) discharge (Briegel et al 1994). He found a normal ACTH response at time of ICU discharge in almost all survivors of septic shock.

Van den Berghe: This seems the same for the thyroid. TSH increases again when the patient recovers.

Singer: We have found that T3 stays high for a long time.

Van den Berghe: That is a peripheral effect. If we talk about the hypothalamus and the pituitary there is a certain degree of recovery. I don't think anyone has studied long term.

Fink: We have two collaborators here of Kevin Tracey's. He wrote a paper five years ago that is buried in the literature (Yang et al 2002). For most of us, if we had written this paper it would have been one of the highlights of our career! He adrenalectomized rats and showed that they were hyperresponsive to endotoxin. He postulated that there was a serum factor in these adrenalectomized animals that was responsible for their hypersensitivity to endotoxin. He spent about six months running the serum from these animals through columns. Ultimately, he isolated a protein that recapitulated the hyperresponsiveness to endotoxin, but he was disappointed that the protein was haemoglobin. Evidently, it is well known that in adrenalectomized animals their red cells are fragile and lyse spontaneously. It is also known that haemoglobin sensitizes macrophages by orders of magnitude to the TNF-releasing effects of lipopolysaccharide (LPS). If he gave normal rats concentrations of haemoglobin that recapitulated what was circulating in the adrenalectomized rats, they were many times more sensitive to endotoxin. Do you think this is an important mechanism accounting for the increased mortality in hypoadrenal humans? Has anyone ever measured circulating haemoglobin levels in humans with septic shock?

Annane: I don't know of this. Obviously we did follow circulating haemoglobin levels in the multicentre clinical trial of low dose corticosteroids for septic shock. Thus, we will get the information on the relationship between haemoglobin levels, response to the ACTH test and mortality from septic shock.

Marshall: You began your paper by talking about how the hypothalamic–pituitary axis responds to stress by inducing cortisol. Biochemically, what is stress?

Annane: Stress is a common experience in our daily life. Yet, we have very little knowledge on how stressful events result in disease.

Marshall: What exactly is happening at a biochemical level that activates the pituitary gland to produce this response? How is the pituitary sensing its environment?

Annane: Activation of the stress system occurs within the CNS in response to various blood borne, neurosensory and limbic signals. The fact that intracerebroventricular injections of corticotrophin-releasing hormone (CRH) mimic the stress response in various animal models, strongly supports the role of the HPA axis in the adaptive response to stressors.

The CRH secretion following LPS challenge includes at least four mechanisms (a) CRH stored in nerve endings can be released by prostaglandins, catecholamines, NO and a number of cytokines (e.g. TNF, IL6); (b) CRH neurons in the paraventricular nucleus of the hypothalamus may be directly activated by cytokines like TNF, IL1 or IL6 and by a number of neuromediators such as NMDA, GABA, serotonin, catecholamines, NO; (c) changes in the pituitary gland facilitate ACTH secretion directly and enhance the effects of CRH; and (d) finally, afferent fibres from both the vagus nerve and the noradrenergic system sense the threat at the tissue levels and activate CRH secretion.

Singer: Is it noradrenaline from the medulla?

Annane: Circulating catecholamines released from the medulla may also contribute to the CRH secretion

Choi: We teach our students from day 1 that the fight or flight response is critical.

Herndon: While there is no simple answer to this, there is a hypothalamic temperature reset that occurs with stress and with sepsis, such that the individuals are struggling for an elevated temperature. This reset is accomplished through secretion of catecholamines and increased substrate cycling in tissues such as muscles and fat. You are asking what the afferent mediators of the hypothalamic temperature reset are. There was considerable effort to study this on the part of Doug Wilmore and his colleagues in the 1970s and 1980s. They found that TNF could do this, as could IL6 (with individual injections into the hypothalamus). But this line of research has hit a dead end. Cytokines and prostanoids were the agents that were investigated in the early 1970s, and when these were injected into mice these were found to cause hypothalamic temperature reset.

Singer: Isn't noradrenaline the first thing that goes up acutely?

Herndon: The catecholamines go up, but so do corticosteroids. The normal response is elevated corticosteroids. These are elevated and stay elevated after burns, for example, for almost a full year post-injury. Corticosteroid production is elevated, even in patients that develop septic shock and transiently have decreased corticosteroid production. The most typical pattern in patients who are truly hypermetabolic and have temperature reset is elevated corticosteroid production.

These patients do not respond greatly to ACTH tolerance tests. Your papers would indicate that even non-responders with elevated levels are at risk. Some would suggest you might treat these patients, but this is counterintuitive, since their levels are already critically high. What do you recommend for someone whose cortisol level is fixed and elevated around 40–60, and then does not go up more than 45 on stimulation? Some have tried to treat these people; I am a little afraid of that.

Annane: If one looks at the paper from Koo et al (2001), it nicely demonstrates that in animals, 20 h after cecal ligation and puncture (CLP)-induced sepsis, plasma cortisol levels are high, but the adrenal cells can no longer produce cortisol. So cortisol levels in plasma are not only related to the rate of production but also to the rate of clearance from plasma and to tissue resistance to cortisol. In addition, during HPA axis activation, adrenocortical cells are more sensitive to ACTH and thus, one may expect that the higher the cortisol levels, the higher the cortisol increment after ACTH injection.

Herndon: We almost need to do kinetic studies to identify the syndrome.

Annane: This was done by Melby & Spink (1958). This paper nicely demonstrated a dramatic impairment in clearance from plasma, in particular in patients with sepsis induced kidney or liver failure.

Van den Berghe: That doesn't answer the question of whether it is enough. Is the elevation high enough?

Herndon: I don't think that question has been answered.

Annane: Adrenocortical cells are actually up-regulating themselves, so the higher the cortisol, the higher the response to ACTH. One may also argue that a patient with an appropriate level of activation of the HPA axis in response to an infection should not progress from sepsis to septic shock.

Singer: An indirect answer to David Herndon's question is provided by the fact that low dose hydrocortisone still produces supraphysiological levels. You can be getting levels two or three times above the endogenous stress response level.

Herndon: The level in patients starts very high, and may not increase too much.

Singer: The treatments we give push them much higher still.

Fink: I used to work in a hospital where we looked after many patients with inflammatory bowel disease. They had been on chronic steroids at home. Occasionally, the doctors failed to give them replacement dose steroids after the operation I had performed on them. I have a fair amount of experience, therefore, of treating patients with acute adrenal insufficiency. When you treat these patients with exogenous hydrocortisone they get better very quickly. They don't take 6–8 h to get better; it is like turning on the lights. But when I treat patients with septic shock with hydrocortisone, it isn't the same. Rather than measuring a bunch of stuff, why not just treat everyone with a little bit of hydrocortisone? If they act like they are adrenally insufficient and the lights come on, then keep doing it. If they don't, don't use it.

Van den Berghe: I'd like to suggest something else. Check whether the patient had received etomidate when they were intubated. One injection could do this for several days.

Annane: Even at low doses, steroids are potently biologically active drugs which should not be given to a patient without a strong rationale. So far, it seems that only patients with septic shock who fail to respond to ACTH (i.e. an increase in cortisol of less than 9 μg/dl after 250 μg of ACTH) benefit from cortisol replacement therapy.

Fink: If they are on lots of noradrenaline, and you give them hydrocortisone, and then their noradrenaline requirement goes away, that is evidence that they need steroids.

Annane: Even a healthy person will become more sensitive to catecholamines following steroids, but this doesn't mean that they need steroids.

References

Briegel J, Kellermann W, Forst H et al 1994 Low-dose hydrocortisone infusion attenuates the systemic inflammatory response syndrome. The Phospholipase A2 Study Group. Clin Investig 72:782–787

Koo DJ, Jackman D, Chaudry IH, Wang P 2001 Adrenal insufficiency during the late stage of polymicrobial sepsis. Crit Care Med 29:618–622

Melby JC, Spink WW 1958 Comparative studies on adrenal cortical function and cortisol metabolism in healthy adults and in patients with shock due to infection. J Clin Invest 37:1791–1798

Messaris E, Memos N, Chatzigianni E et al 2004 Time-dependent mitochondrial-mediated programmed neuronal cell death prolongs survival in sepsis. Crit Care Med 32:1764–1770

Sharshar T, Gray F, Lorin de la Grandmaison G et al 2003 Apoptosis of neurons in cardiovascular autonomic centres triggered by inducible nitric oxide synthase after death from septic shock. Lancet 362:1799–1805

Yang H, Wang H, Bernik TR et al 2002 Globin attenuates the innate immune response to endotoxin. Shock 17:485–490

Modulating the endocrine response in sepsis: insulin and blood glucose control

Ilse Vanhorebeek, Lies Langouche and Greet Van den Berghe[1]

Department of Intensive Care Medicine, Katholieke Universiteit Leuven, B-3000 Leuven, Belgium

Abstract. Hyperglycaemia is a common feature of the critically ill and has been associated with increased mortality. Maintaining normoglycaemia with insulin therapy improves survival and reduces morbidity in prolonged critically ill patients in both surgical and medical intensive care units, as shown by two large randomized controlled studies. Prevention of cellular glucose toxicity by strict glycaemic control appears to play a predominant role, but also other metabolic and non-metabolic effects of insulin appear to contribute to the clinical benefits.

2007 Sepsis—new insights, new therapies. Wiley, Chichester (Novartis Foundation Symposium 280) p 204–222

Patients who are critically ill, either as a result of a septic complication after extensive surgery or trauma, or those who present with organ failure often due to primary sepsis, have a high risk of death and suffer from substantial morbidity. The hypermetabolic stress response that usually follows any type of major trauma or acute illness is associated with hyperglycaemia and insulin resistance, often referred to as 'stress diabetes' or 'diabetes of injury' (McCowen et al 2001, Thorell et al 1999). In critically ill patients, even in those who were not previously diagnosed with diabetes, glucose uptake is reduced in peripheral insulin sensitive tissues, whereas endogenous glucose production is increased, resulting in hyperglycaemia. It has long been generally accepted that a moderate hyperglycaemia in critically ill patients is beneficial to ensure the supply of glucose as a source of energy to organs that do not require insulin for glucose uptake, among which are the brain and the immune system. However, an increasing body of evidence associates the upon-admission degree of hyperglycaemia as well as the duration of hyperglycaemia during critical illness with adverse outcome. The first evidence

---

[1] This paper was presented at the symposium by Greet Van den Berghe, to whom correspondence should be addressed.

against tolerating hyperglycaemia during critical illness came from two recent large, randomized, controlled trials, one in a group of surgical intensive care patients (Van den Berghe et al 2001) and another in strictly medical intensive care patients (Van den Berghe et al 2006). The studies demonstrated that tight blood glucose control with insulin therapy significantly improves morbidity and mortality. Both blood glucose control and glucose-independent actions of insulin appear to contribute to the beneficial effects of the therapy (Van den Berghe et al 2003).

Hyperglycaemia and outcome in critical illness

The development of stress-induced hyperglycaemia is associated with several clinically important problems in a wide array of patients with severe illness or injury. An increasing number of reports associate the upon-admission degree of hyperglycaemia as well as the duration of hyperglycaemia during critical illness with adverse outcome. In patients with severe brain injury, hyperglycaemia was associated with longer duration of hospital stay, a worse neurological status, pupil reactivity, higher intracranial pressures and reduced survival. In severely burned children, the incidence of bacteraemia and fungaemia, the number of skin grafting procedures and the risk of death were higher in hyperglycaemic than in normoglycaemic patients. In trauma patients, elevated glucose levels early after injury have been associated with infectious morbidity, a lengthier intensive care unit (ICU) and hospital stay and increased mortality. Furthermore, this effect appeared to be independent of the associated shock or the severity of injury. Trauma patients with persistent hyperglycaemia had a significantly greater degree of morbidity and mortality. A meta-analysis on myocardial infarction revealed an association between hyperglycaemia and increased risk of congestive heart failure or cardiogenic shock and in-hospital mortality (Capes et al 2000). Higher blood glucose levels predicted a higher risk of death after stroke and a poor functional recovery in those patients who survived (Capes et al 2001). A retrospective review of a heterogeneous group of critically ill patients indicated that even a modest degree of hyperglycaemia occurring after admission to the ICU was associated with a substantial increase in hospital mortality (Krinsley 2003). A retrospective study on non-diabetic paediatric critically ill patients revealed a correlation of hyperglycaemia with a greater in-hospital mortality rate and longer length of stay.

Blood glucose control with intensive insulin therapy

The landmark prospective, randomized, controlled clinical trial of intensive insulin therapy in a large group of patients admitted to the ICU after extensive or complicated surgery or trauma revealed major clinical benefits on morbidity

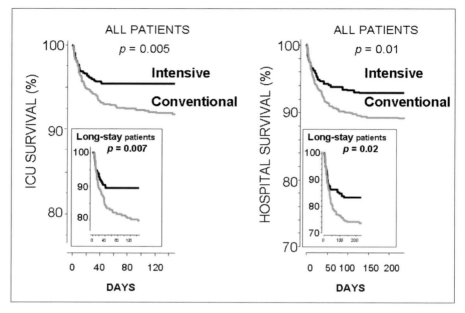

FIG. 1.   Intensive insulin therapy saves lives in the intensive care unit (ICU). Kaplan–Meier
survival plots of patients from the Leuven surgical ICU study who received intensive insulin
treatment (blood glucose maintained below 110 mg/dl; black) or conventional treatment (insulin
administration only when blood glucose exceeded 220 mg/dl; grey) in the ICU. The upper
panels display results from all patients; the lower panels display results for long-stay (>5 days)
ICU patients only. P values were determined with the use of the Mantel-Cox log-rank test.
Adapted with permission from the *Journal of Clinical Investigation* (Van den Berghe 2004).

and mortality (Van den Berghe et al 2001). In the conventional management of
hyperglycaemia, insulin was only administered when blood glucose levels exceeded
220 mg/dl, with the aim of keeping concentrations between 180 and 200 mg/dl,
resulting in mean blood glucose levels of 150–160 mg/dl (hyperglycaemia).
In the intensive insulin therapy group, insulin was administered to the patients
by insulin infusion titrated to maintain blood glucose levels between 80
and 110 mg/dl which resulted in mean blood glucose levels of 90–100 mg/dl
(normoglycaemia). This intervention appeared safe as no hypoglycaemia-
induced adverse events were reported. Maintaining normoglycaemia with insulin
strikingly lowered intensive care mortality by 43% (from 8.0% to 4.6%), the
benefit being most pronounced in the group of patients who required intensive
care for more than 5 days, with a mortality reduction from 20.2% to 10.6%
(Fig. 1). Also in-hospital mortality was lowered from 10.9% to 7.2% in the total
group and from 26.3% to 16.8% in the group of long-stayers. Besides saving

lives, insulin therapy largely prevented several critical illness-associated complications. The development of blood stream infections was reduced by 46%, of acute renal failure requiring dialysis or haemofiltration by 41%, of bacteraemia by 46%, the incidence of critical illness polyneuropathy was reduced by 44%, the number of red blood cell transfusions by 50%. Patients were also less dependent on prolonged mechanical ventilation and needed fewer days in intensive care. Although a large number of patients included in this study recovered from complicated cardiac surgery, the clinical benefits of this therapy were equally present in most other diagnostic subgroups. In the patients with isolated brain injury tight glycaemic control protected the central and peripheral nervous system from secondary insults and improved long-term rehabilitation (Van den Berghe et al 2005). An important confirmation of the clinical benefits of intensive insulin therapy was recently obtained with the demonstration, by a large randomized controlled trial, that the Leuven protocol of glycaemic control with insulin in adult surgical critically ill patients (Van den Berghe et al 2001) was similarly effective in a strictly medical adult ICU patient population (Van den Berghe et al 2006). In this exclusively medical ICU population, in which sepsis is the most common trigger for ICU admission, intensive insulin therapy during ICU stay reduced morbidity among all intention-to-treat medical ICU patients and in those patients who were treated at least for a few days, it improved morbidity and reduced mortality. Morbidity benefits comprised prevention of kidney injury, reduced duration of mechanical ventilation, shorter ICU stay and shorter hospital stay, but not prevention of blood-stream infections. Among the long-stay patients, in-hospital mortality was reduced from 52.5% to 43.0%. These data indicate that the preventive effect on severe infections, observed in the surgical study, is not the key pathway by which mortality is reduced with intensive insulin therapy. Prevention of organ failure appears to be brought about more directly by the intervention.

In 'real-life' intensive care medicine, James Krinsley evaluated the impact of implementing strict blood glucose control in a heterogeneous medical/surgical ICU population (Krinsley 2004). A less strict blood glucose control was aimed for, a regimen chosen primarily to avoid inadvertent hypoglycaemia: in this setting insulin therapy lowered mean blood glucose levels of 152 mg/dl in the baseline period to 131 mg/dl in the protocol period. Comparison with patient data before the implementation of the protocol showed a 29.3% reduction in hospital mortality, and 10.8% decrease in length of ICU stay. Development of new renal insufficiency was 75% lower, and 18.7% fewer patients required red blood cell transfusion. Again, the number of patients acquiring infections did not change significantly, but the incidence was already low at baseline in this patient group (Krinsley 2004). Another small, prospective, randomized, controlled trial by Grey and colleagues conducted in a predominantly surgical ICU, confirmed the beneficial effect of tight blood glucose control on the number of serious infections (Grey & Perdrizet 2004). In this study, insulin therapy was targeted to glucose levels between 80 and 120 mg/dl, which resulted in a mean daily glucose level of 125 mg/dl versus 179 mg/dl in the standard glycaemic control group. A significant reduction in the incidence of total nosocomial infections, including intravascular device, bloodstream, intravascular device-related bloodstream, and surgical site infections was observed in the insulin group compared to the conventional approach (Grey & Perdrizet 2004).

Insulin resistance and hyperglycaemia

The stress imposed by any type of acute illness or injury leads to the development of insulin resistance, glucose intolerance and hyperglycaemia. Hepatic glucose production is up-regulated in the acute phase of critical illness, despite high blood glucose levels and abundantly released insulin. Elevated levels of cytokines, growth hormone, glucagon and cortisol might play a role in the increased gluconeogenesis (Hill & McCallum 1991, Lang et al 1992). Several effects of these hormones oppose the normal action of insulin, resulting in an increased lipolysis and proteolysis which provides substrates for gluconeogenesis. Catecholamines, which are released in response to acute injury, enhance hepatic glycogenolysis and inhibit glycogenesis. Apart from the up-regulated glucose production, glucose uptake mechanisms are also affected during critical illness and contribute to the development of hyperglycaemia. Due to immobilization of the critically ill patient, exercise-stimulated glucose uptake in skeletal muscle is supposedly absent (Rodnick et al 1992). Furthermore, due to impaired insulin-stimulated glucose uptake by the glucose transporter 4 (GLUT4) and due to impaired glycogen synthase activity, glucose uptake in heart, skeletal muscle and adipose tissue is compromised. However, total body glucose uptake is massively increased, but is accounted for by tissues that are not dependent on insulin for glucose uptake, such as brain and blood cells (McCowen et al 2001, Meszaros et al 1987). The higher levels of insulin, impaired peripheral glucose uptake and elevated hepatic glucose production reflect the development of insulin resistance during critical illness.

The mechanism by which insulin therapy lowers blood glucose in critically ill patients is not completely clear. These patients are thought to suffer from both hepatic and skeletal muscle insulin resistance, but data from liver and skeletal muscle biopsies harvested from non-survivors in the Leuven study, suggest that glucose levels are lowered mainly via stimulation of skeletal muscle glucose uptake. Indeed, insulin therapy did increase mRNA levels of GLUT4, which controls insulin-stimulated glucose uptake in muscle, and of hexokinase II, the rate-limiting enzyme in intracellular insulin-stimulated glucose metabolism (Mesotten et al

2004). On the other hand, hepatic insulin resistance in these patients is not overcome by insulin therapy. The hepatic expression of phospoenolpyruvate carboxykinase, the rate-limiting enzyme in gluconeogenesis, and of glucokinase, the rate-limiting enzyme for insulin-mediated glucose uptake and glycogen synthesis, were unaffected by insulin therapy (Mesotten et al 2002, 2004). Moreover, circulating levels of insulin-like growth factor binding protein-1, normally under inhibitory control of insulin, was also refractory to the therapy in the total population of both survivors and non-survivors (Mesotten et al 2004).

Preventing glucose toxicity with intensive insulin therapy

It is striking that during the relatively short period that patients need intensive care, avoiding even a moderate level of hyperglycaemia, on average around 150–160 mg/dl, with insulin improves the most feared complications of critical illness. In critically ill patients, hyperglycaemia thus appears much more acutely toxic than in healthy individuals of whom cells can protect themselves by down-regulating the insulin-independent glucose transporters (Klip et al 1994). This acute toxicity of high levels of glucose in critical illness might be explained by an accelerated cellular glucose overload and more pronounced toxic side effects of glycolysis and oxidative phosphorylation (Van den Berghe 2004).

Hepatocytes, gastrointestinal mucosal cells, pancreatic β cells, renal tubular cells, endothelial cells, immune cells and neurons are insulin-independent for glucose uptake, which is mediated mainly by the glucose transporters GLUT1, GLUT2 or GLUT3. Cytokines, angiotensin II, endothelin 1, vascular endothelial growth factor, transforming growth factor β and hypoxia, all induced in critical illness, have been shown to up-regulate expression and membrane localization of GLUT1 and GLUT3 in different cell types (Pekala et al 1990). This up-regulation might overrule the normal down-regulatory protective response against hyperglycaemia. Moreover, GLUT2 and GLUT3 allow glucose to enter cells directly in equilibrium with the elevated extracellular glucose level which is present in critical illness. Therefore, one would expect increased glucose toxicity in tissues where glucose uptake is mediated by non-insulin-dependent transport. Hyperglycaemia has been linked to the development of increased oxidative stress in diabetes, in part due to enhanced mitochondrial superoxide production (Brownlee 2001). Superoxide interacts with nitric oxide (NO) to form peroxynitrite, a reactive species able to induce tyrosine nitration of proteins which affects their normal function (Aulak et al 2004). During critical illness, cytokine-induced activation of NO synthase increases NO levels, and hypoxia–reperfusion aggravates superoxide production, resulting in more peroxynitrite being generated (Aulak et al 2004). When cells in critically ill patients are overloaded with glucose, high levels of peroxynitrite and superoxide are to be expected, resulting in inhibition

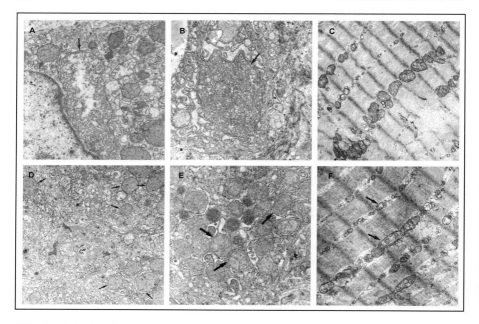

FIG. 2.   Mitochondrial ultrastructure in liver and skeletal muscle of critically ill patients. Electron micrographs show greatly enlarged mitochondria with an increased number of disarrayed cristae and reduced electron density of the matrix in hepatocytes adjacent to normal mitochondria (A,B), contrasting with normal mitochondrial morphology in skeletal muscle (C) of conventionally treated patients. In most of the intensively treated patients hepatocytic mitochondrial ultrastructure was normal (D [c: canaliculus],E), as in all muscle biopsy samples from these patients (F). Original magnification: ×23 000. (Reprinted with permission from Elsevier [Vanhorebeek et al 2005].)

of the glycolytic enzyme GAPDH (Brownlee 2001), and mitochondrial complexes I and IV.

We recently indeed demonstrated that prevention of hyperglycaemia with insulin therapy protected both ultrastructure (Fig. 2) and function of the hepatocytic mitochondrial compartment of critically ill patients, but no obvious morphological or pronounced functional abnormalities were detected in skeletal muscle of critically ill patients (Vanhorebeek et al 2005). Mitochondrial dysfunction with a disturbed energy metabolism is a likely cause of organ failure, the most common cause of death in ICU. Prevention of hyperglycaemia-induced mitochondrial dysfunction in other tissues that allow glucose to enter passively might explain some of the protective effects of intensive insulin therapy in critical illness.

Metabolic and non-metabolic effects of blood glucose control with intensive insulin therapy

Similar to the serum lipid profile of diabetic patients, the lipid metabolism in critically ill patients is strongly deranged. Most characteristic for critical illness is the elevated level of triglycerides together with very low circulating levels of high density lipoprotein (HDL) and low density lipoprotein (LDL) cholesterol. Insulin therapy almost completely reversed the hypertriglyceridaemia and substantially elevated HDL and LDL and the level of cholesterol associated with these lipo-proteins (Mesotten et al 2004). Insulin treatment also has shown to decrease serum triglycerides and free fatty acids in children with burn injury. Multivariate logistic regression analysis revealed that improvement of the dyslipidaemia with insulin therapy explained a significant part of the reduced mortality and organ failure in critically ill patients (Mesotten et al 2004). Given the important role of lipoproteins in transportation of lipid components (cholesterol, triglycerides, phospholipids, lipid-soluble vitamins) and endotoxin scavenging (Harris et al 1990, 1993) a contribution to improved outcome might indeed be expected.

Critically ill patients become severely catabolic, with loss of lean body mass, despite adequate enteral or parenteral nutrition. Intensive insulin therapy might attenuate this catabolic syndrome of prolonged critical illness, as insulin exerts anabolic actions (Agus et al 2004, Gore et al 2004). Intensive insulin treatment indeed resulted in higher total protein content in skeletal muscle of critically ill patients (Vanhorebeek et al 2005) and prevented weight loss in a rabbit model of prolonged critical illness (Weekers et al 2003).

Intensive insulin therapy prevented excessive inflammation, illustrated by decreased C-reactive protein (CRP) and mannose-binding lectin levels (Hansen et al 2003), independent of its preventive effect on infections (Van den Berghe et al 2001). Insulin therapy also attenuated the CRP response in an experimental animal model of prolonged critical illness which was induced by third degree burn injury (Weekers et al 2003). In children with burn injury, administration of insulin resulted in lower pro-inflammatory cytokines and proteins, whereas the anti-inflammatory cascade was stimulated, although these effects were largely seen only late after the traumatic stimulus. Insulin treatment attenuated the inflammatory response in thermally injured rats and endotoxaemic rats and pigs. Next to these anti-inflammatory effects of insulin, prevention of hyperglycaemia may be crucial as well. Hyperglycaemia inactivates immunoglobulins by glycosylation and there-fore contributes to the risk of infection. High glucose levels also negatively affected polymorphonuclear neutrophil function and intracellular bactericidal and opsonic activity (Rassias et al 1999, Rayfield et al 1982). Critically ill rabbits showed an increased phagocytosis capacity of monocytes and their ability to generate an oxidative burst when blood glucose levels were kept normal (Weekers et al 2003).

Critical illness also resembles diabetes mellitus in its hypercoagulation state. In diabetes mellitus vascular endothelium dysfunction, elevated platelet activation and increased clotting factors and inhibition of the fibrinolytic system all might contribute to this hypercoagulation state (Garcia Frade et al 1987, Patrassi et al 1982). Insulin therapy indeed protected the myocardium and improved myocardial function after acute myocardial infarction, during open heart surgery and in congestive heart failure. Prevention of endothelial dysfunction also contributed to the protective effects of insulin therapy in critical illness in part via inhibition of excessive iNOS-induced NO release (Langouche et al 2005) and via reduction of circulating levels of asymmetric dimethylarginine, which inhibits the constitutive enzyme eNOS and hence the production of endothelial nitric oxide (Siroen et al 2005).

Glucose control or insulin?

Multivariate logistic regression analysis of the results of the Leuven study indicated that blood glucose control and not the insulin dose administered statistically explains most of the beneficial effects of insulin therapy on outcome of critical illness (Van den Berghe et al 2003) (Fig. 3). Post-hoc analysis suggested that it is crucial to reduce blood glucose levels below 110 mg/dl for the prevention of morbidity events such as bacteraemia, anaemia and acute renal failure. The level of hyperglycaemia was also an independent risk factor for the development of critical illness polyneuropathy (Van den Berghe et al 2003). Finney et al (2003) confirmed the independent association between hyperglycaemia and adverse outcome in surgical ICU patients. Our recent experiments in an animal model of critical illness, in which we independently manipulated levels of blood glucose and insulin (Ellger et al 2005), confirmed the superior role of strict blood glucose control over the glycaemia-independent effects of insulin, in obtaining the survival benefit as well as most of the morbidity benefits during critical illness.

Conclusions

Hyperglycaemia in critically ill patients is a result of an altered glucose metabolism. Apart from the up-regulated glucose production (both gluconeogenesis and glycogenolysis), insulin-mediated glucose uptake is impaired during critical illness and contributes to the development of hyperglycaemia. The higher levels of insulin, impaired peripheral glucose uptake and elevated hepatic glucose production reflect the development of insulin resistance during critical illness. Hyperglycaemia in critically ill patients has been associated with increased mortality. Simply maintaining normoglycaemia with insulin therapy improves survival and reduces morbidity in surgical and medical ICU patients, as shown by two large

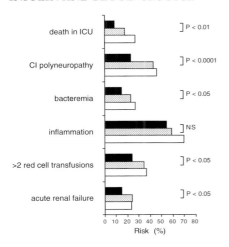
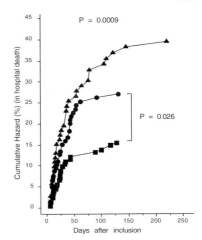

FIG. 3. Stratification of risk of death and morbidity factors for mean blood glucose levels. (*Left panel*) Post-hoc analysis of the percentage of risk of death in ICU, development of critical illness (CI) polyneuropathy, bacteraemia, inflammation (CRP higher than 150 mg/l for more than 3 days), need for more than two red cell transfusions, and acute renal failure requiring haemofiltration/dialysis among long-stay (more than 5 days) patients stratified for mean blood glucose levels. Filled bars represent patients with a mean blood glucose level lower than 110 mg/dl, shaded bars represent patients with a mean blood glucose level between 110 and 15 mg/dl and unfilled bars represent patients with a mean blood glucose level higher than 150 mg/dl. The indicated *P* values were obtained using the χ^2 test. Reproduced with permission from Van den Berghe et al (2003). (*Right panel*) Kaplan–Meier cumulative risk of in-hospital death among long-stay patients with a mean blood glucose level lower than 110 mg/dl (squares), between 110 and 150 mg/dl (circles) and higher than 150 mg/dl (triangles). The *P* value of 0.0009, obtained with Mantel-Cox log-rank test, indicates the significance level of the overall difference in risk of death among the groups, and the *P* value of 0.026 indicates the significance level of the difference between the <110 mg/dl and 110–150 mg/dl groups. Reproduced with permission from Van den Berghe et al (2003).

randomized controlled studies. These results obtained in an investigational setting were also confirmed in 'real-life' intensive care of a heterogeneous patient population admitted to a mixed medical/surgical ICU. Prevention of glucose toxicity by strict glycaemic control appears to be crucial although other metabolic and non-metabolic effects of insulin, independent of glycaemic control, may contribute to the clinical benefits.

Acknowledgements

I. Vanhorebeek and L. Langouche are Postdoctoral Fellows of the FWO Flanders Belgium. G. Van den Berghe holds an unrestrictive Catholic University of Leuven Novo Nordisk Chair of Research. Work supported by the Research council of the Leuven University and the Fund for Scientific Research Flanders, Belgium.

References

Agus MS, Javid PJ, Ryan DP, Jaksic T 2004 Intravenous insulin decreases protein breakdown in infants on extracorporeal membrane oxygenation. J Pediatr Surg 39:839–844

Aulak KS, Koeck T, Crabb JW, Stuehr DJ 2004 Dynamics of protein nitration in cells and mitochondria. Am J Physiol Heart Circ Physiol 286:H30–38

Brownlee M 2001 Biochemistry and molecular cell biology of diabetic complications. Nature 414:813–820

Capes SE, Hunt D, Malmberg K, Gerstein HC 2000 Stress hyperglycaemia and increased risk of death after myocardial infarction in patients with and without diabetes: a systematic overview. Lancet 355:773–778

Capes SE, Hunt D, Malmberg K, Pathak P, Gerstein HC 2001 Stress hyperglycemia and prognosis of stroke in nondiabetic and diabetic patients: a systematic overview. Stroke 32:2426–2432

Ellger B, Debaveye Y, Herijgers P, Van den Berghe G 2005 Impact of maintaining normoglycemia and glycemia-independent insulin-effects in critical illness. Intensive Care Med 31[S1]: S80, Abstract

Finney SJ, Zekveld C, Elia A, Evans TW 2003 Glucose control and mortality in critically ill patients. JAMA 290:2041–2047

Garcia Frade LJ, de la CH, Alava I, Navarro JL, Creighton LJ, Gaffney PJ 1987 Diabetes mellitus as a hypercoagulable state: its relationship with fibrin fragments and vascular damage. Thromb Res 47:533–540

Gore DC, Wolf SE, Sanford AP, Herndon DN, Wolfe RR 2004 Extremity hyperinsulinemia stimulates muscle protein synthesis in severely injured patients. Am J Physiol Endocrinol Metab 286:E529–534

Grey NJ, Perdrizet GA 2004 Reduction of nosocomial infections in the surgical intensive-care unit by strict glycemic control. Endocr Pract 10 Suppl 2:46–52

Hansen TK, Thiel S, Wouters PJ, Christiansen JS, Van den Berghe G 2003 Intensive insulin therapy exerts antiinflammatory effects in critically ill patients and counteracts the adverse effect of low mannose-binding lectin levels. J Clin Endocrinol Metab 88:1082–1088

Harris HW, Grunfeld C, Feingold KR, Rapp JH 1990 Human very low density lipoproteins and chylomicrons can protect against endotoxin-induced death in mice. J Clin Invest 86: 696–702

Harris HW, Grunfeld C, Feingold KR et al 1993 Chylomicrons alter the fate of endotoxin, decreasing tumor necrosis factor release and preventing death. J Clin Invest 91:1028–1034

Hill M, McCallum R 1991 Altered transcriptional regulation of phosphoenolpyruvate carboxykinase in rats following endotoxin treatment. J Clin Invest 88:811–816

Klip A, Tsakiridis T, Marette A, Ortiz PA 1994 Regulation of expression of glucose transporters by glucose: a review of studies in vivo and in cell cultures. FASEB J 8:43–53

Krinsley JS 2003 Association between hyperglycemia and increased hospital mortality in a heterogeneous population of critically ill patients. Mayo Clin Proc 78:1471–1478

Krinsley JS 2004 Effect of an intensive glucose management protocol on the mortality of critically ill adult patients. Mayo Clin Proc 79:992–1000

Lang CH, Dobrescu C, Bagby GJ 1992 Tumor necrosis factor impairs insulin action on peripheral glucose disposal and hepatic glucose output. Endocrinology 130:43–52

Langouche L, Vanhorebeek I, Vlasselaers D et al 2005 Intensive insulin therapy protects the endothelium of critically ill patients. J Clin Invest 115:2277–2286

McCowen KC, Malhotra A, Bistrian BR 2001 Stress-induced hyperglycemia. Crit Care Clin 17:107–124

Mesotten D, Delhanty PJ, Vanderhoydonc F et al 2002 Regulation of insulin-like growth factor binding protein-1 during protracted critical illness. J Clin Endocrinol Metab 87:5516–5523

Mesotten D, Swinnen J V, Vanderhoydonc F, Wouters PJ, Van den Berghe G 2004 Contribution of circulating lipids to the improved outcome of critical illness by glycemic control with intensive insulin therapy. J Clin Endocrinol Metab 89:219–226

Meszaros K, Lang CH, Bagby GJ, Spitzer JJ 1987 Contribution of different organs to increased glucose consumption after endotoxin administration. J Biol Chem 262:10965–10970

Patrassi GM, Vettor R, Padovan D, Girolami A 1982 Contact phase of blood coagulation in diabetes mellitus. Eur J Clin Invest 12:307–311

Pekala P, Marlow M, Heuvelman D, Connolly D 1990 Regulation of hexose transport in aortic endothelial cells by vascular permeability factor and tumor necrosis factor-alpha, but not by insulin. J Biol Chem 265:18051–18054

Rassias AJ, Marrin CA, Arruda J, Whalen PK, Beach M, Yeager MP 1999 Insulin infusion improves neutrophil function in diabetic cardiac surgery patients. Anesth Analg 88:1011–1016

Rayfield EJ, Ault MJ, Keusch GT, Brothers MJ, Nechemias C, Smith H 1982 Infection and diabetes: the case for glucose control. Am J Med 72:439–450

Rodnick KJ, Piper RC, Slot JW, James DE 1992 Interaction of insulin and exercise on glucose transport in muscle. Diabetes Care 15:1679–1689

Siroen MP, van Leeuwen PA, Nijveldt RJ, Teerlink T, Wouters PJ, Van den Berghe G 2005 Modulation of asymmetric dimethylarginine in critically ill patients receiving intensive insulin treatment: a possible explanation of reduced morbidity and mortality? Crit Care Med 33:504–510

Thorell A, Nygren J, Ljungqvist O 1999 Insulin resistance: a marker of surgical stress. Curr Opin Clin Nutr Metab Care 2:69–78

Van den Berghe G 2004 How does blood glucose control with insulin save lives in intensive care? J Clin Invest 114:1187–1195

Van den Berghe G, Wouters P, Weekers F et al 2001 Intensive insulin therapy in critically ill patients. N Engl J Med 345:1359–1367

Van den Berghe G, Wouters PJ, Bouillon R et al 2003 Outcome benefit of intensive insulin therapy in the critically ill: Insulin dose versus glycemic control. Crit Care Med 31:359–366

Van den Berghe G, Schoonheydt K, Becx P, Bruyninckx F, Wouters PJ 2005 Insulin therapy protects the central and peripheral nervous system of intensive care patients. Neurology 64:1348–1353

Van den Berghe G, Wilmer A, Hermans G et al 2006 Intensive insulin therapy in medical intensive care patients. N Engl J Med 354:516–518

Vanhorebeek I, De Vos R, Mesotten D, Wouters PJ, Wolf-Peeters C, Van den Berghe G 2005 Protection of hepatocyte mitochondrial ultrastructure and function by strict blood glucose control with insulin in critically ill patients. Lancet 365:53–59

Weekers F, Giulietti AP, Michalaki M et al 2003 Metabolic, endocrine, and immune effects of stress hyperglycemia in a rabbit model of prolonged critical illness. Endocrinology 144:5329–5338

DISCUSSION

Marshall: Is there any evidence that other strategies to lower glucose might be beneficial?

Van den Berghe: Probably, yes, but there are no data.

Marshall: On the basis of the fact that it looks like it is the patients who are in the intensive care unit (ICU) for more than three days who benefit, is there any downside to waiting until the third day to start the intensive insulin therapy?

Van den Berghe: That's an important question. This determines how we have to deal with the data in clinical practice. The observational data from Tony Furnary, who has studied the effect of blood glucose control in diabetics undergoing coronary bypass surgery, are important in this discussion. He found that the first three days are crucial to get the effect. I don't think the data that are out there support the concept of waiting for three days before starting. The studies that have been done suggest this is something that needs to be prevented early in the disease course, which then shows its impact on outcome after three days.

Singer: Did you do subset analyses in your medical patients to find the ones who had been ill for a while in the ward?

Van den Berghe: No, because most of them probably were ill on the ward for a while.

Radermacher: The German multicentre study on glucose control was abandoned prematurely. The treatment arm didn't show any benefit. I calculated the glucose supplementation from the data in your paper. It is roughly 150–180 g per day for a normal weight adult. In Germany, it is popular to substitute half the glucose amount with xylitol. Xylitol has two advantages: it doesn't affect the blood glucose, and the transport is insulin-independent. From the beginning of this German study it struck me that there was a major difference between what everyone does around the world and what is done in Germany. It could be that just going back to a strategy of administering substrates that replace glucose could have some effect in terms of glycaemic control.

Van den Berghe: I don't agree. If you look at the blood glucose levels, they weren't well controlled and the conventionally treated patients overlapped with the intensively treated patients.

Radermacher: What I mean is that by using xylitol and thus *per se* having lower glucose levels, they missed the opportunity to find something beneficial. Admittedly, it is just a suspicion due to the fact that this practice is relatively common.

Van den Berghe: It is difficult to answer that. From the low numbers of patients in the study (fewer than 500) they looked at 30 and 90 day mortality and didn't see much. It was dramatically underpowered. Perhaps there might have been something had they continued. They stopped because they thought they were doing something bad, with relatively high incidence of hypoglycaemia.

Choi: Clinically, in your 1200 patients, did many of them have a normal glucose level of 100 that did not require any insulin therapy?

Van den Berghe: 2.5% or so.

Choi: Can that help you decide whether it may be an exogenous insult? The reason I mention this is that you described what glucose does with the signalling pathway and insulin. You tried to locate biochemical markers in the muscle and liver with the glucose. Other than nitric oxide (NO), there wasn't much there. AKT is such a pro-survival signal. Did you measure AKT levels in your human samples?

Van den Berghe: Yes. There is something there. We can stimulate the whole insulin metabolic signal in the muscle. Not in the liver. The insulin doses differ by sixfold between the conventionally and intensively treated patients. Yet the insulin serum levels are equal even though the blood glucoses are hugely different. What we are doing is affecting the sensitivity to insulin.

Choi: Why muscle? If it was in liver, people would think this was an explanation. Do we know an example in clinical medicine of muscle being a sink for anything other than for what muscle does?

Fink: It is a sink for glucose.

Griffiths: Is this to do with inactivity of the muscle?

Van den Berghe: Partially, this will contribute, because the most important GLUT4-mediated glucose uptake in the muscle occurs via muscle contraction.

Thiemermann: In 2001/2, we found that that peroxisome proliferator-activated receptor (PPAR)γ agonists decrease myocardial infarct size. (Wayman et al 2002). Then we reported that a number of PPARγ agonists including glitazones and cyclopentanone prostaglandins protect tissues against injury caused by ischaemia–reperfusion or shock. Unfortunately this doesn't really help us in addressing your questions, because these are acute models of disease which involve hypoglycaemic animals, and all of the PPARγ agonists used have been found to have profound anti-inflammatory effects. These effects are so potent, that clinical trials with rosiglitazone are being conducted in patients with psoriasis. This doesn't help us with the glucose versus anti-inflammation problem. I was impressed with the reduction in iNOS induction, which you observed. Do you want to speculate on how hyperglycaemia drives iNOS induction?

Van den Berghe: It's via NF-κB according to the literature.

Thiemermann: So you believe that lowering plasma glucose will result in a reduced activation of NF-κB.

Fink: Have you looked for markers of redox stress by measuring exhaled ethane?

Van den Berghe: No.

Szabó: What is it about the high sugar that would make things worse? One of my interests lies in the field of diabetic complications. If we make animals diabetic and give them a low dose of endotoxin, the high sugar seems to potentiate some cytokine responses (but not all of them). Is this part of the story?

Van den Berghe: We measured a whole battery of cytokines, and there is no effect.

Szabó: When we made these animals streptozocin diabetic and gave them a low dose of endotoxin, this didn't really affect cardiac function in normal animals. But the cardiac function seemed to go down in the animals that had higher sugar. Do you have any data for troponin or other cardiac markers: is there a difference in the clinical setting?

Van den Berghe: Not for the clinical data. We are currently studying children who are undergoing surgery for congenital heart diseases. We are focusing on the heart there. The rabbit data show that there are effects.

Szabó: The reactive oxygen species (ROS) story is also important here. We can do some measurements in this direction if you send us samples; we can stain any kinds of tissue sections. By the way, there is this very interesting story of glucose memory, which people in the field of diabetic complications are getting very excited about. If you put endothelial cells in high sugar and then return them to normal sugar, they still think they are in high sugar, with up-regulated inflammatory pathways and reactive species.

Van den Berghe: I agree. The advice given by the editorial that we don't have to worry and can wait to start treatment is not evidence based.

Griffiths: You can think of a mechanism for why high glucose can affect the cardiac contractility. One of the mistakes of looking at the mechanics of Myosin ATPase turnover has been doing studies at lower temperatures. When the studies are done at 37 °C ROS has much greater effects on the actin–myosin interaction.

Fink: This is a hard thing to do, but it's important: you need to ask the question, why did these people die? The patients need to be bifurcated into at least two groups. One group died despite the best efforts of their doctors. Then there was a group who died a programmed death that was doctor-based. One mechanism to explain all your findings could be based on your neurosurgical data. In other words, if the tight glucose control preserves cerebral function in these patients, the doctors and family are going to be less likely to want to pull the plug than if the patient has been comatose for 10 days.

Van den Berghe: We looked at the causes of death, and asked the senior physicians to write it down each time. It looked as if in all the categories of deaths they were fewer. It wasn't as if they were all in one group. In the surgical study it appeared to be the septic organ failure group.

Griffiths: Some of them would have left ICU and then died later.

Fink: When I look at the survival curves from both studies, the treatment effect is during the ICU phase. After this, the survival curves are parallel. At least in the ICUs at the University of Pittsburgh, there are very few deaths that are not programmed. One of the clues that tells the doctor and family that it is time to give up is when the patient no longer responds to stuff.

Van den Berghe: Neurotoxicity is very important.

Fink: Later we will address the role of the CNS in controlling inflammatory responses.

Choi: With regard to insulin resistance, did you have enough type 1 and 2 diabetics in the medical ICU to see whether this could help you, if you believe that type 2 is more resistant to insulin production than type 1?

Van den Berghe: 17% were known to be diabetic in the medical study. Most of the elderly patients are type 2 diabetics. The numbers were too small to look at this as a subgroup. It didn't correlate with their glucose levels on admission.

Choi: Did you measure insulin levels on admission?

Van den Berghe: Yes.

Singer: All the attention is focusing on before three days, but I'd like to turn this the other way. You showed that the big difference was on late death. What did the late deaths die of? Was there a cardiac element?

Van den Berghe: No, it wasn't cardiac death. The majority of patients die through non-recovery from the multiple organ failure.

Singer: Didn't a fair number of deaths occur after patients left the ICU?

Van den Berghe: Yes, but more or less the same numbers in both groups.

Herndon: These are remarkable studies that are going to impact mortality this decade in ICUs from sepsis. Do you think it is too late to do a randomized multi-centre study? Your results have been so dramatic and standards of care are already affected by what you have done. If it is not too late, which questions need to be answered early and late? How could we plan a study to answer all these questions if it were to be done?

Van den Berghe: What is the evidence so far? We now have two randomized controlled trials. They are not blinded because it is impossible to blind them. They are single centre studies, performed at one hospital, albeit in two departments with different staff. We have substantial morbidity effects in these two trials on the intention to treat basis. There is a mortality benefit in the surgical study on the intention to treat and the long-stay, and a mortality benefit in the medical study when patients are treated for at least three days. If you just look at the criteria of recommendations and the level of evidence, I see these as a level A recommendation, but Derek Angus, for example, wouldn't agree with me. People have to decide for themselves.

Marshall: There is an ongoing study—a collaboration between the Australians and the Canadians—that will recruit 6000 patients to study this question. The other question that arises is: what is the maximal level of glucose that should be tolerated? The Surviving Sepsis Campaign suggests that it should be controlled to 150 mg/dl or less.

Van den Berghe: That is not correct. Our control group has blood glucose levels of 150–160 mg/dl. And bringing that down to <110 mg/dl works. The target clearly is not 150 mg/dl.

Fink: Right now the only evidence is for 110 mg/dl.

Herndon: Since there are these ongoing randomized trials, what questions need to be answered, from what you have already done?

Van den Berghe: If one is critical about the available data, perhaps we still need to repeat the trial in a multicentre way, in units that apply different nutritional strategies. Regarding the hypoglycaemia issue, how can one study the impact of hypoglycaemia in a randomized controlled trial? It should be picked up quickly and treated adequately, but one couldn't do a study where you didn't do this. The level is an important question. If you want to study the impact of 150 mg/dl versus 130 mg/dl, and versus 110 mg/dl, you need cardiology-size studies. With the study that is planned, involving some 6000 patients, we won't be able to answer that. Adequately powered studies addressing the level of blood glucose control would need tens of thousands of patients.

Fink: Apart from the hypoglycaemia issue, if 110 is good, is 90 even better?

Van den Berghe: The polyneuropathy data suggest that it is. There is a linear correlation between the blood glucose level and the toxicity to the neurons, even going to the hypoglycaemic range. If you ask diabetologists, patients with the lowest neurotoxicity are the ones that have the frequent hypoglycaemia.

Griffiths: One of the great issues I see when I look at multicentre studies is whether they have been able to follow a process of care. This isn't a single treatment; it is a complex process of care to implement. You had highly trained people to implement this process. It is fantastic, but when people transfer this into multicentre studies, this is a challenge. It is immensely more difficult to test a complex process of care than testing a single-shot intervention. The other point I want to raise is that I agree that it is about electrophysiology. There are many membrane physiologies that need to be addressed. It isn't just the nerves and nervous system; it is probably other issues of membrane physiology that are being affected.

Pugin: There are patients who will remain stable at 110, and they are easy to clamp at this level, and there are patients who will go up and down. In the end the mean will be 110. Have you looked at this?

Van den Berghe: We are doing this as we speak. It is quite complicated to analyse all these profiles. For the surgical study we didn't have the data electronically, but we do have this for the medical study.

Pugin: What is your feeling?

Van den Berghe: The short excursions are probably also toxic.

Fink: This seems like an area where technology could help us. Glucose clamping using closed loop feedback should be here.

Szabó: *In vitro* studies show that if endothelial cells are put in high sugar they tolerate it better than fluctuating levels (Piconi et al 2004).

Herndon: One other thing you might want to consider is duration of treatment. I know you stopped your intensive therapy as people went up to the wards they received conventional therapy. In patients that are heavily stressed, cortisol remains elevated for prolonged periods. Wasting and catabolic injury also continue for a long time, too. Strategies that would prolong this philosophy might be useful.

Van den Berghe: I agree with you. There should be studies on this issue. It could theoretically be that when patients are only treated for a few days they may do worse because their blood glucose goes up again thereafter.

Radermacher: To support Richard Griffiths' comment on multicentre studies, you need a type of learning curve before going into any study like this. Your team is well trained and well educated in delivering care. In the German study, I suspect the learning curve in many of the centres was part of the study. This could have caused the overlap seen. Any multicentre study which doesn't take this into account has a great risk of failing and then destroying what is a good concept.

Van den Berghe: We didn't have a specialized team. We just did it with the nurses that took care of the patients (one nurse for two patients is the standard in our ICUs). But they were educated and trained.

Annane: So far more than 1000 patients have been enrolled in the ongoing European GLUCOCONTROL study. Though, there are more than 30 sites in 11 different countries, it has turned out not to be a problem.

Radermacher: But it requested a training phase, at least theoretically.

Annane: The training phase was very short (1 month). In addition, in most of the participating centres the nurse to patient ratio was about one to three, on average. Do you think that there might be different responses to glucose control in different types of critical illness? Do patients with sepsis respond as well as those with other diseases? This may be a reason that the German study failed, because they studied only septic patients.

Van den Berghe: That's a difficult question because in our study we didn't use sepsis as an inclusion criterion. We wanted this to be a standard of care issue. Of course, a lot of the medical ICU patients were septic when they entered the ICU, but we didn't use this as a diagnosis. The cardiac surgery population responds best relatively, because there is a lot to prevent there: the more the patient would die just of the complications, the more the effect is going to be. In this way, the sickest patients would benefit less. The medical ICU has a relatively smaller mortality reduction, but still we save a huge number of patients.

Annane: The potential higher risk of hypoglycaemia in patients with sepsis may be related to a high glucose consumption by the bacteria. It is common to have severe septic shock patients with low blood glucose for this reason.

Van den Berghe: It is a rare complication of sepsis but it does happen.

References

Piconi L, Quagliaro L, Da Ros R et al 2004 Intermittent high glucose enhances ICAM-1, VCAM-1, E-selectin and interleukin-6 expression in human umbilical endothelial cells in culture: the role of poly(ADP-ribose) polymerase. J Thromb Haemost 2:1453–1459

Wayman NS, Hattori Y, McDonald MC et al 2002 Ligands of the peroxisome proliferator-activated receptors (PPAR-gamma and PPAR-alpha) reduce myocardial infarct size. FASEB J 16:1027–1040

The neuronal strategy for inflammation

Luis Ulloa and Ping Wang*

*Feinstein Institute of Biomedical Research, *Department of Surgery, North Shore University Hospital, 350 Community Drive, Manhasset, NY 11030, USA*

Abstract. Severe sepsis, a leading cause of death in hospitalized patients, is one of the most dramatic examples of the pathological potential of inflammation. Since inflammation contributes to multiple clinical scenarios, it may not be surprising that diverse infectious and inflammatory disorders converge in the pathogenesis of severe sepsis. The physiological regulation of the immune responses by the nervous system represents effective anti-inflammatory mechanisms that can be exploited against inflammatory disorders. Recent studies indicate that acetylcholine, the principal cholinergic neurotransmitter, also functions as an immune cytokine that prevents macrophage activation through a 'nicotinic anti-inflammatory pathway'. Nicotine is more efficient than acetylcholine at inhibiting the NF-κB pathway and attenuating the production of proinflammatory cytokines from macrophages through a mechanism dependent on the α7-nicotinic acetylcholine receptor (α7nAChR). Treatment with nicotinic agonists attenuated systemic inflammation and improved survival in experimental sepsis in a clinically relevant time frame. Nicotine has already been used in clinical trials, but its clinical potential is limited by its collateral toxicity. Similar to the development of selective agonists for adrenergic receptors, selective nicotinic agonists for the α7nAChR may represent a promising pharmacological strategy against infectious and inflammatory diseases.

2007 Sepsis—new insights, new therapies. Wiley, Chichester (Novartis Foundation Symposium 280) p 223–237

Inflammation is a fundamental physiological process critical for survival, but at the same time, it is a major cause of human morbidity and mortality. One of the most dramatic examples of the pathological potential of inflammation is severe sepsis, the leading cause of mortality in critically ill patients. In the USA alone, severe sepsis affects over 750000 patients a year, and it accounts for 9.3% of overall deaths annually (Martin et al 2003, Hotchkiss & Karl 2003). Sepsis is defined by the clinical signs of systemic immune responses to infection. However, these clinical symptoms and the most characteristic clinical scenarios of sepsis, including the refractory arterial hypotension (septic shock) and multiple organ failure (severe sepsis), are not specific to infection and can also be produced by the immune responses of the host to injury or trauma (Cohen 2002, Ulloa 2005). In fact, despite the use of antibiotics, severe sepsis remains one of the most common causes of death in hospitalized patients, in part because antibiotics

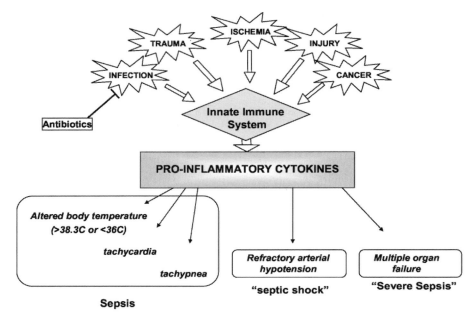

FIG. 1.   The pathogenesis of severe sepsis may not be exclusive to infections. Sepsis is defined by the clinical signs of systemic immune responses to infection. However, this clinical symptoms and the most characteristic clinical scenarios of sepsis including the refractory arterial hypotension (septic shock), and multiple organ failure (severe sepsis) are not specific to infection and can also be produced by the immune responses of the host to injury or trauma. Trauma, haemorrhage, shock, ischaemia and cancer can also cause systemic inflammatory responses leading to cardiovascular dysfunction and multiple organ failure similar to that described in severe sepsis. Currently there is a major interest in analysing the pathological potential of specific pro-inflammatory cytokines and their contribution to infectious and inflammatory disorders.

cannot control inflammation and systemic inflammation is not exclusive to infection (Fig. 1). Trauma, haemorrhage, shock, ischaemia and cancer can also cause systemic inflammatory responses leading to cardiovascular dysfunction and multiple organ failure similar to that described in severe sepsis. These inflammatory responses are characterized by an overwhelming production of pro-inflammatory cytokines that can become more dangerous than the original stimuli (Riedemann et al 2003, Rice & Bernard 2005). This clinical outcome is especially notable in severe sepsis, where the excessive production of proinflammatory cytokines causes cardiovascular dysfunction, capillary leakage, tissue injury and lethal multiple organ failure.

Among other pro-inflammatory cytokines, tumour necrosis factor (TNF)α, interleukins (ILs), and high mobility group box (HMGB)1 play a critical role in the pathogenesis of sepsis (Wang et al 1999, Ulloa & Tracey 2005). Recent studies indicate that TNFα is a major myocardial depressant factor, and a prototype inflammatory mediator of 'septic shock'. Administration of TNFα causes cardiovascular shock, hypotension, intravascular coagulopathy, and the characteristic haemorrhagic necrosis observed in 'septic shock'. Neutralization of TNFα prevents endotoxic- or bacteraemic-induced shock, even when endotoxin or bacteria persist in the circulation (Tracey & Cerami 1994). According to their causative effects, experimental strategies neutralizing these cytokines (monoclonal anti-TNFα antibodies, IL1 receptor antagonists, and TNFα–receptor fusion proteins) are successful therapeutic approaches to prevent tissue damage in several inflammatory disorders including rheumatoid arthritis and Crohn's disease (Feldmann 2002). However, these strategies have limited effects in sepsis, and failed to receive the approval of the Food and Drug Administration for the treatment of patients with severe sepsis (Abraham et al 1998). Although the reason for this challenging conundrum remains controversial, a potential explanation is that TNFα is not the only cytokine contributing to sepsis and therapeutic strategies against sepsis may require the inhibition of several pro-inflammatory cytokines (Ulloa et al 1999, Perl et al 2006). In agreement with this hypothesis, recent studies indicated that the administration of other proinflammatory cytokines such as HMGB1 recapitulated the most characteristic clinical signs of 'severe sepsis' including derangement of the intestinal barrier function, acute lung injury, multiple organ failure, and abrupt cardiac standstill (Wang et al 1999, Ulloa & Messmer 2006). Since the nervous system is the principal regulator of the immune system, neuronal anti-inflammatory strategies may represent comprehensive systems to control the production of different inflammatory cytokines and stop the pathological progression of sepsis (Miksa et al 2005, Ulloa 2005).

Neuronal strategy for inflammation

Recent studies indicated that the parasympathetic nervous system can control the immune system as a part of the composite physiological process of ingestion. The parasympathetic nervous system, which controls heart rate, hormone secretion, gastrointestinal peristalsis and digestion during ingestion, can also modulate the immune system to prevent an inflammatory response to commensal flora and dietary components. Ingestion of dietary fat stimulates cholecystokinin receptors and activates an anti-inflammatory mechanism mediated by the vagus nerve (Luyer et al 2005). The physiological implications of this mechanism are not limited to ingestion, and the parasympathetic nervous system can modulate inflammation in a variety of physiological scenarios including infection, trauma and injury. This physiological anti-inflammatory mechanism has a major clinical relevance because it can be exploited for the treatment of infectious and inflammatory disorders. Indeed, a growing number of studies indicate that the vagus nerve mediates the anti-inflammatory potential of a variety of pharmacological compounds such as non-steroidal anti-inflammatory drugs, semapimod, and melanocortin peptides (Ulloa 2005). Similar to cholecystokinin, melanocortin peptides and some non-steroidal anti-inflammatory drugs appear to control the production of pro-inflammatory cytokines through an anti-inflammatory mechanism mediated by the vagus nerve. As examples, semapimod and ACTH(1–24) activate efferent vagus nerve and limit circulating serum TNFα levels during endotoxaemia through a mechanism dependent on the vagus nerve because bilateral cervical vagotomy abrogates their anti-inflammatory potential. These anti-inflammatory effects are clinically significant because they confer protection against experimental sepsis by attenuating systemic inflammation and the subsequent cardiovascular dysfunction and multiple organ failure. These studies evidence a previously unrecognized role of the parasympathetic nervous system in mediating the action of pharmacological anti-inflammatory agents and thus, this mechanism can have a translational potential for the treatment of infectious and inflammatory disorders.

We recently discovered that acetylcholine, the principal neurotransmitter of the parasympathetic nervous system, can control the production of pro-inflammatory cytokines from macrophages (Wang et al 2004). Since acetylcholine signals through either muscarinic (G protein-coupled receptors) or nicotinic (ligand-gated ion channels) receptors (Miyazawa et al 2003), selective cholinergic agonists and antagonists were used to identify the receptors involved in the control of macrophage activation (Fig. 2). Muscarine slightly inhibited macrophage activation at supraphysiological levels, but nicotine was more efficient than acetylcholine at inhibiting the production of pro-inflammatory cytokines from macrophages (Wang et al 2004). These effects were specific for pro-inflammatory cytokines and neither acetylcholine nor nicotine inhibited the production of anti-inflammatory cytokines such as IL10. Although acetylcholine is historically referred to as a neurotransmitter, it can also function as an immune cytokine and may represent a common ancestral mediator in cellular biology. Acetylcholine is synthesized by both neurons and immune cells and serves as link for neural-immune coordination (Ulloa 2005). From a pharmacological perspective, the antiinflammatory effects of acetylcholine on macrophages seem to be mediated through nicotinic receptors, and nicotine is a more selective pharmacological agonist to control the production of pro-inflammatory cytokines.

Nicotinic acetylcholine receptors (nAChRs) are a family of ligand-gated ion channels composed of subunits that form homo- or heteropentameric receptors with distinct pharmacological properties. The nicotinic subunits identified include 10 α (α1–10), four β (β1–β4) and γ, δ and ε subunits. According to the structural organization, nAChRs are classified in muscle (composed of five different types

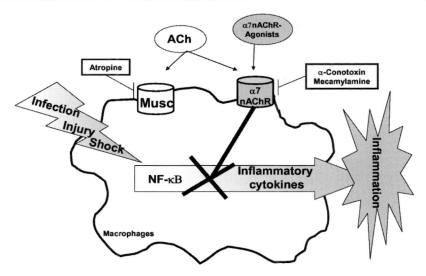

FIG. 2. Acetylcholine inhibits macrophage activation through a comprehensive 'nicotinic anti-inflammatory pathway'. Although acetylcholine is historically referred to as a neuro-transmitter, it can also function as an immune cytokine and may represent a common ancestral mediator in cellular biology. This mechanism implies a comprehensive 'nicotinic anti-inflammatory pathway' because nicotine is more efficient than acetylcholine at inhibiting macrophage activation, and it is dependent on the α7-nicotinic acetylcholine receptor (α7nAChR). A critical consideration is that selective α7nAChR agonists can avoid the toxicity of nicotine and provide a therapeutic anti-inflammatory potential for the treatment of infectious and inflammatory diseases.

of subunits) and neuronal (composed of α and β subunits) receptors that have been associated with neuromuscular junctions and neuronal synapses, respectively. Neuronal nAChRs can be subclassified according to their affinity for nicotine and α-bungarotoxin. Receptors that bind nicotine with high affinity contain α2–α6 as ligand binding subunits, and require β-subunits for proper activation. A second class of receptors (α7–α10) binds nicotine with low affinity and has high affinity for α-bungarotoxin. α7 subunits can form homopentameric receptors, and this α7nAChR is the only α-bungarotoxin binding receptor identified in mammalian brain, as α8 subunit appears to be expressed only in chick, and α9,10 subunit expression is limited to mechanosensory cochlear hair cells and the pituitary (Drisdel & Green 2000). In a similar approach, the presence of nAChRs in human macrophages was first suggested by using α-bungarotoxin and confirmed by RT-PCR. These studies indicate that macrophages are deficient in α9nAChR because they express mRNA for the α1 and α7 but not for α9 subunits (Wang et al 2003). Similar experiments failed to detect mRNA for the δ subunit (a necessary component of the α1-bearing nAChR) suggesting that human macrophages are deficient in functional α1-bearing nAChR. Western blot analysis revealed that the α7 protein expressed in macrophages has a relative molecular mass of 55 kDa that is identical to that described in neurons. The identity of the α7 subunit expressed on macrophages was confirmed by cloning and sequencing, and it is identical to the α7 subunit expressed in neurons. Together, these results indicate that human macrophages lack functional α1nAChR and α9nAChR, and that nicotinic modulation of macrophage activation is mediated by α7nAChRs.

Both acetylcholine and nicotine inhibit the production of pro-inflammatory cytokines from macrophages through a nicotinic signalling dependent on α7nAChRs (Wang et al 2004). The specific depletion of α7nAChRs in macrophages, using phosphorothioate antisense oligonucleotides, re-established the production of pro-inflammatory cytokines even in the presence of acetylcholine. Control sense oligonucleotides to α7nAChR and antisense oligonucleotides against similar regions in α1nAChR did not significantly affect the inhibitory potential of acetylcholine or nicotine in macrophages. Macrophages derived from α7nAChR knockout mice were also refractory to cholinergic agonists, and produced TNFα even in the presence of acetylcholine or nicotine. From a physiological perspective, mice lacking the α7nAChR develop normally and show no gross anatomical defects, but they are more susceptible to systemic inflammation and lethal endotoxaemia (Orr-Urtreger et al 1997). Endotoxin significantly causes higher levels of circulating TNFα, IL1 and IL6 in α7nAChR-deficient mice than in wild-type mice (Wang et al 2003), suggesting that this receptor can trigger a comprehensive 'nicotinic anti-inflammatory pathway' able to control the production of a variety of pro-inflammatory cytokines from macrophages.

The nicotinic anti-inflammatory pathway

Stimulation of macrophages with bacterial products induces the transcription of a number of pro-inflammatory cytokines (TNFα, IL1, IL6, IL18), and both acetylcholine and nicotine inhibit the production of these cytokines through a post-transcriptional mechanism without affecting their intracellular mRNA levels. This anti-inflammatory mechanism is especially relevant because, unlike the other cytokines, HMGB1 protein synthesis is required for survival, and thus, nicotine did not affect the intracellular levels of this factor (Wang et al 1999, Ulloa & Messmer 2006). HMGB1-deficient mice die within hours after birth, in part due to deficiency in gene expression induced by transcriptional factors such as glucocorticoid receptors (Calogero et al 1999). Endotoxin and other inflammatory stimuli activate macrophages and induce HMGB1 extracellular secretion. Extracellular HMGB1 functions as a pro-inflammatory cytokine that contributes to the pathogenesis of different inflammatory disorders including rheumatoid arthritis and severe sepsis (Ulloa et al 2003, Ulloa & Messmer 2006). Treatment with endotoxin and/or nicotine did not affect HMGB1 mRNA or total HMGB1 protein levels in macrophages. However, nicotine can halt HMGB1 secretion from macrophages by inhibiting its translocation from the nucleus to the cytoplasm, a critical step for its extracellular secretion. General inhibitors of protein synthesis (such as a cycloheximide) do not block HMGB1 secretion, suggesting that nicotine may regulate HMGB1 secretion through a posttranscriptional mechanism. Since HMGB1 secretion and binding to DNA may be modulated by post-translational regulation (Bianchi 2004), nicotine may impinge directly on macrophage activation by modulating HMGB1 acetylation or phosphorylation. Recent studies suggest that acetylcholine and nicotine inhibit the production of proinflammatory cytokines from macrophages by preventing the activation of the NF-κB pathway. Nicotine prevented the endotoxin-induced activation of the NF-κB pathway through a mechanism dependent on the α7nAChR because specific inhibition of this receptor in macrophages restored the endotoxin-induced activation of the NF-κB pathway even in the presence of nicotine (Wang et al 2004, Ulloa 2005). These results have been confirmed in other cell types and nicotine inhibits the NF-κB pathway in human U937 monocytic (Sugano et al 1998), and HuMVECs endothelial cells (Saeed et al 2005). These studies indicate that nicotine prevents LPS-induced nuclear translocation of the NF-κB complexes by preserving cytoplasmic levels of the I-κB inhibitors. However, it is unknown whether nicotine activates the transcription of specific I-κB inhibitors or inhibits an upstream mediator preventing I-κB ubiquitination and subsequent degradation. These studies are of special interest because nicotinic agonists inhibit macrophage activation through a mechanism that resembles vagus nerve stimulation (Ulloa 2005). Nicotinic agonists act on the α7nAChR to inhibit the NF-κB pathway and attenuate TNFα production in macrophages (Wang et al 2004). In a similar fashion, vagus nerve stimulation acts on the α7nAChR to inhibit the NF-κB pathway and attenuate TNFα production during endotoxaemia (Guarini et al 2004). Stimulation of the vagus nerve blunts the NF-κB signalling by preserving the I-κBα inhibitor protein levels in the liver. Likewise, nicotine blunts the NF-κB signalling by preserving the I-κBα inhibitor in human monocytic and endothelial cells. Although these studies refer to different experimental models (vagus nerve stimulation was analysed in haemorrhagic shock in rats, whereas the human monocytic and endothelial cells were activated with endotoxin), they also represent the critical contribution of NF-κB and TNFα to diverse clinical scenarios and inflammatory disorders. According to this reasoning, it may not be surprising that nicotine has already been used in clinical trials to control inflammation in a variety of clinical scenarios.

The therapeutic use of the anti-inflammatory potential of nicotine has been proposed for the treatment of a large number of diseases ranging from neurological diseases to inflammatory bowel disorders such as ulcerative colitis. To date, ulcerative colitis is the only condition for which controlled trials have provided evidence of the anti-inflammatory potential of nicotine. Most patients with ulcerative colitis are non-smokers, and patients with a history of smoking usually acquire their disease after they have stopped smoking. Patients who smoke intermittently often experience improvement in their colitis symptoms during the periods when they are smoking. Available treatments for ulcerative colitis are far from satisfactory and new strategies are needed. There are only two major treatments approved by the FDA, mesalamine and glucocorticoids, either of which may be poorly tolerated or ineffective in regular use. The addition of transdermal nicotine to conventional therapy improves significantly symptoms in patients with ulcerative colitis for six weeks in a randomized, double-blind study. Seventeen of the 30 patients that finished the nicotine treatment had complete remissions, as compared with nine of the 37 patients in the placebo group (Pullan et al 1994). However, five out of 35 patients in the initial nicotine group withdrew from treatment because of intolerable side effects. The most common side effects were nausea, lightheadedness, headache, sleep disturbance and dizziness. These studies indicate that the anti-inflammatory potential of this mechanism is limited by the collateral toxicity of nicotine. A critical consideration is that selective α7nAChR agonists can avoid the toxicity of nicotine and provide a therapeutic anti-inflammatory potential for the treatment of infectious and inflammatory diseases.

Selective α7nAChR agonists have been designed to activate the neurons of the central nervous system in patients with Alzheimer's disease. Among other compounds, nefiracetam (N-[2,6-dimethylphenyl]-2-[2-oxo-1-pyrrolidinyl]acetamide) and GTS-21 (3-[(2,4-dimethoxy)benzylidene]-anabaseine dihydrochloride) are selective agonists designed to activate the α7nAChR in the cerebral cortex and hippocampus, which are the most affected areas in Alzheimer's patients (Kitagawa et al 2003). GTS-21 can protect neurons against damage induced by amyloid peptides suggesting that α7nAChRs may have a protective neuronal role *in vitro*. However, clinical trials in patients with Alzheimer's disease suggest that GTS21 induces a limited effect on the CNS because of its limited ability to cross the blood–brain barrier. An interesting consideration is that from an immunological perspective, this characteristic is an advantage, it avoids potential secondary effects of GTS21. In fact, GTS21 has no effect on locomotor activity in mice or dopamine turnover in rats indicating that it appears to have a less toxic effect than nicotine. Furthermore, patients tolerated well doses of up to 450 mg/day, and there were no clinically significant differences in adverse events between the treatment groups.

Concluding remarks

Acetylcholine, the principal neurotransmitter of the parasympathetic nervous system, can control the production of pro-inflammatory cytokines from macrophages, and temper systemic inflammation during sepsis. This novel mechanism implies a comprehensive 'nicotinic antiinflammatory pathway' because nicotine is more efficient than acetylcholine at inhibiting macrophage activation, and it is dependent on the α7nAChR. Recent studies suggest that the specific activation of the α7nAChR can be sufficient to mimic the anti-inflammatory effects of nicotine. This hypothesis is consistent with recent studies indicating that specific nicotinic acetylcholine receptors mediate specific physiological effects of nicotine. For instance, specific activation of α4nAChR or α5nAChR is sufficient for tolerance and sensitization or allodynia, respectively (Tapper et al 2004, Vincler et al 2005). Nicotine has already been used in clinical trials to control inflammation and prevent the pathogenesis of ulcerative colitis. However, the anti-inflammatory potential of this mechanism is limited by the collateral toxicity of nicotine. Similar to the development of alpha- and beta-agonists for adrenergic receptors, the design of selective α7nAChR agonists may avoid the toxicity of nicotine and represent a promising pharmacological strategy to control systemic inflammation in infectious and inflammatory diseases. This mechanism has a major interest because it regulates the NF-κB pathway inducing a comprehensive anti-inflammatory potential against a variety of pro-inflammatory cytokines. These studies represent a clinical challenge because the NF-κB contributes to the production and cytotoxicity of proinflammatory cytokines, but it also appears to protect parenchyma cells from cytotoxic reagents and cell death. For instance, inhibition of NF-κB after partial hepatectomy resulted in massive hepatocyte apoptosis associated with impaired liver function and decreased survival (Iimuro et al 1998). Treatment with anti-HMGB1 antibodies, that prevented hepatic injury in response to ischaemic insult, enhanced activation of the NF-κB pathway *in vivo* (Tsung et al 2005). However, anti-HMGB1 antibodies abrogated the activation of NF-κB in HMGB1-challenged enterocytes and prevented intestinal derangements (Sappington et al 2002). These studies suggest that unless the therapy is specifically targeted to cytokine-producing cells, inhibition of NF-κB activity may not generate an overall beneficial effect, especially in tissue injuries such as hepatic. Future studies should determine the therapeutic anti-inflammatory potential of selective α7nAChR-agonists and whether they can provide a means to inhibit NF-κB activity in specific cytokine-producing cells such as macrophages.

References

Abraham E, Anzueto A, Gutierrez G et al 1998 Double-blind randomised controlled trial of monoclonal antibody to human tumour necrosis factor in treatment of septic shock. Norasept ii study group. Lancet 351:929–933

Bianchi ME 2004 Significant re location: how to use chromatin and/or abundant proteins as messages of life and death. Trends Cell Biol 14:287–293

Calogero S, Grassi F, Aguzzi A et al 1999 The lack of chromosomal protein Hmg1 does not disrupt cell growth but causes lethal hypoglycaemia in newborn mice. Nat Genet 22:276–280

Cohen J 2002 The immunopathogenesis of sepsis. Nature 420:885–891

Drisdel RC, Green WN 2000 Neuronal-bungarotoxin receptors are 7-subunit homomers. J Neurosci 20:133–139

Feldmann M 2002 Development of anti-TNF-α therapy for rheumatoid arthritis. Nat Rev Immunol 2:364–371

Guarini S, Cainazzo MM, Giuliani D et al 2004 Adrenocorticotropin reverses hemorrhagic shock in anesthetized rats through the rapid activation of a vagal anti-inflammatory pathway. Cardiovasc Res 63:357–365

Hotchkiss RS, Karl IE 2003 The pathophysiology and treatment of sepsis. N Engl J Med 348:138–150

Huston J, Ochani M, Liao H et al 2006 Splenectomy inactivates the cholinergic anti-inflammatory pathways during lethal endotoxemia and polymicrobial sepsis. J Exp Med 203:1623–1628

Iimuro Y, Nishiura T, Hellerbrand C et al 1998 NFkappaB prevents apoptosis and liver dysfunction during liver regeneration. J Clin Invest 101:802–811

Kitagawa H, Takenouchi T, Azuma R et al 2003 Safety, pharmacokinetics, and effects on cognitive function of multiple doses of GTS-21 in healthy, male volunteers. Neuropsychopharmacology 28:542–551

Luyer MD, Greve JW, Hadfoune M et al 2005 Nutritional stimulation of cholecystokinin receptors inhibits inflammation via the vagus nerve. J Exp Med 202:1023–1029

Martin GS, Mannino DM, Eaton S et al 2003 The epidemiology of sepsis in the United States from 1979 through 2000. N Engl J Med 348:1546–1554

Miksa M, Wu R, Zhou M, Wang P 2005 Sympathetic excitotoxicity in sepsis: pro-inflammatory priming of macrophages by norepinephrine. Front Biosci 10:2217–2229

Miyazawa A, Fujiyoshi Y, Unwin N 2003 Structure and gating mechanism of the acetylcholine receptor pore. Nature 423:949–955

Orr-Urtreger A, Goldner FM, Saeki M et al 1997 Mice deficient in the 7 neuronal nicotinic acetylcholine receptor lack-bungarotoxin binding sites and hippocampal fast nicotinic currents. J Neurosci 17:9165–9171

Perl M, Chung CS, Garber M, Huang X, Ayala A 2006 Contribution of anti-inflammatory/immune suppressive processes to the pathology of sepsis. Front Biosci 11:272–299

Pullan RD, Rhodes J, Ganesh S et al 1994 Transdermal nicotine for active ulcerative colitis. N Engl J Med 330:811–815

Rice TW, Bernard GR 2005 Therapeutic intervention and targets for sepsis. Annu Rev Med 56:225–248

Riedemann NC, Guo RF, Ward PA 2003 Novel strategies for the treatment of sepsis. Nat Med 9:517–524

Saeed RW, Varma S, Peng-Nemeroff T et al 2005 Cholinergic stimulation blocks endothelial cell activation and leukocyte recruitment during inflammation. J Exp Med 201:1113–1123

Sappington PL, Yang R, Yang H et al 2002 HMGB1 B box increases the permeability of Caco-2 enterocytic monolayers and impairs intestinal barrier function in mice. Gastroenterology 123:790–802

Sugano N, Shimada K, Ito K, Murai S 1998 Nicotine inhibits the production of inflammatory mediators in U937 cells through modulation of nuclear factor-kappaB activation. Biochem Biophys Res Commun 252:25–28

Tapper AR, McKinney SL, Nashmi R et al 2004 Nicotine activation of alpha4 receptors: sufficient for reward, tolerance, and sensitization. Science 306:1029–1032

Tracey KJ, Cerami A 1994 Tumor necrosis factor: a pleiotropic cytokine and therapeutic target. Annu Rev Med 45:491–503

Tsung A, Sahai R, Tanaka H et al 2005 The nuclear factor HMGB1 mediates hepatic injury after murine liver ischemia-reperfusion. J Exp Med 201:1135–1143

Ulloa L 2005 The vagus nerve and the nicotinic anti-inflammatory pathway. Nat Rev Drug Discov 4:673–684

Ulloa L, Tracey KJ 2005 The 'cytokine profile': a code for sepsis. Trends Mol Med 11:56–63

Ulloa L, Messmer D 2006 High-mobility group box 1 (HMGB1) protein: friend and foe. Cytokine Growth Factor Rev 17:189–201

Ulloa L, Doody J, Massague J 1999 Inhibition of transforming growth factor-beta/SMAD signalling by the interferon-gamma/STAT pathway. Nature 397:710–713

Ulloa L, Batliwalla FM, Andersson U et al 2003 High mobility group box chromosomal protein 1 as a nuclear protein, cytokine, and potential therapeutic target in arthritis. Arthritis Rheum 48:876–881

Vincler MA, Eisenach JC 2005 Knock down of the alpha 5 nicotinic acetylcholine receptor in spinal nerve-ligated rats alleviates mechanical allodynia. Pharmacol Biochem Behav 80:135–143

Wang H, Bloom O, Zhang M et al 1999 HMG-1 as a late mediator of endotoxin lethality in mice. Science 285:248–251

Wang H, Yu M, Ochani M et al 2003 Nicotinic acetylcholine receptor alpha7 subunit is an essential regulator of inflammation. Nature 421:384–388

Wang H, Liao H, Ochani M et al 2004 Cholinergic agonists inhibit HMGB1 release and improve survival in experimental sepsis. Nat Med 10:1216–1221

DISCUSSION

Marshall: The fact that you can abolish the effect with an antisense suggests that the $\alpha7$ receptor is dynamically regulated. Do you know anything about the regulation of the synthesis of the $\alpha7$ receptor?

Ulloa: That is an important consideration, and we haven't looked yet at the regulation or production of the receptor, or its sensitization.

Thiemermann: Is there much else known about GTS21? If it is available, you may have tried it in other conditions.

Ulloa: GTS21 is a selective nicotinic agonist that was designed to target neuronal $\alpha7$ nicotinic receptors in the brain of patients with Alzheimer's disease. Clinical trials using GTS21 for the treatment of Alzheimer's disease were unsuccessful. Most of the studies related to GTS21 were performed in neurons and very little is known about its effects in other cell types including macrophages. An interesting consideration is that some authors propose that GTS21 failed the clinical trials in Alzheimer's disease because it may have limited ability to cross the blood–brain barrier. If so, this is an interesting consideration because this feature can be an advantage to target peripheral inflammation and avoid side and collateral effects in the brain.

Radermacher: When you look at the data on pharmacological stimulation of the vagus, does sympathetic blockade using epidural anaesthesia have any impact on the HMGB1 release?

Ulloa: In our experimental models, we have found that different anaesthetics modify the inflammatory response and affect the anti-inflammatory potential of the vagus nerve. Indeed, there is a wide diversity of compounds that can induce a pharmacological activation of the vagus nerve. A growing number of studies indicate that non-steroidal anti-inflammatory drugs, semapimod, and melanocortin peptides have an anti-inflammatory potential, that is at least in part, mediated by the vagus nerve (Ulloa 2005). This is an exciting new field and we did not have the opportunity to study the effect of sympathetic compounds. However, we expect a coordination between the sympathetic system and the vagus nerve. The sympathetic system has an anti-inflammatory potential that may contribute to the anti-inflammatory mechanism of the vagus nerve.

Szabó: We have been playing with this from a different angle. Some years ago we had a few studies looking at lipopolysaccharide (LPS)-stimulated macrophages, testing the effect of adrenergic compounds. We found that β agonists were also able to suppress inflammatory responses (Szabo et al 1997). This was primarily by cAMP pathway. Even dopamine acts like this. When we normally think about the sympathetic/parasympathetic system, these two in many cases transmit opposing effects. From your data it seems that the parasympathetic activation has some kind of anti-inflammatory effect, but many other data suggest that the sympathetic activation can also have anti-inflammatory effects, so it seems to me that they don't actually oppose each other in this respect.

Ulloa: Both systems are probably working alongside each other *in vivo.* The vagus nerve affects the sympathetic nervous system, and modulates the production of catecholamines. In a similar way, nicotinic agonists also appear to affect the production of catecholamines. We will have to determine whether the sympathetic nervous system may contribute to the anti-inflammatory potential of nicotinic agonists.

Szabo: There is a paper we have published where we found that nicotine inhibits type 1 diabetes (Mabley et al 2002). We could never really place it anywhere or make a connection with anything we know about. The islet cell destruction could have some similar mechanism to what you talked about here.

Fink: This is one of the great stories in immunology over the last few years. But like everything, there are some pieces missing. One of the pieces that hasn't been published yet, but which I know you have done, is vagal nerve stimulation in animals with carageenan-induced paw swelling. When you stimulate the vagal nerve in these mice after injecting carageenan, they don't develop the swelling. Vagal nerve stimulation is having an anti-inflammatory effect to a place where the vagal nerve doesn't go. How does this happen?

Ulloa: This study published by Dr Metz indicates that nicotinic agonists inhibit the NF-κB pathway in endothelial cells (Saeed et al 2005), results that are in agreement with our previous studies indicating that nicotinic agonists inhibit the activation of the NF-κB pathway in macrophages (Wang et al 2004). At a physiological level, this study also indicated that vagal stimulation prevented inflammation in the carrageenan air pouch model. Although it is difficult to explain these results because the vagus nerve does not innervate the feet, we believe that one potential explanation is that the vagus nerve is controlling the production and maturation of immune cells in the thymus and the spleen. If so, vagus nerve can induce a systemic anti-inflammatory potential and modulate leukocyte recruitment during inflammation. Indeed we are publishing an article (Houston et al 2006) indicating that the innervation of the spleen by the vagus nerve can be critical to the control of systemic inflammation.

Fink: It's an important observation. It says to me that vagal nerve stimulation has some primary effects because of the innervation of cells by the vagus. But the vagus nerve doesn't innervate most of the macrophages in your body! It certainly doesn't innervate your feet. This suggests that the main mechanism involves an intermediate step, whether it is in the spleen or somewhere else. This suggests that there is another drug target here. There is a mediator that comes between the vagal nerve stimulation and the immune cell.

Marshall: The vagus probably does innervate the largest population of macrophages in the body, in the liver.

Fink: No one has taken a picture, though, of a vagal nerve touching a macrophage.

Marshall: Is there a soluble factor in those animals, which, when added to culture will have an effect? Why is it that patients who have had a vagotomy do not appear to be adversely affected when they become septic?

Ulloa: In order to demonstrate a physical synapse between the vagus nerve and macrophages, we spent almost a year trying to get a picture of the vagus nerve connecting Kupffer cells in the liver. Although we know that the vagus nerve innervates the liver we couldn't capture that physical connection.

Marshall: There is a vagal branch to the liver.

Fink: I think it stops at the capsule. When you slice the liver there aren't vagal afferents going into the stuff.

Marshall: What about a vagotomy? This would seem to suggest that the worst thing you could do for someone would be a vagotomy, but this used to be a common procedure.

Ulloa: Vagotomy increases the susceptibility of rodents to endotoxaemia and sepsis. However, we haven't seen any epidemiological studies supporting that hypothesis in humans.

Radermacher: On the other hand, this could be a hint about why patients after oesophageal resection often do so badly. You most often inevitably damage the vagal nerve in this procedure.

Marshall: Maybe it is the lung.

Fink: Everyone has always assumed that the reason oesophageal surgery is risky is because the oesophagus doesn't have a serosa. But perhaps it is because almost all the time it involves vagotomy.

Singer: On the practical issues, anaesthetists often give glycopyrolate to block the vagus, and they might use inotropes. Do you think all of these things are actually causing harm?

Radermacher: On the other hand, you normally administer anaesthetics, which is what I was referring to with my comment about epidural anaesthesia. It is not stimulating the vagus directly, but a good, well done epidural anaesthesia will block the sympathetic system and consequently result in increased vagal tone. Surgeons sometimes complain that when the sympathetic blockade is instituted, there is a contraction of the intestine *in situ*, which makes it harder to do sutures. This is interpreted as a sign of a rebalancing in favour of the vagal nerve. In your measurements on the HMGB1 plasma levels, is there a difference between people who had an epidural and those who didn't?

Fink: We haven't looked at that. I agree that activation of the α7 receptor clearly blocks NF-κB activation and HMGB1 secretion. But I think these facts are unrelated. We have used three completely different approaches to block NF-κB activation, including molecular approaches. The α7 agonists do a lot of things to the cell, and not all of them converge on HMGB1 secretion. In other words, there may be more than one signalling pathway in the cell that is affected.

Ulloa: I agree with those results. Our results are very similar, nicotinic agonists prevent the activation of the NF-κB, but we don't know yet, whether this is a critical step to inhibit HMGB1 release.

Singer: Do opioids have any effect?

Fink: Absolutely. There is a literature that dates back to the 1980s showing that there are morphine receptors on neutrophils (Sharp et al 1985). There are morphine receptors of at least a couple of different types on macrophages. The opioid part of the neuro/immuno pharmacology was much better developed until recently than the vagal nerve part, although I think the vagal nerve part is a lot more interesting. The notion was that this was why stress is immunosuppressive. If you do cold restraint stress on mice and then measure delayed-type hypersensitivity (DTH) responses or proinflammatory cytokine release, they are all depressed. This was thought to be because of endogenous opioid release.

Radermacher: It is well known that the more recent opioids have a marked vagal activity beyond their effects as anaesthetics or narcotics.

Gilroy: Do all macrophages respond in an anti-inflammatory manner to nicotine?

Ulloa: That is a good question. Our studies indicated that peritoneal macrophages are the best at responding to nicotinic agonists. Circulating macrophages didn't appear to be very good. The effects of nicotinic agonists is especially controversial in alveolar macrophages depending on the cell line analyzed. While nicotine attenuates both TNF and IL10 production in murine alveolar macrophage AMJ2-C11 cells, nicotine attenuates TNF but not IL10 production in murine alveolar macrophage MH-S cells. The expression of the α7nAChR wasn't confirmed in these MH-S cells, but it was confirmed in other cell lines including alveolar type II cells and free alveolar macrophages.

Gilroy: You also mentioned that monocytes that make their way to the lung during inflammation tend to be different to those which make their way to the peritoneal cavity. If you took out inflammatory monocyte-derived macrophages that went to the lung, would they also be deficient in their ability to respond to nicotine?

Ulloa: We haven't done that experiment. However, vagal nerve stimulation attenuates TNF production in most of the organs but not in the lung. We should now perform a similar experiment with nicotinic agonists.

Pugin: Acetylcholine is very short-lived in body fluids. Is it fair to say that it is not the antagonist that we are looking for?

Ulloa: When we are looking for the systemic pathway that might be mediated by the vagal nerve, acetylcholine is unstable and probably not the best chemical candidate. One possibility is that a breakdown product of acetylcholine or nicotine can also provide an anti-inflammatory potential. Indeed, a treatment with nicotine provides a prophylactic potential in endotoxaemia even when it is administered long before the LPS injection.

Fink: Is choline immunosuppressive?

Ulloa: Yes, choline is not as efficient as nicotine or other nicotinic agonists and it also attenuates the production of pro-inflammatory cytokines from macrophages (Ulloa & Messmer 2006).

References

Huston J, Ochani M, Liao H et al 2006 Splenectomy inactivates the cholinergic anti-inflammatory pathway during lethal endotoxemia and polymicrobial sepsis. J Exp Med 203:1623–1628

Mabley JG, Pacher P, Southan GJ, Salzman AL, Szabo C 2002 Nicotine reduces the incidence of type I diabetes in mice. J Pharmacol Exp Ther 300:876–881

Saeed RW, Varma S, Peng-Nemeroff T et al 2005 Cholinergic stimulation blocks endothelial cell activation and leukocyte recruitment during inflammation. J Exp Med 201:1113–1123

Sharp BM, Keane WF, Suh HJ, Gekker G, Tsukayama D, Peterson PK 1985 Opioid peptides rapidly stimulate superoxide production by human polymorphonuclear leukocytes and macrophages. Endocrinology 117:793–795

Szabo C, Hasko G, Zingarelli B et al 1997 Isoproterenol regulates tumour necrosis factor, interleukin-10, interleukin-6 and nitric oxide production and protects against the development of vascular hyporeactivity in endotoxaemia. Immunology 90:95–100

Ulloa L 2005 The vagus nerve and the nicotinic anti-inflammatory pathway. Nat Rev Drug Discov 4:673–684

Ulloa L, Messmer D 2006 High-mobility group box 1 (HMGB1) protein: friend and foe Cytokine Growth Factor Rev 17:189–201

Wang H, Liao H, Ochani M et al 2004 Cholinergic agonists inhibit HMGB1 release and improve survival in experimental sepsis. Nat Med 10:1216–1221

Beta-blockade in burns

C. T. Pereira, M. G. Jeschke and D. N. Herndon[1]

Shriners Hospitals for Children, 815 Market Street, Galveston, Texas 77550-2725 and The University of Texas Medical Branch, 301 University Boulevard, Galveston, Texas 77555-0527, USA

Abstract. A significant proportion of the mortality and morbidity of severe burns is attributable to the ensuing hypermetabolic response that typically lasts for at least 9–12 months post-injury. This is associated with impaired wound healing, increased infection risks, erosion of lean body mass, hampered rehabilitation and delayed reintegration of burn survivors into society. The endocrine status is markedly altered during this period with an initial and then sustained increase in proinflammatory 'stress' hormones such as cortisol and other glucocorticoids, and catecholamines including epinephrine and norepinephrine by the adrenal medulla and cortex. These hormones exert catabolic effects leading to muscle wasting, the intensity of which depends upon the percentage of total body surface area (TBSA) involved, as well as the time elapsed since initial injury. Pharmacological and non-pharmacological strategies may be used to reverse the catabolic effect of thermal injury. Of these, β-adrenergic blockade with propranolol has been the most efficacious anti-catabolic therapy in the treatment of burns. The underlying mechanism of action of propranolol is still unclear, however its effect appears to occur due to an increased protein synthesis in the face of a persistent protein breakdown and reduced peripheral lipolysis. This article aims to review the current understanding of catecholamines in postburn muscle wasting and focuses on the clinical and metabolic effects of β-blockade in severe burns.

2007 Sepsis—new insights, new therapies. Wiley, Chichester (Novartis Foundation Symposium 280) p 238–251

The greatest achievement in severe burn management over the past two decades has been the prompt excision and immediate closure of burn wounds. This has favourably affected mortality and morbidity from severe thermal injury. However, despite this major advance, patients are subject to a persistent hypermetabolic response and catabolism which is more severe and sustained than any other form of trauma. It can begin as early as day 5 post-injury and last at least nine months thereafter (Reiss et al 1956, Hart et al 2000). Its intensity is directly proportional to the percentage of total body surface area (TBSA) involved, as well as the time elapsed since initial injury. Thus the resting metabolic rates in burn patients

---

[1]This paper was presented at the Symposium by D. N. Herndon, to whom correspondence should be addressed.

increase in a curvilinear fashion ranging from near normal for burns less than 10% total body surface area (TBSA) to twice normal in burns over 40% TBSA. In patients with burn injuries greater than 40% TBSA, the resting metabolic rate at a thermally neutral temperature (33 °C) reaches 180% of the basal rate during acute admission, 150% at full healing of the burn wound and 140%, 120% and 110% at 6 months, 9 months and 12 months post injury, respectively (Hart et al 2000).

Muscle wasting, defined as the unintentional loss of 5–10% of muscle mass, occurs when there is an imbalance between protein synthesis and degradation. Post-burn metabolic derangements lead to an amplification of lean muscle protein breakdown in both the acute and convalescent phases of burn injury (Jahoor et al 1998). Enhanced oxygen consumption occurs secondary to increased energy expenditure in the major visceral organs and tissues. This results from significant aberrations in the major ATP consumption pathways that control the increased protein turnover; enhanced gluconeogenesis, elevated urea production and substrate cycling that occur in severely burned patients (Yu et al 1999). A substrate cycle exists when opposing, non-equilibrium reactions catalysed by different enzymes are active simultaneously. Stable isotope tracer studies have demonstrated that significant increases occur in total rates of gluconeogenic and triglyceride-fatty acid cycling (250% and 450% respectively) (Hart et al 2000). Alanine and other three-carbon amino acids that are released due to continuing degradation of peripheral muscle are also used as substrate for the increased gluconeogenic drive. The continuing protein degradation is disconcerting since animal research studies and isolated observations in starving human beings have demonstrated that loss of a quarter of total body nitrogen can be fatal. This limit can easily be reached in 3–4 weeks in untreated burned patients where daily losses of 20–25 g/m^2 per day occur if patients do not receive maximal nutritional support (Rutan & Herndon 1990). The aim of clinical care is to ensure both the survival and maximal rehabilitation of the severely burned patient in the shortest possible period of hospitalization. Facilitating an early return to normal function can be achieved if the loss of nitrogen is restricted during the acute flow phase and the protein stores can be replenished during convalescence to facilitate an early return to normal function. Evidence-based improvements in surgical and nursing care, such as early excision and closure, prompt treatment of sepsis, maintenance of ambient temperature to 33 °C and vigorous nutritional support have been shown to attenuate persistent protein catabolism that occurs following severe burns. However, they cannot in isolation completely reverse this phenomenon, requiring therefore further investigation into more innovative and effective techniques if we are to prevent the loss of lean body mass and growth delay in severely burned children (Rutan & Herndon 1990). New and innovative methods to modulate post-burn hormonal imbalances using anabolic agents such as growth hormone (GH), insulin, insulin-like growth factor (IGF)1, IGF1 and IGF binding protein 3 (IGFBP3) combinations, oxandrolone, or testosterone and anticatabolic agents such as adrenergic antagonists (propranolol or metoprolol), have been the subject of intensive study (Herndon & Tompkins 2004). Of these, the attenuation of muscle catabolism has become the principle target of efforts to modify hypermetabolic physiology owing to its deleterious effects both during the acute and convalescent phase of burn recovery.

Molecular mechanisms regulating muscle proteolysis

The mechanisms causing muscle-specific atrophy are undoubtedly complex, but some insights into the mechanisms have been provided recently. Understanding this is important if we are to produce efficient techniques to effectively attenuate muscle-wasting trajectories. Growth factors such as IGF1 and proinflammatory cytokines such as tumour necrosis factor (TNF)α have been implicated in playing a role in post-burn muscle atrophy (Fang et al 2002, Baracos et al 1983). Reduction in circulating and muscle IGF1 concentrations occurs in most catabolic situations (Heszele & Price 2004). Preventing this decline via systemic infusions alleviates post-burn muscle wasting (Herndon et al 1999). Studies in many different rodent models of muscle wasting have indicated that the ubiquitin–proteasome pathway is the main pathway associated with accelerated proteolysis induced by burns and excess glucocorticoids (Mitch & Goldberg 1996, Chai et al 2002). Ubiquitin (7.6 kDa) is a small molecular weight polypeptide whose conjugation to protein substances takes place through a sequence of reactions requiring the hydrolysis of ATP. Prevailing evidence suggests that the targeting of proteins for destruction by ubiquitin conjugation is regulated during atrophy. The conjugation of ubiquitin to proteins occurs in a series of steps involving distinct enzymes or complexes. The key enzymes in this process are the E3 ubiquitin ligases, which act as the substrate recognition component of the ubiquitin conjugation recognition component of the ubiquitin conjugation machinery and prevent proteins from undergoing non-specific modification. Notably, three E3s are uniquely expressed in muscle: MAFbx/atrogin-1, MuRF1 and E3α-II (Gomez et al 2001, Bodine et al 2001, Kwak et al 2004). Little is known about the substrates of these E3 ligases, except that atrogin 1 targets MyoD in skeletal muscle (Tintignac et al 2005) while MuRF1 targets troponin I in cardiomyocytes (Kedar et al 2004). Recent studies have demonstrated that IGF1 inhibits the expression of atrogin 1, and to some extent MuRF-1, in myotubes and muscle (Dehoux et al 2004, Sacheck et al 2004). Inhibition of phosphoinositide 3-kinase (PI3K) prevents the anabolic effects of IGF1 (or insulin) in cultured muscle cells (Dehoux et al 2004, Sacheck et al 2004). Another consequence of activating the PI3K pathway is the Akt-dependent phosphorylation of FOXO proteins, which regulates the transcription of metabolic genes. Mutating the Akt phosphorylation sites in FOXO prevents the increased transcription of MAFbx/atogin 1 and MuRF1, while overexpressing it suppresses atrogin 1 expression (Sandri et al 2004). FOXO proteins also regulate muscle mass through actions other than on genes for protein degradation, such as genes for muscle cell growth and differentiation and metabolism (Sandri et al 2004). Hormones such as glucocorticoids and possibly catecholamines exert their catabolic effect by interfering with the phosphorylation of FOXO and the expression of MAFbx/atogin 1 and MuRF1 (Sandri et al 2004). Evidence indicates that IGF1 and insulin also inhibit muscle proteolysis via FOXO-independent mechanisms. Yasuhara et al (1999, 2000) showed that cytochrome c is released from mitochondria into the cytosol within 1 hour after burn due to altered mitrochondrial membrane potential. Ceramide, a key apoptotic second messenger, increases leading the activation of stress-activated protein kinase (a downstream-signalling kinase of ceramide), leading ultimately to activation of caspase 1, 3 and 9. These changes occurred in muscle distant to the burn wound. Further, postburn insulin resistance is secondary to an impaired postreceptor insulin signalling mechanism (Yashura et al 2000). PI3K, via its activation of a further downstream molecule, Akt, is a key anti-apoptotic factor. Burns induce an increased Ca^{2+} availability in skeletal muscle (Sayeed 2000). The PI3K pathway is sensitive to Ca^{2+} in that enhanced cytosolic Ca^{2+} can suppress PI3K activation (Sayeed 2000). It is conceivable, therefore, that the apoptosis observed in burns is related to impaired growth factor (insulin) signalling. How anabolic hormones such as insulin/IGF1 suppress caspase 3 activity in skeletal muscle is not well understood.

The nuclear factor kappa B (NF-κB) is another signalling system implicated in the regulation of skeletal muscle mass. The NF-κB family of transcription factors have been linked to muscle atrophy caused by burns (Shea et al 2003). MyoD and cyclin D genes are targeted by NF-κB, which are responsible for muscle cell differentiation and activating some segments of the ubiquitin–proteasome pathway (Shea et al 2003). Thus the role of NF-κB in muscle atrophy goes beyond the role of proinflammatory cytokines such as TNFα.

IGF1 and insulin acting through the PI3K pathway are therefore important regulators of muscle mass. A reduction in PI3K activity increases the FOXO-dependent transcription of muscle-specific E3 ubiquitin ligases and caspase-dependent cleavage of myofibrillar proteins. Other signalling proteins such as the inhibitor of NF-κB kinase/NF-κB system are also important determinants of muscle mass. It is likely that the proportionate role of any given pathway depends upon the pathophysiological circumstances, mechanism of injury, hormonal milieu and distance from the burn wound. Further studies are required to clarify the relative contribution of different ubiquitin ligases to muscle wasting under different conditions.

Rationale for use of β-blockade in burn management

Role of catecholamines in post-burn hypermetabolism

Endotoxin, IL1 and 6, platelet-activating factor, TNF, arachidonic acid metabolites via the cyclooxygenase and lipooxygenase pathways, reactive oxygen species, neutrophil-adherence complexes, nitric oxide (NO) and the complement and coagulation cascades have all been implicated in the post-burn hypermetabolic response (Sheridan 2001). The release of these mediators is thought to be triggered by a combination of factors, including a change in hypothalamic function with coincident increases in stress hormone levels; impairment of the gastrointestinal mucosal barrier with bacterial translocation; and wound infection and heat loss through trans-eschar fluid evaporation. Of these mediators, the complex change in hormonal milieu post-burn, especially of catecholamines, has been securely implicated in animal as well as human studies as a primary mediator (Wilmore et al 1974, Herndon 1981). Post-injury increase in oxygen consumption was blunted to 7–15% after adrenalectomy, with steroid support having little effect; it was blunted to 16% when catecholamine stores were depleted with a monoamine oxidase inhibitor, reserpine; the response was blunted to 11–19% when prostaglandin synthesis or effect was blocked by the competitive inhibitors indomethacin, RO2-5720 and meclofenamate. This suggests that catecholamines but not thyroid hormone or steroids, are the primary efferent mediator by which the hypothalamus effects central metabolic reset (Herndon 1981). Goodall et al (1957) have shown urinary excretion of catecholamines to be elevated in proportion to increases in metabolic rate subsequent to increasing burn size. This increase can be as much as 10 times and correlates well with the elevated metabolic rate, suggesting that the metabolic response to burn trauma 'escapes' the usual refractory state produced with chronic exposure to catecholamines. Aprille et al (1979) showed that adenylate cyclase was resistant to desensitization by chronic exposure to catecholamines in a murine burn model, suggesting that chronic elevations of catecholamines evoke regulatory mechanisms in target cells to circumvent the desensitization which would otherwise occur consequent to acute exposures to catecholamines. Thus changes in receptor density and efficacy may provoke additional metabolic modulation in the burned patient.

Metabolic effects of catecholamines

The main metabolic effects of adrenergic agents refer to increased glucose production, enhanced Cori cycle and glucose-alanine cycle activity and hyperglycaemia. Increased catecholamine output also stimulates both amino acid and lactate acid efflux from muscle and fat breakdown and release from lipocytes. It increases glucagon secretion, which in turn promotes hepatic gluconeogenesis. This occurs especially when the increase is relative to insulin (Aprille et al 1979). This ratio appears central to the regulation of skeletal muscle uptake and release of amino acids, relatively low levels of insulin favouring release. Glucose and insulin support in burn patients does not decrease hypermetabolism but does preserve body mass, reverses nitrogen balance, and retains energy stores (Wilmore et al 1971). Thus catecholamines play a key role in the initiation of the various cascades leading to post-burn hypermetabolism. Once initiated these cascades, their mediators and their by-products appear to stimulate the persistent and increased metabolic rate seen after severe burn injury. Blocking the triggering of these cascades at the onset by blocking the action of catecholamines at the receptor level could attenuate this response and improve clinical outcomes. Blockade of β-adrenergic stimulation after severe burns decreases supraphysiological thermogenesis (Herndon et al 1988), tachycardia, cardiac work (Barron et al 1997) and resting energy expenditure (Breitenstein et al 1990).

Modulation of post-burn catecholamine response

Alterations in protein kinetics that are responsible for the increased loss of nitrogen following severe trauma occur as a result of two distinct phenomenon, (a) increase in protein breakdown and (b) decrease in protein synthesis (Jahoor et al 1988). Protein kinetics studies in burned patients suggest that the flow phase post-burn is associated with an inability of the protein synthetic rate to keep up with the elevated rate of protein degradation. The anabolic response of convalescence on the other hand is due to the protein synthetic rate exceeding protein degradation (Jahoor et al 1988). This is an important finding since it demonstrates that it is possible to achieve a protein anabolic state in the face of an elevated protein breakdown. Several studies have been conducted on the use of β-blockade to modulate the post-burn response in the short term (Herndon et al 1988, Barron et al 1997, Breitenstein et al 1990). Since β-blockade has been shown to decrease resting energy expenditure after burns (Breitenstein et al 1990), we conducted clinical trials on the long-term use of propranolol based on the hypothesis that the propranolol-induced reduction in resting energy expenditure in the short-term would translate to decreased rate of muscle-protein catabolism in the long-term. Twenty-five children with acute and severe burns (>40% TBSA) and similar demographics were studied in a randomized trial (Herndon et al 2001). Thirteen received oral propranolol for at least two weeks and 12 served as untreated controls. The dose of propranolol was adjusted to decrease the resting heart rate by 20% from each patient's base-line value. We have shown previously that this is safe (Baron et al 1997) and does not reduce the ability of patients with burns to respond to cold-induced stress (Honeycutt et al 1992). Resting energy expenditures and skeletal-muscle protein kinetics were measured before and after two

weeks of β-blockade (or no treatment, in controls). Body composition was measured serially throughout hospitalization. β-blockade reduced heart rates and
resting energy expenditure in the propranolol group as compared with controls.
Net muscle-protein balance was increased by 82% over baseline values in the
propranolol group whereas it decreased by 27% in the control group. The fat-free
mass, as measured by whole-body potassium scanning did not change substantially in the propranolol group, whereas it decreased significantly in the control
group. Stable-isotope data showed acceleration in the rate of protein synthesis in
the propranolol-treated patients. It is the myofibrillar protein that constitutes the
majority of protein undergoing breakdown and causing net protein loss. The
underlying mechanism is still unclear. However, our studies indicate that propranolol induces an increase in the intracellular recycling of free amino acids. In
the process of substrate reuse, free intracellular amino acids derived from stimulated protein breakdown were incorporated back into bound protein without
leaving the myocyte (Herndon et al 2001). We showed that propranolol did not
change the inward transport of protein but did increase the efficiency of protein
synthesis in muscle. Net balance of protein increased due to an increase in protein
synthesis in the face of continued protein breakdown. This correlated well with
the finding that the increase in expression of genes involved in protein synthesis
such as HSP70 (GRP-78KD-NM005347), which plays a significant role in the
recovery of mRNA translation during the stress response, eukaryotic initiation
factor 2 cycling and ribosomal mRNA loading. The expression of fructose-1,6-
bisphosphatase 2 (Y12235), encoding a key regulatory enzyme of gluconeogenesis
that catalyses the hydrolysis of fructose-1,6-bisphosphatase to generate fructose-
6-phosphate and inorganic phosphate, was suppressed nearly threefold in propranolol-treated children (Herndon et al 2003). Further, gene expression profiles
and protein balance studies in skeletal muscle of burned children done at our
institute, after β-blockade (propranolol), have shown a significant up-regulation
in genes involved in muscle metabolism and down-regulation of an important
enzyme involved in gluconeogenesis and insulin resistance compared with burned
children receiving placebo (Herndon et al 2003). Propranolol appears to improve
lean body mass by increasing the efficiency of protein synthesis in muscle rather
than by increasing the inward transport of protein. It does this by inducing an
increase in the intracellular recycling of free amino acids, thus recycling the free
intracellular amino acids derived from protein breakdown, back into bound
protein. It also up-regulates genes involved in muscle metabolism and down-
regulates genes involved in gluconeogenesis, thereby decreasing the catabolic
drive.

We have previously documented an increased lipolysis secondary to elevated
catecholamines in severely burned children (Aarsland et al 1996). Increased lipolysis, results in an increased plasma fatty acid level, which leads to an increased

storage of fatty acids within the splanchnic bed. As delivery of fatty acids to the liver increases, uptake increases proportionately. However, the rate of hepatic fatty acid oxidation is inhibited by the hyperglycaemia/hyperinsulinaemia often present in burn patients, without affecting uptake. Fatty acids taken up by the liver are channelled away from oxidation and towards triacylglycerol (TAG) synthesis. The release of hepatic TAG into the blood (via VLDL-TAG) is inhibited in burn patients. Thus hepatic fat accumulation results from an imbalance between fatty acid uptake, oxidation, and release via very-low-density lipoprotein (VLDL)-triacylglycerols (Herndon et al 1994, Aarsland et al 1996). Nutritional support is ineffective in avoiding fatty livers in burn patients since the amount of hepatic fat storage in critically ill patients is a function of the seriousness of the illness, presumably because the extent of stimulation of lipolysis is related to the seriousness of the illness. Hence pharmacological management may be necessary to preserve the integrity of the liver. We have shown that β-blockade (propranolol) lowers peripheral lipolysis and increases the efficiency of the liver in secreting fatty acids in burned children receiving growth hormone (Aarsland et al 1996). Further, propranolol decreased splanchnic fatty acid storage in burned children receiving high carbohydrate diets (Morio et al 2002). No inhibition of lipolysis was noted in this study, probably because the high-carbohydrate diet had already maximally inhibited lipolysis. Since the major effect of propranolol was a decrease in splanchnic blood flow, the low rate of lipolysis in propranolol treated patients could be explained by the reduced inflow of fatty acids into the splanchnic bed.

Overall, the anabolic effects of propranolol treatment appear to occur due to an increased protein synthesis in the face of a persistent protein breakdown and reduced peripheral lipolysis. Further propranolol may benefit burn patients by decreasing hepatic TAG storage and maintaining the integrity of liver function.

Implications for the future

Patients with burns below 40% TBSA are rarely hypermetabolic unless septic. Those with burns above 40% are always catabolic, effecting metabolic derangements that persist for at least a year after injury in most body tissues, especially skeletal muscle. Muscle catabolism is a principle therapeutic target, due to its direct effects on survival in the acute phase and its indirect effects on rehabilitation in the convalescent phase. Burn associated catabolism cannot be completely reversed, but may be manipulated by non-pharmacological and pharmacological means (anabolic and anti-catabolic) (Herndon & Tompkins 2004). It should be noted that anabolic agents are only beneficial for patients who are catabolic. Anticatabolic agents, such as propranolol, during acute care and rehabilitation greatly assist therapeutic minimization of loss of lean body mass and linear growth delay, and are effective in both septic and non-septic burned patients (Hart et al

2001). The underlying mechanism of action of propranolol is still unclear. It is possible that its effect occurs directly via its effects on the protein flux machinery either at the level of the gene through up-regulation of protein synthetic genes in muscles or at the level of the amino acid cycles by increasing capture of free intracellular amino acids into bound protein. It could also work via indirect modulations of the signal transduction pathways and cell receptor responsiveness leading to decreased insulin resistance and reduced regional blood flow.

Hypermetabolic physiology probably had survival value as it is well retained across mammalian species. However in the current modern medical era, it is widely accepted to have maladaptive features that may actually impair recovery. An incomplete understanding of the cellular and subcellular biology of injury physiology has limited our ability to modify it. Continuing research efforts in the molecular mechanisms behind hypermetabolic physiology will lead to an enhanced ability to control it and is likely to translate to improved clinical outcomes for our patients.

References

Aarsland A, Chinkes D, Wolfe RR et al 1996 Beta-blockade lowers peripheral lipolysis in burn patients receiving growth hormone. Rate of hepatic very low-density lipoprotein triglyceride secretion remains unchanged. Ann Surg 223:777–787

Aprille JR, Aikawa N, Bell TC, Bode HH, Malamud DF 1979 Adenylate cyclase after burn injury: resistance to desensitization by catecholamines. J Trauma 19:812–818

Baracos V, Rodermann HP, Dinarello CA, Goldberg AL 1983 Stimulation of muscle protein degradation and prostaglandin E2 release by leukocytic pyrogen (interleukin-1). A mechanism for the increased degradation of muscle proteins during fever. New Engl J Med 308:553–558

Baron PW, Barrow RE, Pierre EJ, Herndon DN 1997 Prolonged use of propranolol safely decreases cardiac work in burned children. J Burn Care Rehabil 18:223–227

Bodine SC, Latres E, Baumhueter S et al 2001 Identification of ubiquitin ligases required for skeletal muscle atrophy. Science 23:1704–1708

Breitenstein E, Chiolero RL, Jequier E, Dayer P, Krupp S, Schutz Y 1990 Effects of beta-blockade on energy metabolism following burns. Burns 16:259–264

Chai J, Wu Y, Sheng Z 2002 The relationship between skeletal muscle proteolysis and ubiquitin-proteasome proteolytic pathway in burned rats. Burns 8:527–533

Dehoux M, Van Beneden R, Pasko N et al 2004 Role of the insulin-like growth factor I decline in the induction of atrogin-1/MAFbx during fasting and diabetes. Endocrinology 145:4806–4812

Fang CH, Li BG, Wray CJ, Hasselgren PO 2002 Insulin-like growth factor-I inhibits lysosomal and proteasome-dependent proteolysis in skeletal muscle after burn injury. J Burn Care Rehabil 23:318–325

Gomes MD, Lecker SH, Jagoe RT, Navon A, Goldberg AL 2001 Atrogin-1, a muscle specific F-box protein highly expressed during muscle atrophy. Proc Natl Acad Sci USA 98: 14440–14445

Goodall MC, Stone C, Haynes BW Jr 1957 Urinary output of adrenaline and nonadrenaline in severe thermal burns. Ann Surg 145:479

Hart DW, Wolf SE, Mlcak R et al 2000 Persistence of muscle catabolism after severe burn. Surgery 128:312–319

Hart DW, Wolf SE, Chinkes DL, Wolfe RR 2001 Anabolic strategies after severe burn. Ann Surg 233:556–564

Herndon DN 1981 Mediators of metabolism. J Trauma 21:701–705

Herndon DN, Tompkins RG 2004 Support of the metabolic response to burn injury. Lancet 363:1895–1902

Herndon DN, Barrow RE, Rutan TC, Minifee P, Jahoor F, Wolfe RR 1988 Effect of propranolol administration on hemodynamic and metabolic responses of burned pediatric patients. Ann Surg 208:484–492

Herndon DN, Nguyen TT, Wolfe RR et al 1994 Lipolysis in burned patients is stimulated by the beta 2-receptor for catecholamines. Arch Surg 129:1301–1304

Herndon DN, Ramzy PI, DebRoy MA et al 1999 Muscle protein catabolism after severe burn: the effect of IGF-1 over IGF BP3 treatment. Ann Surg 229:713–722

Herndon DN, Hart DW, Wolfe SE, Chinkes DL, Wolfe RR 2001 Reversal of catabolism by beta-blockade after severe burns. New Engl J Med 345:1223–1229

Herndon DN, Dasu MRK, Wolfe RR, Barrow RE 2003 Gene expression profiles and protein balance in skeletal muscle of burned children after α-adrenergic blockade. Am J Physiol Endocrinol. Metab 285:E783–789

Heszele MF, Price SR 2004 Insulin-like growth factor I: the yin and yang of muscle atrophy. Endocrinology 145:4803–4805

Honeycutt D, Barrow RE, Herndon DN 1992 Cold stress response in patients with severe burns after beta-blockade. J Burn Care Rehabil 13:181–186

Jahoor F, Desai MH, Herndon DN, Wolfe RR 1998 Dynamics of protein anabolic response to burn injury. Metabolism 37:330–337

Kedar V, McDonough H, Arya R, Li HH, Rockman HA, Patterson C 2004 Muscle-specific RING finger 1 is a bona fide ubiquitin ligase that degrades cardiac troponin I. Proc Natl Acad Sci USA 101:18135–18140

Kwak KS, Zhou X, Solomon V et al 2004 Regulation of protein catabolism by muscle-specific and cytokine-inducible ubiquitin ligase E3alpha-II during cancer cachexia. Cancer Res 15:8193–8198

Mitch WE, Goldberg AL 1996 Mechanisms of muscle wasting. The role of the ubiquitin-proteasome pathway. New Engl J Med 335:1897–1905

Morio B, Irtun O, Herndon DN, Wolfe RR 2002 Propranolol decreases splanchnic triacylglycerol storage in burn patients receiving a high-carbohydrate diet. Ann Surg 236:218–225

Reiss W, Pearson E, Artz CP 1956 The metabolic response to burns. J Clin Invest 35:62–77

Rutan RL, Herndon DN 1990 Growth delay in post-burn pediatric patients. Arch Surg 125:392–395

Sacheck JM, Ohtsuka A, McLary SC, Goldberg AL 2004 IGF-I stimulates muscle growth by suppressing protein breakdown and expression of atrophy-related ubiquitin ligases, atrogin-1 and MuRF-1. Am J Physiol Endocrinol Metab 287:E591–601

Sandri M, Sandri C, Gilbert A et al 2004 Foxo transcription factors induce the atrophy-related ubiquitin ligase atrogin-1 and cause skeletal muscle atrophy. Cell 117:399–412

Sayeed MM 2000 Signaling mechanisms of altered cellular responses in trauma, burn and sepsis. Arch Surg 135:1432–1442

Shea JE, Bowman BM, Miller SC 2003 Alterations in skeletal and mineral metabolism following thermal injuries. J Musculo Neuronal Interaction 3:214–222

Sheridan RL 2001 A great constitutional disturbance. New Engl J Med 34:1271–1272

Tintignac LA, Lagirand J, Batonnet S, Sirri V, Leibovitch MP, Leibovitch SA 2005 Degradation of MyoD mediated by the SCF (MAFbx) ubiquitin ligase. J Biol Chem 280:2847–2856

Wilmore DW, Curreri PW, Spitzer KW 1971 Supranormal diet in thermally injured patients. Surg Gynecol Obstet 132:881

Wilmore DW, Long JM, Mason AD Jr, Skreen RW, Pruit BA Jr 1974 Catecholamines: mediator of the hypermetabolic response to thermal injury. Ann Surg 180:653–669

Yasuhara S, Perez ME, Kanakubo E et al 1999 Burn injury induces skeletal muscle apoptosis and the activation of caspase pathways in rats. J Burn Care Rehabil 20:462–470

Yasuhara S, Perez ME, Kanakubo E et al 2000 Skeletal muscle apoptosis after burns is associated with activation of proapoptotic signals. Am J Physiol Endocrinol Metab 279: E1114–11121

Yu YM, Tompkins RG, Ryan CM, Young VR 1999 The metabolic basis of the increase in energy expenditure in severely burned patients. J Parenter Enteral Nutr 23:160–168

DISCUSSION

Griffiths: One of the things that has greatly impressed me in this series of work is that it addresses a long term problem, but the elegance is that it is a titratable treatment. This is like the glucose story: it is something the clinicians can address, because the right amount can be administered to the right people due to this marker of suppressed heart rate.

Herndon: Physicians are uncanny in their ability to take a pulse. Propranolol can be titrated to the pulse rate.

Griffiths: The pulse is a beautiful marker of this hypermetabolism which we can make use of.

Fink: I have been following your part of this story most closely since your report about the effects of recombinant growth hormone (GH) and the effects of propranolol (Herndon et al 2001, Ramirez et al 1998). I am struck by the fact that so much of what you are advocating for these (mostly paediatric) burn patients is the opposite of what we are doing for adult intensive care unit (ICU) patients. You are advocating β-blockade; we use catecholamines to support the cardiovascular system. You advocate using anabolic hormones; we talk about using oestrogens as anti-inflammatory agents. You advocate using rhGH, but the Takala et al (1999) study would suggest that in an adult critical care patient, this is positively lethal. Is this because children with burns are different from adult patients, or are we doing something wrong? One area where there is consistency is what Greet Van den Berghe is recommending, which is giving lots of insulin, an anabolic hormone with what you are recommending.

Herndon: There is a tremendous age effect. The interaction of age with the hypermetabolic response can't be understated. You get very old very quickly in relationship to a burn. Whereas a 98% burn is survived half the time in children under the age of 14, a 50% burn is 50% lethal in people over 50. Many therapies that can be tolerated in children can't be tolerated in adults. I think the physiological responses and cascades that occur are essentially the same, it is just that the therapies can't be tolerated as well.

Singer: I have a slightly tongue-in-cheek question: how much of the β-blockade effect is helping the cholinergic sympathetic/parasympathetic balance, and how much is preventing glucose toxicity?

Herndon: It has both effects. Using a β blocker does improve glucose control indirectly. It directly affects parasympathetic tone.

Singer: Can you speculate on proportions? Is one mode or mechanism predominant?

Herndon: β-blockade is a large bat that is changing a basic physiological mediator that affects grossly many different systems. I don't think we can point to any particular effect as being dominant.

Singer: Do you give corticosteroids to your patients?

Herndon: They are used in conditions in which adrenal insufficiency is expected. ACTH challenge tests are done to identify which patients should receive those therapies. It is rare that this occurs, but it does.

Singer: Is that when they are 'septic' or hyperdynamic or vasodilated?

Herndon: Hypotenstion is usually the trigger to do the test.

Singer: Do you then stop the β blockers?

Herndon: Yes.

Fink: β blockers have been shown to be beneficial in all kinds of conditions. But the ones that are relevant to what we all do include perioperatively in high-risk surgical patients, outpatient management of severe congestive heart failure, outpatient management of patients after myocardial infarction and burn patients. Except for our patients who are hypotensive and needing cardiovascular support, do you think it would be reasonable to consider a clinical trial of β-blockade as a standard therapeutic intervention in haemodynamically stable critically ill adults?

Herndon: Yes. In particular for any patient who is tachycardic, you can make a sound physiological argument that by decreasing pathological tachycardia this decreases cardiac work. The other metabolic benefits of the treatment would more than justify a trial.

Griffiths: The β-blockade isn't starting until about two weeks into these childrens' illness. In a sense, these are super-repairing machines. When you are dealing with the elderly, we are struggling in the first periods with the failures of the systems, and our little repair machines that we are dealing with may not be switching on. The use of the β-blockade may not be within that timeframe—perhaps even longer than 2 weeks later.

Radermacher: With respect to the hypotensive children, did you look at vasopressin levels? Instead of stopping β blockade, did you consider using vasopressin in order to support the blood pressure? This may not help the heart itself, but combining the β blockade for that purpose and treating the hypotension with something else could change the paradigm of haemodynamic support.

Hendon: That's a good point. Vasopressin is effective in those rare patients who do become hypotensive. Pathological tachycardia should always be treated with β blockade. You will improve cardiac output by decreasing tachycardia. I haven't thought about combining the two.

Evans: What do you think about other long-term inflammatory problems, such as TB or HIV, where there is considerable long-term muscle wasting?

Herndon: I feel that chronic administration of anabolic agents and agents that decrease sympathetic tone will be standard treatments in diseases like HIV or chronic wasting diseases.

Szabó: Is there a β receptor subtype difference in the metabolic effects versus the cardiovascular effects?

Herndon: The primary cardiac effect is a β1 effect, decreasing heart rate. The reason we use the combined β1/β2 blocker is that the β2 effect abolishes lipolysis. It would perhaps be wiser to use selective blocking agents if they were available. β3 blocking agents haven't yet reached market and would need to be tested separately.

Szabó: If the problem is just peripheral vasodilation, there are probably five or six agents that could be used instead of catechols. Some of these are overcoming this NO-mediated resistance. There are probably other ways of driving the heart, too. So why is it that this is still the standard of care?

Herndon: The tachycardia was the first thing we tried to control. This is the reason the β-blocking agents were so useful perioperatively in decreasing myocardial infarction. They slow down the heart rate. The peripheral vascular tone effects are secondary to that. A β1-blocking agent is more specific for the heart alone, and those are the kinds of β blockers that were used in the perioperative cardiac trials. Our interest extended to preventing peripheral lipolysis.

Singer: The worry is that just because we can use something different, it doesn't mean it is safer. With vasopressin, sometimes the patients do a Lazarus, but other times you just see horrible necrotic fingers and toes. We don't understand half of what we are doing pharmacologically.

Van den Berghe: The unifying mechanism for the insulin effects, the β blocker effects and the potential deleterious effects of GH is the lipolysis. Insulin and β blockers prevent it, while GH is lipolytic. Your GH studies showed that the children had an increased liver size. This is fine for children, whose β cells are able to compensate. But for adults this may be a problem.

Herndon: I too have thought that the lipids were the common pathway. They are understudied. The dyskinesia of lipids is fairly important in critical illness.

Singer: Do you use insulin a lot in your children?

Herndon: Absolutely. Propranolol and insulin are additive.

Singer: Do you use it for sugar control, or over and above? Does everyone get it?

Herndon: We began studying it as an anabolic agent, and gave hyperinsulinaemic euglycaemic clamps through acute hospitalisation in children, before even studying propranolol. It is a useful therapy in this patient population.

References

Herndon DN, Hart DW, Wolf SE, Chinkes DL, Wolfe RR 2001 Reversal of catabolism by beta-blockade after severe burns. N Engl J Med 345:1223–1229

Ramirez RJ, Wolf SE, Barrow RE, Herndon DN 1998 Growth hormone treatment in pediatric burns: a safe therapeutic approach. Ann Surg 228:439–448

Takala J, Ruokonen E, Webster NR et al 1999 Increased mortality associated with growth hormone treatment in critically ill adults. N Engl J Med 341:785–792

System interactions

Mervyn Singer

Bloomsbury Institute of Intensive Care Medicine, Dept of Medicine and Wolfson Institute of Biomedical Research, University College London, Gower Street, London WC1E 6BT, UK

Abstract. The paradigm of sepsis as an excessive inflammatory response to infection should now be extended to include activation and/or depression of numerous systems within the body. These include neural, immune, hormonal, bioenergetic and metabolic pathways. The levels of activity of these systems vary both with illness severity and over time. Perturbation of the components of each pathway is independently associated with a heightened mortality risk yet interactions and temporal relationships remain poorly understood. A better delineation of this intricate network and an enhanced ability to monitor these changes should lead to improved targeting of interventions and an avoidance of potentially harmful therapeutic strategies. In addition, greater recognition of the deleterious covert effects on these systems of many therapies currently established as standard management, for example inotropes, antibiotics and sedatives, should hopefully minimise the iatrogenic contribution to mortality and morbidity.

2007 Sepsis—new insights, new therapies. Wiley, Chichester (Novartis Foundation Symposium 280) p 252–265

Sepsis is currently defined as an exaggerated and systemic inflammatory response to infection (Bone et al 1992). The bulk of sepsis research in the past few decades has been primarily geared towards inflammatory and immune aspects, however the present definition fails to take into account the major involvement of most (if not all) other systems within the body, including neural, endocrine, coagulant, bioenergetic and metabolic. The degrees of perturbation of these pathways have all been independently associated with worse clinical outcomes and little attention has been paid towards interactions between these different systems. This article attempts to bring together current knowledge and to speculate as to how targeted therapeutic modulation may impact positively upon morbidity and mortality.

Adaptive or maladaptive?

The oldest fossil evidence for anatomically modern humans dates back approximately 130 000 years. Our species has thus been long exposed to a variety of thermal, infectious, traumatic and malnutritonal insults. Clearly, we have evolved sophisticated defence mechanisms to cope with such insults and, by a natural selection process, the more hardy individuals have survived to foster successive generations. In health, we live in perfect symbiosis with several kilograms of bacteria that also serve to protect against exogenous flora. Basic mechanisms such as fever and sympathetic activation are important intrinsic responses that protect against a stressful insult such as bacterial infection (Romanosky & Szekely 1998). Cross-talk is mandatory so that these activated pathways can communicate and coordinate their response to facilitate survival. Importantly, there has to be negative feedback and regulatory control mechanisms to prevent excessive and prolonged systems activation (or suppression).

The current mainstream view of sepsis is that this regulatory control is lacking, probably due to an as yet undefined genetic predisposition, allowing an exaggerated and amplified inflammatory response to infection (or other insult) that is out of proportion to the body's needs (Hotchkiss & Karl 2003). This is then considered to lead to the development of multiple organ failure and, in 20–60% of cases, to the death of the individual. While there is certainly an element of truth, this stance rather neglects certain salient details that enable this condition to be potentially viewed in a different light. Unless patients have specific genetic mutations leading to conditions such as complement deficiency or agranulocytosis, and thus an increased predisposition to infection, it is highly unusual for the same individual to present with recurrent episodes of septic shock or multi-organ failure following a further infectious episode. A fascinating paradox of multi-organ failure is the strikingly normal histological appearance of these severely dysfunctional organs with surprisingly little evidence of cell death (Hotchkiss et al 1999). Furthermore, the high likelihood of recovery of organ function in survivors (Noble et al 2001) is in contrast to organ-specific disease such as glomerulonephritis. This does imply that the response to a severe and prolonged inflammatory insult may be adaptive rather than maladaptive; the individual may move from an initial 'offensive' strategy at the onset of infection to one of organ shutdown in the hope of riding out the insult without permanently compromising organ function and thus enabling long-term survival. Until the near-recent introduction of long-term mechanical organ support, for example renal dialysis, severe and long-standing organ failure had to be fatal. Thus the patient can withstand a short period of anuria lasting several days, but longer-term survival is incumbent on relatively prompt recovery of organ function.

The iatrogenic component

We perhaps naively and arrogantly consider medical developments to have started in earnest within the last century or so, with replacement of herbal and quack remedies and the barber surgeons by sophisticated and highly-engineered new drugs and devices, and well-trained and educated staff. However, scrutiny of outcomes of injured soldiers from historical battles show remarkably good survival rates (Singer & Glynne 2005). For example, of the 102 injured sailors on HMS Victory who survived the battle and immediate aftermath of the Battle of Trafalgar in 1805, only six subsequently died of their wounds. Yet ten amputations were performed onboard the ship, under less than ideal conditions, and deaths from gangrene and tetanus were reported. Though these sailors were likely to have been relatively young and fit, nutritional deficiency and poor hygiene and sanitation were the norm. It could be argued that we have lost a lot of our natural immunity by living in today's more sterile and sanitized environment and are thus less well able to respond to a severe extrinsic insult. We should also consider the impact of modern medical management—for example, the crucial skin barrier is penetrated by numerous cannulae and drains; the patient receives sedatives that will blunt the neurosympathetic response and modulate hormonal, immune and mitochondrial function; inotropes are given that will exogenously increase catecholamine levels with effects on metabolism, inflammation and bacterial growth; high levels of oxygen are administered with the attendant risk of further oxidant injury; corticosteroids are given to suppress the inflammatory response; other people's antigenic blood is transfused; and so forth (Singer & Glynne 2005). Greater cognizance of the effects of our interventions on all the various aspects of the acute and prolonged stress response to injury may either lessen the initial severity or shorten the duration of organ dysfunction.

The early 'acute phase' response

Clearly, the onset of infection cannot be accurately timed unless it occurs directly during an intervention such as intraoperative bowel perforation or nephrolithotripsy, or is performed within a research study. Using experimental animal models of sepsis or volunteer endotoxaemia studies, an acute inflammatory response can, in a dose-dependent fashion, be detected within the first few hours (Michie et al 1988). Clinical evidence of temperature change and sympathetic stimulation (tachycardia, blood pressure alterations, sweating) accompany non-specific symptoms such as malaise and fatigue. Metabolic rate and oxygen consumption increase, pro-inflammatory cytokines such as tumour necrosis factor (TNF)α and interleukin 1 can be detected in the plasma, and levels of stress hormones such as cortisol, catecholamines and vasopressin rise. White cell, platelet and endothelial activation leads to increased production of proteases, oxidants, vasoactive mediators (e.g. nitric oxide, prostaglandins, thromboxanes), and thrombin. Positive feedback from these products stimulates further inflammatory mediator release, thus amplifying and perpetuating the cycle.

The down-regulation phase

As well as effects on gene expression (*q.v.*), there is direct damage and/or inhibition of target cells involved in normal functioning of both the end-organs and effector pathways. Apart from the development of multiple organ failure, which occurs without cell death being a major feature (Hotchkiss et al 1999), there is a down-regulation of all the pathways that are initially activated (Hotchkiss & Karl 2003). This appears to commence within hours-to-days of the initiating insult. The degree of down-regulation has been individually associated with worse outcomes, e.g. immunosuppression (Tschaikowsky et al 2002), bioenergetic-metabolic shutdown (Brealey et al 2002), and various hormonal deficiency syndromes, e.g. corticosteroid insufficiency (Annane et al 2000), low T3 syndrome (Kaptein et al 1982), and hypoleptinaemia (Bornstein et al 1998). However, little research to date has attempted to determine the temporal relationships between these different pathways and any common causative factors. This phase of critical illness is associated with marked catabolism, manifest as muscle wasting, and which is considerably in excess of that caused by starvation alone. This occurs despite concerted attempts to feed the patient, either enterally or parenterally.

The recovery phase

A further fascinating paradox of multi-organ failure is the ability in surviving patients of their organs to recover (relatively) normal functioning such that life-long dependency on an organ support device is unnecessary (Noble et al 2001). Clearly, the relative absence of cell death is a fundamental ingredient to enable recovery as many cell types are poorly regenerative. Indeed, we have hypothesized that multi-organ failure is a process analogous to hibernation or aestivation and may actually represent a protective, adaptive response to enable the individual to cope with severe, prolonged inflammation after the initial offensive approach has been overwhelmed (Singer et al 2004). Even the severe muscle wasting may be explained in similar terms. From an evolutionary standpoint, the septic individual would have been unlikely to be able to hunt or forage thus body stores of fat and protein provide an important endogenous source of substrate to enable essential metabolic activity to continue. The recovery period is, however, rather variable (days to months) and evidence of systemic inflammation has often long abated. This is, in part, related to secondary nosocomial infections that are more likely to occur in the immunosuppressed milieu of multi-organ failure and which can contribute to further bouts of inflammation. We have also argued that many of our routinely used medications, including antibiotics and sedatives, will suppress mitochondrial function and biogenesis (Singer & Glynne 2005). The lack of sufficient energy production will thus prevent the restoration of metabolic activity needed to maintain normal cellular processes.

The recovery period is characterized by evidence of mitochondrial biogenesis (Suliman et al 2004) and an increase in metabolic activity, overshooting values seen in health (Kreymann et al 1993), that will enable anabolic processes such as protein synthesis to proceed.

Changes in phenotype

Other than direct effects on target proteins or damage to the organ itself, there are marked temporal changes in phenotype during sepsis that are presumed to lead to significant differences in protein encoded. Post-transcriptional modifications remain to be determined, however studies utilizing multiarray analysis are now appearing that demonstrate an effect on gene expression. A recent study (Calvano et al 2005) assessed changes in leukocyte gene expression patterns over a 24 h period in volunteers given a single dose of endotoxin, thus allowing precise timing of the initiating inflammatory insult. Of 44 000 probe sets, the signal intensity of 5093 probe sets (representing 3714 unique genes) was significantly affected. A minority of probe sets were induced by 2 h; over half showed *reduced* abundance at 2–9 h but returned to baseline by 24 h; while the remainder showed a delayed response, peaking at 4–9 h but returning to baseline by 24 h. Expression of various pro-inflammatory cytokines and chemokines (e.g. TNF, IL1α, IL1β, IL8, MCP1) reached a maximum at 2–4 h post-endotoxin, consistent with an early activation of innate immunity. The 4–6 h period post-endotoxin appeared critical, with increased expression of a number of transcription factors that both initiate (e.g. STAT, CREB and CEBP gene families) and limit (e.g. SOCS3 and IKBK genes) the innate immune response. There was also increased mRNA abundance of secreted and membrane-associated proteins that limit the inflammatory response, including those encoding TNF soluble receptor, IL1 receptor antagonist and IL10. As active secretory cells, leukocytes devote a substantial amount of energy expenditure to protein synthesis. Of note, alongside suppression of genes involved in energy production (e.g. components of mitochondrial respiratory chain complexes I, III and V), there was down-regulation of genes encoding for both protein synthesis and protein degradation. The response to endotoxin administration in these blood leukocytes can thus be viewed as an integrated cell-wide response, propagating and resolving over time in a self-limiting fashion. Importantly, this study also demonstrates how leukocytes exposed to inflammatory stimuli are likely to have an altered capacity to sustain subsequent immune challenges.

Nitric oxide

Nitric oxide (NO) is an important intercellular signalling molecule involved in regulating diverse physiological and pathophysiological mechanisms in the nervous, cardiovascular, immunological and other systems with effects on smooth muscle relaxation, neurotransmission, platelet aggregation, host defence, immunity and inflammation. It also has a crucial influence in modulating energy production (Brown & Borutaite 2002). Excess production of NO, produced predominantly by the inducible isoform of NO synthase (iNOS), plays a critical role in sepsis (Titheradge 1999). Though poorly defined *in vivo,* the consequent effects are likely to depend on both the degree and duration of NO production, with totally opposing actions (stimulatory and inhibitory) being reported in the same system. NO affects: (i) the *inflammatory response* with both pro- and anti-inflammatory effects ascribed; (ii) *cell-mediated immunity*—NO has a powerful and ubiquitous immunosuppressive role in a variety of inflammatory models (Grimm et al 2002); (iii) *cell death*—NO is reported to both incite and protect against apoptosis and necrosis (Vodovotz et al 2004); (iv) *vascular smooth muscle*—causing excess relaxation and hyporeactivity (decreased responsiveness to [endogenous and exogenous] catecholamines) (O'Brien et al 2001), thus resulting in the clinical condition of septic shock, affecting blood pressure and tissue perfusion; (v) *mitochondrial respiration*—ATP production, which is integral to fuelling cellular metabolism, is impaired (Brealey et al 2002); and (vi) *endocrine function*—at all levels of the hypothalamic–pituitary hormone-secreting organ axis. Depending on dose, duration and site of action, NO has both stimulatory and inhibitory effects on hormone production (including cortisol, thyroxine, prolactin and sex hormones). For example, endogenous NO has been shown to decrease ACTH (Gadek-Michalska & Bugajski 2004) and vasopressin release in endotoxic shock (Carnio et al 2005). However, dose-dependent and differential effects of endotoxin have also been noted, with high doses stimulating CRF and vasopressin release from the hypothalamus, whereas low doses inhibited pituitary release of ACTH and vasopressin (Rivier 2003). NO has been shown to be integral for ACTH-stimulated release of corticosterone from the adrenal gland (Mohn et al 2005) but, on the other hand, it also inhibited release of catecholamines from sympathetic nerves and the adrenal medulla, and decreased the biological activity of catecholamines (Macarthur et al 1995). Positive and negative feedback also occurs for NO production. For example, NO directly inhibits its own synthase (Griscavage et al 1995) while, in endotoxaemia, eNOS-derived NO is integral in stimulating iNOS induction (Vo et al 2005). Thyroid status also has effects on NO production, for example, hypothalamic expression of NOS was significantly reduced in hypothyroidism (Ueta et al 1995), whereas liver and skeletal muscle mitochondrial NOS activities were significantly increased, correlating inversely with both serum T3 levels and oxygen uptake (Carreras et al 2001). The capacity for vascular nitric oxide (NO) formation and the ability of the vasculature to respond to NO was also found to be decreased in low thyroid states (McAllister et al 2005). This effect of thyroid hormones on NO production may be highly pertinent in view of the low T3 syndrome induced by sepsis (see below).

Endocrine–metabolic–bioenergetic interactions

Setting aside the multiple actions of NO, there are also multiple interactions between the different systems. For example, in health, most hormones will impact directly on metabolism, for example insulin, androgens and growth hormone have largely anabolic effects while 'stress' hormones such as adrenaline, glucagon and cortisol are predominantly catabolic, at least in the short-term. Catecholamine effects are dose-dependent: plasma levels of $0.05–0.1\,ng/ml$ are associated with an increase in heart rate; lipolysis and blood pressure elevation occur at $0.075–0.125\,ng/ml$ while hyperglycaemia, ketogenesis and glycolysis occur at $0.1–0.2\,ng/ml$ (Clutter et al 1980). There are specific organ effects, for example, oxygen consumption in heart, skeletal muscle, liver, kidney and gut is markedly stimulated by the thyroid hormones T3 and T4, whereas brain, spleen and gonads are metabolically less responsive (Barker & Klitgaard 1952, Barker & Schwartz 1953). Normal levels of T3 are required for protein synthesis, lipolysis and fuel utilization by muscle, and for normal secretion and action of growth hormone. Many hormones also impact on mitochondrial function in health, for example, oxidative phosphorylation activity (insulin, thyroid, catecholamines), efficiency and uncoupling (thyroid, growth hormone, testosterone), free radical formation and lipid peroxidation (insulin, dehydroepiandrosterone) and biogenesis (leptin). Short-term dosing of corticosteroids increased rat skeletal muscle mitochondrial mass and respiratory complex activity, while chronic administration had the opposite effect (Weber et al 2002).

During sepsis and other critical illness, there are well-recognized perturbations in endocrine, metabolic and bioenergetic activity, as described earlier. Taking thyroid hormone as an example, the magnitude of the low T3 ('sick euthyroid') syndrome will distinguish eventual non-survivors from survivors, even on admission to intensive care (Kaptein et al 1982). Cytokines are implicated in its causation through inhibiting TSH release, thyroid iodide uptake, thyrocyte growth, synthesis and release of thyroid hormones and inhibition of 5′-deiodinase activity (Papanicolaou 2000). Girvent et al (1998) studied 66 elderly patients undergoing emergency surgery; 34 had a sick euthyroid (low T3/high rT3) state and this was associated with higher APACHE II scores, higher plasma levels of cortisol, norepinephrine and IL6, and an increased mortality (20% vs. 0%) Delivery-dependent oxygen consumption in septic patients was also inversely related to plasma concentrations of T3 and T4, though not to lactate, epinephrine, norepinephrine, dopamine or cortisol (Palazzo & Suter 1991).

Impairment of an additional and important control mechanism has recently been described in sepsis, namely neural control and modulation of inflammation (Tracey 2002). Autonomic dysfunction is a well-recognized phenomenon in sepsis and produces a sympathetic/parasympathetic imbalance. The decrease in parasympathetic outflow (the 'cholinergic anti-inflammatory pathway') leads to increased cytokine activation. Recent experimental studies using cholinergic agonists resulted in improved survival in a mouse sepsis model (Wang et al 2004).

Therapeutic interventions

The complexity of these interactions and the varying response depending on the phase of the septic process have been under-appreciated in many clinical trials. Contrary to expectation, trials involving replacement of thyroid hormone (Acker et al 2000) or growth hormone (Takala et al 1999), TNF antagonism, (Fisher et al 1996), NOS blockade (Lopez et al 2004) and high doses of the sympatho-mimetic agent, dobutamine (Hayes et al 1994) have all resulted in significant harm to the critically ill patient. With the benefit of hindsight, we can recognize the considerable degree of naivety attached to the design of these studies but they certainly highlight the importance of ensuring correct dosing and timing of administration. Positive outcome studies have been achieved with hormonal manipulation. Although mortality was improved through the use of corticosteroids in patients with septic shock (Annane et al 2002), concerns have been since expressed regarding an increased incidence of neuromyopathy and delayed functional recovery post-acute respiratory distress syndrome (ARDS) (Herridge et al 2003), possibly related to the mitochondrial effects of long-term corticosteroids (Weber et al 2002). β-adrenergic blockade with propranolol in paediatric burn patients had a significant effect in reducing the catabolic response and improving recovery (Herndon et al 2001). Intensive insulin therapy with tight glycaemic control also resulted in improved survival rates and reductions in morbidity (van den Berghe et al 2001). The precise mechanism(s) through which benefit is achieved still remain uncertain, but protective effects on mitochondrial function and structure, endothelial damage and alterations in lipid profile have all been shown (van den Berghe 2004).

Conclusions

In conclusion, sepsis and multi-organ failure is a consequence of a highly intricate whole body response to prolonged inflammation involving multiple pathways at both transcriptional and post-transcriptional levels. These effects will vary over time and with severity, and will be strongly influenced by concurrent therapies that may superficially carry little relevance to the pathway being affected. Clearly, evolution dictates that many of these changes must be adaptive, otherwise survival could not occur in the hardiest individuals. Our enthusiasm to modulate these pathways may thus be in conflict to these adaptive efforts. We thus need to better understand the mechanisms, their interactions and temporal relationships, and how and when to intervene, to either pre-emptively prevent decline, or to hasten recovery.

References

Acker CG, Singh AR, Flick RP, Bernardini J, Greenberg A, Johnson JP 2000 A trial of thyroxine in acute renal failure. Kidney Int 57:293–298

Annane D, Sebille V, Troche G, Raphael JC, Gajdos P, Bellissant E 2000 A 3-level prognostic classification in septic shock based on cortisol levels and cortisol response to corticotropin. JAMA 283:1038–1045

Annane D, Sebille V, Charpentier C et al 2002 Effect of treatment with low doses of hydrocortisone and fludrocortisone on mortality in patients with septic shock. JAMA 288: 862–871

Barker SB, Klitgaard HM 1952 Metabolism of tissues excised from thyroxine-injected rats. Am J Physiol 170:81–86

Barker SB, Schwartz HS 1953 Further studies on metabolism of tissues from thyroxine injected rats. Proc Soc Exp Biol Med 83:500–502

Brealey D, Brand M, Hargreaves I et al 2002 Association between mitochondrial dysfunction and severity and outcome of septic shock. Lancet 360:219–223

Bone RC, Balk RA, Cerra FB et al 1992 Definitions for sepsis and organ failure and guidelines for the use of innovative therapies in sepsis. The ACCP/SCCM Consensus Conference Committee. American college of chest physicians/society of critical care medicine. Chest 101: 1644–1655

Bornstein SR, Licinio J, Tauchnitz R et al 1998 Plasma leptin levels are increased in survivors of acute sepsis: associated loss of diurnal rhythm, in cortisol and leptin secretion. J Clin Endocrinol Metab 83:280–283

Brown GC, Borutaite V 2002 Nitric oxide inhibition of mitochondrial respiration and its role in cell death. Free Rad Biol Med 33:1440–1450

Calvano SE, Xiao W, Richards DR et al 2005 A network-based analysis of systemic inflammation in humans. Nature 437:1032–1037

Carnio EC, Stabile AM, Batalhao ME et al 2005 Vasopressin release during endotoxaemic shock in mice lacking inducible nitric oxide synthase. Pflugers Arch 450:390–394

Carreras MC, Peralta JG, Converso DP et al 2001 Modulation of liver mitochondrial NOS is implicated in thyroid-dependent regulation of O_2 uptake. Am J Physiol Heart Circ Physiol 281:H2282–2288

Clutter WE, Bier DM, Shah SD, Cryer PE 1980 Epinephrine plasma metabolic clearance rates and physiologic thresholds for metabolic and hemodynamic action in man. J Clin Invest 66:94–101

Fisher CJ Jr, Agosti JM, Opal SM et al 1996 Treatment of septic shock with the tumor necrosis factor receptor:Fc fusion protein. The soluble TNF receptor sepsis study group. N Engl J Med 334:1697–1702

Gadek-Michalska A, Bugajski J 2004 Role of prostaglandins and nitric oxide in the lipopolysaccharide-induced ACTH and corticosterone response. J Physiol Pharmacol 55:663–675

Girvent M, Maestro S, Hernandez R et al 1998 Euthyroid sick syndrome, associated endocrine abnormalities, and outcome in elderly patients undergoing emergency operation. Surgery 123:560–567

Grimm M, Spiecker M, De Caterina R, Shin WS, Liao JK 2002 Inhibition of major histocompatibility complex class II gene transcription by nitric oxide and antioxidants. J Biol Chem 277:26460–26467

Griscavage JM, Hobbs AJ, Ignarro LJ 1995 Negative modulation of nitric oxide synthase by nitric oxide and nitroso compounds. Adv Pharmacol 34:215–234

Hayes MA, Timmins AC, Yau EH, Palazzo M, Hinds CJ, Watson D 1994 Elevation of systemic oxygen delivery in the treatment of critically ill patients. N Engl J Med 330:1717–1722

Herndon DN, Hart DW, Wolf SE, Chinkes DL, Wolfe RR 2001 Reversal of catabolism by beta-blockade after severe burns. N Engl J Med 345:1223–1229

Herridge MS, Cheung AM, Tansey CM 2003 For the Canadian critical care trials group 2003 One-year outcomes in survivors of the acute respiratory distress syndrome. N Engl J Med 348:683–693

Hotchkiss RS, Karl IE 2003 The pathophysiology and treatment of sepsis. N Engl J Med 348:138–150

Hotchkiss RS, Swanson PE, Freeman BD et al 1999 Apoptotic cell death in patients with sepsis, shock, and multiple organ dysfunction. Crit Care Med 27:1230–1251

Kaptein EM, Weiner JM, Robinson WJ et al 1982 Relationship of altered thyroid hormone indices to survival in nonthyroidal illnesses. Clin Endocrinol 16:565–574

Kreymann G, Grosser S, Buggisch P, Gottschall C, Matthaei S, Greten H 1993 Oxygen consumption and resting metabolic rate in sepsis, sepsis syndrome, and septic shock. Crit Care Med 21:1012–1019

Lopez A, Lorente JA, Steingrub J et al 2004 Multiple-center, randomized, placebo-controlled, double-blind study of the nitric oxide synthase inhibitor 546C88: effect on survival in patients with septic shock. Crit Care Med 32:21–30

Macarthur H, Mattammal MB, Westfall TC 1995 A new perspective on the inhibitory role of nitric oxide in sympathetic neurotransmission. Biochem Biophys Res Commun 216:686–692

McAllister RM, Albarracin I, Price EM, Smith TK, Turk JR, Wyatt KD 2005 Thyroid status and nitric oxide in rat arterial vessels. J Endocrinol 185:111–119

Michie HR, Manogue KR, Spriggs DR et al 1988 Detection of circulating tumor necrosis factor after endotoxin administration. N Engl J Med 318:1481–1486

Mohn CE, Fernandez-Solari J, De Laurentiis A et al 2005 The rapid release of corticosterone from the adrenal induced by ACTH is mediated by nitric oxide acting by prostaglandin E2. Proc Natl Acad Sci USA 102:6213–6218

Noble JS, MacKirdy FN, Donaldson SI, Howie JC 2001 Renal and respiratory failure in Scottish ICUs. Anaesthesia 56:124–129

O'Brien AJ, Wilson AJ, Singer M, Clapp L 2001 Temporal variation in endotoxin-induced vascular hyporeactivity in a rat mesenteric artery organ culture model. Br J Pharmacol 133:351–360

Palazzo MG, Suter PM 1991 Delivery dependent oxygen consumption in patients with septic shock: daily variations, relationship with outcome and the sick-euthyroid syndrome. Intensive Care Med 17:325–329

Papanicolaou DA 2000 Euthyroid sick syndrome and the role of cytokines. Rev Endocr Metab Disord 1:43–48

Rivier C 2003 Role of nitric oxide in regulating the rat hypothalamic-pituitary-adrenal axis response to endotoxemia. Ann NY Acad Sci 992:72–85

Romanovsky AA, Szekely M 1998 Fever and hypothermia: two adaptive thermoregulatory responses to systemic inflammation. Med Hypotheses 50:219–226

Singer M, Glynne P 2005 Treating critical illness: the importance of first doing no harm. PLOS Med 2:e167

Singer M, De Santis V, Vitale D, Jeffcoate W 2004 Multiorgan failure is an adaptive, endocrine-mediated, metabolic response to overwhelming systemic inflammation. Lancet 364:545–548

Suliman HB, Welty-Wolf KE, Carraway M, Tatro L, Piantadosi CA 2004 Lipopolysaccharide induces oxidative cardiac mitochondrial damage and biogenesis. Cardiovasc Res 64: 279–288

Takala J, Ruokonen E, Webster NR et al 1999 Increased mortality associated with growth hormone treatment in critically ill adults. N Engl J Med 341:785–792

Titheradge MA 1999 Nitric oxide in septic shock. Biochim Biophys Acta 1411:437–455

Tracey KJ 2002 The inflammatory reflex. Nature 420:853–859

Tschaikowsky K, Hedwig-Geissing M, Schiele A, Bremer F, Schywalsky M, Schuttler J 2002 Coincidence of pro- and anti-inflammatory responses in the early phase of severe sepsis: Longitudinal study of mononuclear histocompatibility leukocyte antigen-DR expression, procalcitonin, C-reactive protein, and changes in T-cell subsets in septic and postoperative patients. Crit Care Med 30:1015–1023

Ueta Y, Levy A, Chowdrey HS, Lightman SL 1995 Hypothalamic nitric oxide synthase gene expression is regulated by thyroid hormones. Endocrinology 136:4182–4187

Van den Berghe G 2004 How does blood glucose control with insulin save lives in intensive care? J Clin Invest 114:1187–1195

Van den Berghe G, Wouters P, Weekers F et al 2001 Intensive insulin therapy in the critically ill patients. N Engl J Med 345:1359–1367

Vo PA, Lad B, Tomlinson JA, Francis S, Ahluwalia A 2005 Autoregulatory role of endothelium-derived nitric oxide (NO) on lipopolysaccharide-induced vascular inducible NO synthase expression and function. J Biol Chem 280:7236–7243

Vodovotz Y, Kim PK, Bagci EZ et al 2004 Inflammatory modulation of hepatocyte apoptosis by nitric oxide: in vivo, in vitro, and in silico studies. Curr Mol Med 4:753–762

Wang H, Liao H, Ochani M et al 2004 Cholinergic agonists inhibit HMGB1 release and improve survival in experimental sepsis. Nat Med 10:1216–1221

Weber K, Bruck P, Mikes Z, Kupper JH, Klingenspor M, Wiesner RJ 2002 Glucocorticoid hormone stimulate mitochondrial biogenesis specifically in skeletal muscle. Endocrinology 143:177–184

DISCUSSION

Griffiths: My prejudices on this are that mitochondria in different organ tissues are quite different. Some may be extremely susceptible others not. If you look at skeletal muscle, exercise physiology has taught us that the mitochondria here are very strong and adaptable increasing or reducing their number related to activity very quickly. Fatigue in the true physiological sense of contractile function (the inability to sustain force or work rate) is unrelated to the mitochondrial activity directly but more to excitation contraction coupling. It might be that we could have impaired mitochondria number and this could affect someone's ability to keep climbing the stairs in old age, but the failure of the force generation in sepsis is likely to be more related to excitation-contraction failure and disturbed membrane physiology. Many of the changes you see in the mitochondria in muscle could be simply related to the acute alteration of function of that tissue, and the substrates that are being delivered to it.

Singer: For this reason we try to develop the long-term models so we can look at other organs, to see how the changes in muscle relate to them. Greet Van den

Berghe echoed this perfectly: even in the conventionally treated group, the liver was affected far more than muscle. We are finding this in our rat model. Because the muscle is accessible in patients, we can look at this. We can't study the liver like this. People are looking at white cells and monocytes and are finding that there are changes in the mitochondria. Didier Payen has results linking immune suppression with energy failure in monocytes, so there are parallels. I think some tissues are better adapted than others, but the overall message I still think holds true.

Wang: We have some relevant unpublished data in collaboration with Dr Kevin J. Tracey from several years ago. We were trying to understand how HMGB1 killed animals. The experiment we did was to infuse recombinant HMGB1 into rats, and then harvested different organs, looking for any pathological changes using electron microscopy. The only organ in which we found any changes was the kidney. The changes were in the inner membrane of the mitochondria, which is somehow disrupted and hardly seen under electron microscope. We do not know if this explains how HMGB1 killed animals.

Singer: Was the liver alright? Does HMGB1 get into the liver?

Wang: We didn't see similar changes in the mitochondrial structure in the liver. If you culture cells with recombinant HMGB1, it is likely that the protein can get into the cells. *In vivo*, we don't know.

Piantadosi: It is enough that the combination of tumour necrosis factor (TNF) and nitric oxide (NO) can lead to damage from peroxynitrite generation. Mervyn Singer mentioned already the inhibition of complex IV, so if you couple this with a TNF stress, it wrecks mitochondria. Then the issue becomes one of damage control. Feeding substrate to complex IV damaged mitochondria won't work in the long run.

Singer: Isn't it the timing, though?

Piantadosi: We don't understand the timing issues here, in terms of how, what and when to feed. Understanding the mitochondrial pathogenesis and recovery strategies will prove important.

Fink: In this field we are all guilty of being like blind people examining the elephant. The part of the elephant Mervyn Singer has chosen to study is the mitochondria. Greet Van den Berghe is studying the endocrine system. But when patients get septic to the extent that the cells in their body are the elephant, the whole cell gets sick. The notion that there is just one organelle or mechanism of cytopathology is probably wrong. We have published a series of papers in the last five years looking at epithelial cells subjected to cytokine stress in a variety of organs, both *in vivo* and *in vitro*. The part of the elephant that we have been looking at is the tight junction between these adjacent epithelial cells. It is deranged. This is because the proteins that form the tight junction don't go to the right place. In some cases too much of the protein is made; in other cases not enough. Whatever the cytopathological mechanisms are, in the lung, liver, gut and probably the kidney, the tight junctions don't form. But if you look elsewhere you can find evidence for the transporters for bile components in the liver that don't insert themselves into the membrane properly. In polarized cells, appropriate distribution of proteins that should localize themselves to the apical membrane and not appear in the basolateral membrane get deranged. The point I am trying to make is that this pathology we call sepsis messes up a lot of different things. As a laboratory head I can only focus on one part of the elephant, but I have to be open to the idea that there are lots of other parts of the elephant that are sick too.

Singer: I agree with you, and this is why I mentioned all the studies at the beginning, showing that different bits can be modulated with effect. The question is how, by modulating all these different bits, do we get this effect? Modulating one thing has to have effects on the other bits of the system.

Fink: In Greet's paper (Vanhorebeek et al 2005) the pictures of the liver mitochondria are striking. Those mitochondria are toast, but the hepatocytes are not dead. In Hotchkiss' paper (Hotchkiss et al 1999), hepatocellular necrosis is a few percent of the liver, and hepatocellular apoptosis is essentially non-existent. The hepatic parenchyma is not normal at the electron microscopic level, and it is not just the mitochondria that are screwed up. At the light microscope level it is screwed up because of fatty infiltration, but the hepatocytes aren't dead. If the hepatocytes get most of their ATP turnover from mitochondria, and their mitochondria have been toasted, what is going on?

Singer: Hibernation.

Van den Berghe: I don't know, but they are not fully toasted. They are not gone yet. As you say, there is no sign of apoptosis or necrosis, and I am not sure if it is reversible or not. We will have to do animal models and investigate a time effect as well as see whether it recovers or not.

Piantadosi: Our notions about the relationship between the mitochondria and the cell are over-simplified. The mitochondrion is a great communicator. You can't have too many: the more mitochondria a cell or tissue has, the better protected it is—provided the mitochondria don't release Ca^{2+} or over-produce free radicals. I view them as the central regulator of cell metabolism, which underpins every cell process. We wouldn't be giant multicellular eukaryotes without mitochondria. We didn't develop until the endosymbiote came into the cell. We need a more sophisticated view of what mitochondria do: they don't just supply ATP. ATP is the currency of the cell and it is regulated, and so there is a priority system, and some processes are sacrificed or shifted to power-saving mode when the cell is sick.

Fink: In terms of cellular economy, ATP is used for six things. Protein synthesis, nucleic acid synthesis, pumping Na^+ and K^+, urea synthesis, glycogen synthesis and protein breakdown. Have you measured these six things from your septic animals? When we have looked at it in cell culture, nucleic acid synthesis is way up, protein synthesis is way up, urea synthesis is way up. My sense is that ATP turnover is up and not down.

Singer: Imitation is the greatest form of flattery: we took your paper, evolved it and stretched it out, using a different cell line (you used Caco cells and we used macrophages). Essentially, we found exactly what you did early on, but once it stretched out everything then down-regulated. There was early mitochondrial damage, but the glycolysis was keeping things going, and accelerating as part of the fight phase. Later on, everything was down-regulating, and the ATP turnover was dropping hours before the ATP level fell, which was a prelude to the death of the cell. However, if we got there early enough and intervened by washing away the endotoxin, they recovered.

Piantadosi: I agree. Stressed cells often survive as long as the mitochondria are healthy. There is plenty of ADP around, and this is a regulator of respiration. When you crank up the ATP utilization, ADP is there for phosphorylation. Oxygen and substrate keep things going as long as mitochondrial function is healthy. In sepsis, at some point the stress is so severe, eventually mitochondrial damage becomes limiting and the cell has to use a different strategy.

References

Hotchkiss RS, Swanson PE, Freeman BD et al 1999 Apoptotic cell death in patients with sepsis, shock, and multiple organ dysfunction. Crit Care Med 27:1230–1251

Vanhorebeek I, De Vos R, Mesotten D, Wouters PJ, De Wolf-Peeters C, Van den Berghe G 2005 Protection of hepatocyte mitochondrial ultrastructure and function by strict blood glucose control with insulin in critically ill patients. Lancet 365:53–59

Protecting the permeability pore and mitochondrial biogenesis

C. A. Piantadosi, M. S. Carraway, D. W. Haden and H. B. Suliman

Box 3315, Room 0570 DHS, Duke University Medical Center, Durham, NC 27710, USA

Abstract. Recent evidence links the pathogenesis of multiple organ dysfunction syndrome (MODS) in sepsis to mitochondrial damage. Our hypothesis is that cellular mechanisms maintaining mitochondrial function must be protected in order to prevent MODS. Recent animal experiments indicate that host defences which target and kill microbes, in part via reactive oxygen and nitrogen production, also injure mitochondria, thus activating mitochondrial cell death pathways. To limit such collateral damage, the cell up-regulates and imports into mitochondria several nuclear-encoded proteins for antioxidant defence and mitochondrial DNA (mtDNA) replication. Fully integrated responses lead to mitochondrial biogenesis, which may alter cellular phenotype to avoid mitochondrial permeability transition, apoptosis, or energy failure. Key to the cell's vulnerability to oxidant generation by the innate immune response is the mtDNA content. MtDNA depletion is opposed by oxidation-reduction (redox) signals that communicate the extent of mitochondrial damage to the nucleus. Molecular studies suggest that redox mechanisms activate two biogenic transcription factors, nuclear respiratory factors 1 and 2, which forestall a deterioration of oxidative phosphorylation during infection. Biogenic failure or an intrinsic biogenic arrest could hasten degradation of mitochondrial function and drive the cell to apoptosis or necrosis. By implication, novel protective strategies for biogenesis hold promise for the prevention of MODS.

2007 Sepsis—new insights, new therapies. Wiley, Chichester (Novartis Foundation Symposium 280) p 266–280

The activation of innate immunity in sepsis, especially the elaboration of specific cytokine mediators, causes damage to the host's cells and tissues. Under prolonged or severe conditions, this damage may become widespread and bring about the multiple organ dysfunction syndrome (MODS) (Hotchkiss et al 2000). Recent work on MODS has implicated disordered oxygen utilization (dysoxia) in its pathogenesis (Fink 2002), and clinically detectable mitochondrial dysfunction correlates with a poor outcome in sepsis (Brealey et al 2002). This paper briefly reviews some emerging concepts of how mitochondrial function changes and adapts to the pro-inflammatory milieu of sepsis and their implications for mitochondrial regulation of cell death.

During sepsis-induced inflammation, cell survival requires the full support of energy metabolism, and damage to mitochondria may initiate apoptosis, trigger necrosis, or both, by several mechanisms. These mechanisms manifest biochemically through oxidation, nitration, or nitrosation of mitochondrial structural components, causing failure of the energy supply or activation of the core apoptotic pathway (Su 2002). The latter pathway is regulated by the calcium-dependent mitochondrial permeability transition pore (PTP) and by Bcl-2 family proteins in macromolecular aggregates that link mitochondrial function to apoptosome formation (Green & Kroemer 2004). In addition, the cell reacts to the stress of sepsis with protective mechanisms that help prevent mitochondrial damage or that replace damaged organelles with better adapted ones.

The mitochondria of both immune and non-immune cells appear to be damaged in sepsis, but this paper primarily focuses on the mitochondria of non-immune cells in tissues with high metabolic needs. Of the systemic organs affected by MODS, the liver has an important place. The liver is not just metabolically active, but clears circulating portal and systemic bacteria and bacterial products (Su 2002) and activation of resident Kupffer cells (KCs) initiates the acute-phase response. This response invokes a potent pro-inflammatory cascade in which tumour necrosis factor (TNF)α, nitric oxide (NO) and other cytokines are important (Tracey et al 1986, Kurose et al 1996). Some of these factors activate receptor and/or non-receptor pathways which regulate mitochondrial function and have major roles in determining cell survival (Kurose et al 1996).

The innate response to microbes is initiated by activation of membrane-bound Toll-like receptors (TLRs) (Takeda et al 2003, Matsumura et al 2000). To respond to bacteria, TLR2 and TLR4 in conjunction with CD14 share a common pathway through Toll-IL1R (TIR) signalling domains and the adapter molecule, MyD88, to activate nuclear factor κB (NF-κB) and its downstream inflammatory gene expression (Poltorak et al 1998, Yang et al 2000). For instance, TLR4 binds to endotoxin lipopolysaccharide (LPS) to initiate the critical defence against Gram-negative bacteria (Poltorak et al 1998, Yang et al 2000), while TLR2 facilitates Gram-positive bacteria recognition (Takeuchi et al 1999) and influences specificity for Gram-negative organisms. These innate defences are largely responsible for producing the factors that contribute to mitochondrial damage in sepsis.

Mitochondrial oxidative and nitrosative stress in sepsis

Mitochondria normally generate small amounts of reactive oxygen species (ROS) as a by-product of metabolism, but this can increase dramatically in cytokine-activated cells. An important aspect of this inflammatory response is attributable to induction of iNOS, reactive nitrogen species (RNS) production, and the interaction of NO with cytochrome c oxidase (Lemasters et al 1999). NO reversibly inhibits respiration and increases the ROS leak rate by the respiratory chain, which may selectively damage mitochondria. A case in point is the up-regulation of mitochondrial antioxidant defences in the early phase response exemplified by the coordinated regulation of TNFα and the major mitochondrial antioxidant enzyme, superoxide dismutase 2 (MnSOD) in response to LPS (Tsan et al 2001).

About a decade ago, our group came to realize that the manifestations of oxidative stress in sepsis were not reflected in standard assessments of mitochondrial function, such as ATP production and respiratory control ratio. Thus, mitochondrial ROS production doubles or triples without a measurable effect on oxidative phosphorylation. In short, oxidant damage to non-respiratory mitochondrial constituents precedes a decline in respiratory capacity by *in vitro* measures (Taylor et al 1995). Different patterns of respiration were also detected in liver mitochondria and hepatocytes (Kantrow et al 1997), and electron microscopy revealed dazzling heterogeneity of mitochondrial structure in the liver, heart, and skeletal muscle, in various mammalian species in sepsis including primates (Welty-Wolf et al 1996, Suliman et al 2003a).

The first clue to an explanation for these apparently disparate findings came from mitochondrial isolation techniques based on density centrifugation developed 50 years ago. These techniques yield intact organelles, which serve well in working out basic aspects of normal mitochondrial physiology. However, the value of those methods in recovering organelles that tend to be swollen is limited, and they have not provided specific insights in sepsis research. For instance, in the liver in sepsis, subpopulations of damage-resistant mitochondria, or those adapted to the new levels of metabolic stress, are recovered to the exclusion of swollen or badly damaged organelles. In hepatocytes isolated from rodents with sepsis, however, maximal respiration rates are lower and cyanide-resistant respiration rates are higher compared with control hepatocytes, suggesting that energy metabolism is supported by the function of fewer 'healthy' mitochondria (Kantrow et al 1997). These data, in the context that the mitochondrial yield falls in sepsis, imply an alteration in mitochondrial phenotype and function. This background provided a foundation for our work on mitochondrial biogenesis.

Mitochondrial biogenesis and sepsis

In searching for keys to the cell's vulnerability to oxidant generation we settled on the idea that mtDNA content would be important to evaluate because mtDNA is predisposed to oxidative damage. MtDNA is present in low copy number, lacks protective histones, and is found in proximity to respiratory chain components that generate ROS. Persistent mtDNA damage may lead to impairment of mitochondrial genome transcription and oxidative phosphorylation (Clayton 1984,

Suliman et al 2003a, Ballinger et al 2000). Indeed, mtDNA was found to be depleted transiently in the livers and hearts of rodents given injurious but sublethal doses of heat-killed bacteria (Suliman et al 2003a, 2004, Ballinger et al 2000).

The cell's ability to maintain oxidative phosphorylation depends on the replication of mtDNA, which is also necessary for mitochondrial biogenesis. This process requires coordinated interactions between the nuclear and mitochondrial genomes. Mitochondrial biogenesis thus depends on the expression of nuclear-encoded regulatory proteins that are imported into existing mitochondria. For instance, replication and transcription of the circular double-stranded mtDNA is under nuclear control via mitochondrial transcription factor A, (Tfam or mtTFA) a high mobility group-box protein that binds the light and heavy strand promoter regions. Also required are the single stranded binding protein (mtSSB), a co-activator, mtTFB, and a dedicated DNA polymerase (pol γ) (Grosschedl et al 1994, Larsson et al 1998). Tfam expression is regulated by two nuclear transcription factors, nuclear respiratory factors 1 and 2 (NRF1 and 2), which respond to changes in the redox environment, and a master co-activator PGC1α, which responds to NO through guanylate cyclase. In short, mtDNA replication and mitochondrial biogenesis require bidirectional cell communication: mitochondrion to nucleus (retrograde) and nucleus to mitochondrion (anterograde). These concepts are illustrated in Fig. 1.

Based on observations that NO and ROS can damage mtDNA, we proposed that intense innate immune activation induces damage to mtDNA in sepsis. Furthermore, this problem coexists within the complex interplay of iNOS and ROS production as redox signals for the regulation of mitochondrial biogenesis (Suliman et al 2003b). In studies of wild-type (Wt), TLR4$^{-/-}$, TLR2$^{-/-}$ and TLR2/4$^{-/-}$ double knockout mice, we found that TLR4 activation depletes mtDNA through the activation of iNOS in concert with the elaboration of TNFα (Suliman et al 2005). However, an intact TLR4 signalling response was also required to express Tfam and restore mtDNA content. In other words, TLR4-null mice are more resistant than Wt to mitochondrial damage by Gram negative bacteria, but resolution of damage in the TLR4 null strains is impaired relative to TLR4-competent strains. This was demonstrated by failed induction of Tfam (Suliman et al 2005), a central regulator of mtDNA transcription, replication, and biogenesis.

It is important to mention that TLR4 signalling also activates the pro-survival kinase Akt (Suliman et al 2005). This kinase is known to enhance NF-κB-dependent gene expression via p65 phosphorylation (Madrid et al 2000, 2001). Although NF-κB activity is a target of this kinase, NF-κB also regulates *Akt* transcription through p65 binding (Madrid et al 2000, 2001). In TLR4$^{-/-}$ mice, Akt phosphorylation after exposure to Gram negative bacteria is impaired, which offered an explanation for the failure of Tfam expression, e.g. Akt

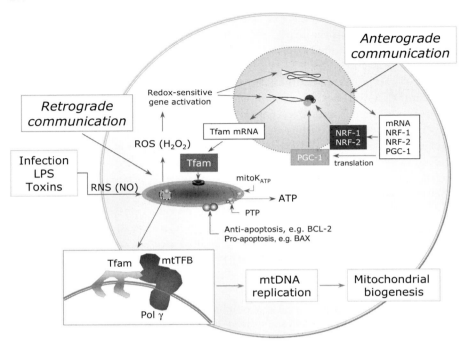

FIG. 1.   Simplified illustration of the communication between the nucleus and mitochondrion needed for mitochondrial biogenesis. New mitochondria are normally made under primarily nuclear control, for instance in the presence of growth factors (anterograde communication). When mitochondria are damaged by sepsis, signals from the mitochondrion, such as hydrogen peroxide, can stimulate signalling pathways that activate genes for biogenesis (retrograde communication). Tfam, mitochondrial transcription factor A; NRF, nuclear respiratory factors 1 and 2; PGC1, peroxisome proliferator-activated receptor γ co-activator 1α; mtTFB, mitochondrial transcription factor B; Pol γ, DNA polymerase γ; PTP, permeability transition pore; MitoK$_{ATP}$, mitochondrial potassium channel.

phosphorylates NRF1. But the significant point is that TLR4 activation not only stimulates ROS and RNS damage but participates in coordinate Tfam induction and mitochondrial biogenic responses stemming perhaps from NF-κB and Akt. The implication is that Tfam expression anticipates mtDNA damage and thereby protects mtDNA replication in sepsis. If confirmed, this may also indicate that biogenesis can forestall a critical degradation in mitochondrial function.

Mitochondrial permeability in sepsis

Mitochondria damaged by ROS production become dysfunctional, and this may further increase their oxidant output. Such a vicious cycle, sometimes loosely

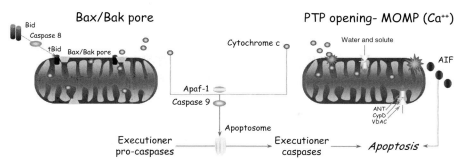

FIG. 2. Simple diagram of the mitochondrial pathways and checkpoints for initiation of programmed cell death. Two pore pathways are illustrated: the left shows formation of the Bax/Bak pore and the right shows the Ca^{2+}-dependent permeability transition pore (PTP), which causes mitochondrial outer membrane permeabilization (MOMP). Both pores allow the release of cytochrome c and formation of the apoptosome, which is responsible for cleaving the executioner pro-caspases. A third mechanism, the release of apoptosis-inducing factor (AIF) results in direct activation of endonucleases. VDAC, voltage-dependent anion channel; ANT, adenine nucleotide translocase; CyP, cyclophilin D.

known as ROS-induced ROS release, is likely to favour PTP opening and apoptosis (Di Lisi et al 2003). Moreover, certain types of mitochondrial damage cause the ATP synthase (complex V) to reverse and actually consume ATP, leading to the rapid depletion of high energy stores. Ostensibly, such a mechanism could be interpreted as a way to preserve ion homeostasis in a last ditch effort by the cell to survive. Indeed, loss of ion homeostasis is an additional process through which mitochondria drive cellular injury towards necrosis or apoptosis. Certain mitochondrial ion channels also have been proposed to contribute to mitochondrial dysfunction, including the K_{ATP} channel and the anion channel of the inner membrane (IMAC) that can interact with endoplasmic reticulum and mitochondrial calcium pools.

There is a growing body of evidence for a role for the mitoK$_{ATP}$ channel in the preconditioning of neuronal and cardiac cells against ischaemia and apoptosis (Ardehali et al 2005). The identity of the channel has been in dispute, but it was recently reported that a macromolecular complex of five proteins (mitochondrial ATP-binding cassette protein 1, the phosphate carrier, adenine nucleotide translocase [ANT], ATP synthase and succinic dehydrogenase [SDH]) confers mitoK$_{ATP}$ channel activity in liver mitochondria (Ardehali et al 2005). The links between this complex, the permeability transition pore (PTP), whose exact composition is also still somewhat uncertain (e.g. VDAC, cyclophilin D, ANT and hexokinase) (Su 2002, Kokoszka et al 2004), and the macromolecular complexes of the Bcl-2 protein family, remain under investigation (see Fig. 2). Moreover, there is significant cross-talk between the cell receptor-mediated and mitochondrial initiation pathways, and this has been observed in sepsis, especially in immune cell apoptosis (Wesche-Soldato et al 2005).

On this basis, it would be interesting to know how the mitochondria of septic animals respond functionally to specific apoptogenic stimuli, such as Ca^{2+}. Our prediction was that the oxidative stress of sepsis, like ROS generation *in vitro*, would bestow sensitivity to PTP and promote apoptosis, which would be consistent with the majority of the pathological observations of the disease (Hotchkiss et al 2000, Wesche-Soldato et al 2005). Interestingly, however, liver mitochondria isolated after caecal ligation and puncture actually show resistance to MPT and cytochrome *c* release (Kantrow et al 2000). It is important to recall that mitochondria harvested by cell fractionation are comprised of subpopulations of 'healthy' organelles. In the case of sepsis there seemed, at least superficially, to be a dichotomy: PTP function had either been damaged or had been protected against opening in sepsis. On the other hand, this may be yet another indication of heterogeneity of mitochondrial phenotypes under inflammation. If we can identify the phenotypes and the factors that regulate them, we should be able to capitalize on the current pharmacological interest in blocking the PTP in order to suppress pathological cell death appropriately in sepsis.

Conclusions and future directions

There is still an important conceptual horizon beyond which little is known. This entails the relationship between the cell's decision to survive and maintain functional mitochondria or to undergo apoptosis. The classical idea that mitochondrial damage disrupts ATP production and Ca^{2+} homeostasis and leads to cell death by necrosis is an accurate description of a subset of organ pathologies in which the injury is rapid and profound, such as cardiac or cerebral ischaemia-reperfusion. But for watershed or penumbral territories, and for diseases such as sepsis and MODS in which apoptosis has a pivotal status, this model is too simple. Take for example the multi-faceted role of Ca^{2+}, which in free intracellular excess triggers the opening of the mitochondrial PTP. This not only releases proteins necessary for apoptosome assembly, such as cytochrome *c*, but dissipates the membrane potential and causes metabolic failure. Because ATP is required for apoptosis, the commitment of a cell to an apoptotic program does not always lead to an orderly death; instead, the program can be short-circuited resulting in what has been called necroptosis (Green & Kroemer 2004).

The observation that necrosis tends to promote inflammation while apoptosis does not, provides the body with a reason to favour apoptosis over necrosis or necroptosis in sepsis. The ability to maintain control of the inflammatory response is the advantage of having cells that when damaged beyond the point of recovery run an apoptotic program to completion. This gives rise to the view that an intact

Mitochondrial Biogenesis in Sepsis

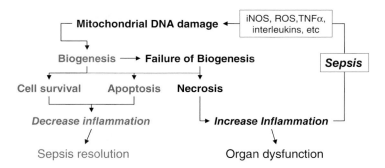

FIG. 3.   Integrated hypothesis for the role of mitochondrial biogenesis in sepsis. Mitochondrial components such as mtDNA are damaged by the host immune response in sepsis, which initiates repair mechanisms including biogenesis. The inflammatory response can be perpetuated in a vicious cycle by failure of biogenesis and the cell's ability to maintain an adequate complement of mitochondria.

mitochondrial biogenic response maximizes the probability that ATP will be available not just for cell survival, but to complete the orderly disposal of the cell, if necessary. Thus, biogenesis would oppose necrosis on at least two levels. This backdrop, however, comes with an outlay of energy because ATP is required to recycle damaged mitochondria through the processes of autophagy and biogenesis. Thus, the injured cell is faced with deciding if its biogenic capacity is up to the task of restoring it to homeostasis (Fig. 3).

If the latter concepts are valid for sepsis, one should be able to predict a rise and fall in biogenesis under two conditions. The first would occur as a tissue recovers from a transient septic insult and the second when an injury overwhelms cell defence and causes irreversible mitochondrial damage. In both cases, the biogenic response should precede the conclusive outcome, for instance, cell proliferation in the first case and apoptosis or necrosis in the second. In the first case, biogenesis marker expression does precede the appearance of cell proliferation markers in the liver, heart and brain as they recover from inflammatory or oxidative injury to the mitochondria (Suliman et al 2003a, 2004). More recently, we have found that an initial wave of hepatic mitochondrial biogenesis in the first two days of persistent staphylococcal sepsis in mice is supplanted by a falloff in biogenic marker expression at day three and by the appearance of widespread apoptosis at day seven (Fig. 4). It is not yet clear whether this phenomenon represents biogenic failure or a biogenic arrest mechanism regulated by endogenous repression.

In conclusion, activation of inflammation in sepsis leads to both the desired innate immune response and unwanted host cell damage. Inflammation stimulates

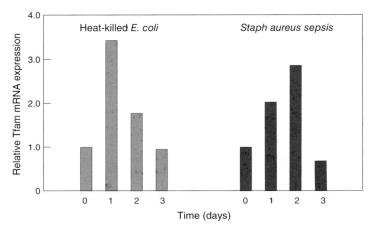

FIG. 4.   Increase in the hepatic expression of mitochondrial transcription factor A (Tfam) with two types of septic insults in mice. Left graph shows the mRNA response to a single injection of heat-killed *Escherichia coli*; the right graph shows the mRNA response to persistent *Staphylococcus aureus* sepsis in a fibrin clot model. Both stresses stimulate the expression of Tfam (as well as other markers of biogenesis that are not shown). The model on the left results in complete histological resolution of organ damage by 7 days while that on the right shows widespread apoptosis at 7 days.

ROS production, especially by mitochondria, and the consequences of NO induction in particular, although vital to the antimicrobial defense, promote oxidative damage to mitochondria, e.g. from mtDNA depletion. Prolonged oxidative stress in mitochondria compromises their ability to support cell survival not just by providing the energy to avoid necrosis, but also by regulating apoptosis. In particular, sepsis leads to early mtDNA damage, which impairs mitochondrial transcription and the capacity for oxidative phosphorylation. The cell compensates with mitochondrial biogenesis, exemplified, for instance, by the synthesis and importation of mitochondrial transcription factor A (Tfam). This response signifies a unique physiological strain that diverts the cell's support to mitochondria, and on closer evaluation, suggests the hypothesis that inability to maintain biogenesis is predictive of cell death. As useful corollaries, it will be important to know whether regulation of biogenesis is linked to apoptosis as well as whether failure of biogenesis is a harbinger of cell necrosis and the perpetuation of inflammation.

References

Ardehali H, Chen Z, Ko Y, Mejia-Alvarez R, Marban E 2005 Multiprotein complex containing succinate dehydrogenase confers mitochondrial ATP-sensitive K channel activity. Proc Nat Acad Sci USA 101:11880–11885

Ballinger SW, Patterson C, Yan CN et al 2000 Hydrogen peroxide- and peroxynitrite-induced mitochondrial DNA damage and dysfunction in vascular endothelial and smooth muscle cells. Circ Res 86:960–966

Brealey D, Brand M, Hargreaves I et al 2002 Association between mitochondrial dysfunction and severity and outcome of septic shock. Lancet 360:219–223

Clayton DA 1984 Transcription of the mammalian mitochondrial genome. Ann Rev Biochem 53:573–594

Di Lisi F, Canton M, Menabo R, Dodoni G, Bernardi P 2003 Mitochondria and reperfusion injury. Bas Res Cardiol 98:235–241

Ekstrand MI, Falkenberg M, Rantanen A et al 2004 Mitochondrial transcription factor A regulates mtDNA copy number in mammals. Hum Mol Genet 13:935–944

Fink MP 2002 Bench-to-bedside review: Cytopathic hypoxia. Crit Care (London) 6:491–499

Green DR, Kroemer G 2004 The pathophysiology of mitochondrial cell death. Science 305:626–629

Grosschedl R, Giese K, Pagel J 1994 HMG domain proteins: architectural elements in the assembly of nucleoprotein structures. Trends Genet 10:94–99

Hotchkiss RS, Schmieg Jr RE, Swanson PE et al 2000 Rapid onset of intestinal epithelial and lymphocyte apoptotic cell death in patients with trauma and shock. Crit Care Med 28:3207–3217

Kantrow SP, Taylor DE, Carraway MS, Piantadosi CA 1997 Oxidative metabolism in rat hepatocytes and mitochondria during sepsis. Arch Biochem Biophys 345:278–288

Kantrow SP, Tatro LG, Piantadosi CA 2000 Oxidative stress and adenine nucleotide control of mitochondrial permeability transition. Free Rad Biol Med 28:251–260

Kokoszka JE, Waymire KG, Levy SE et al 2004 The ADP/ATP translocator is not essential for the mitochondrial permeability transition pore. Nature 427:461–465

Kurose I, Miura S, Higuchi H et al 1996 Increased nitric oxide synthase activity as a cause of mitochondrial dysfunction in rat hepatocytes: roles for tumor necrosis factor alpha. Hepatol 24:1185–1192

Larsson NG, Wang J, Wilhelmsson H et al 1998 Mitochondrial transcription factor A is necessary for mtDNA maintenance and embryogenesis in mice. Nat Genet 18:231–236

Lemasters JJ, Qian T, Bradham CA et al 1999 Mitochondrial dysfunction in the pathogenesis of necrotic and apoptotic cell death. J Bioenerg Biomembr 31:305–319

Madrid LV, Wang CY, Guttridge DC, Schottelius AJ, Baldwin AS Jr, Mayo MW 2000 Akt suppresses apoptosis by stimulating the transactivation potential of the RelA/p65 subunit of NF-κB. Mol Cell Biol 20:1626–1638

Madrid LV, Mayo MW, Reuther JY, Baldwin AS Jr 2001 Akt stimulates the transactivation potential of the RelA/p65 Subunit of NF-kappa B through utilization of the Ikappa B kinase and activation of the mitogen-activated protein kinase p38. J Biol Chem 276:18934–18940

Matsumura T, Ito A, Takii T, Hayashi H, Onozaki K 2000 Endotoxin and cytokine regulation of Toll-like receptor (TLR) 2 and TLR4 gene expression in murine liver and hepatocytes. J Interferon Cytokine Res 20:915–921

Poltorak A, He X, Smirnova I et al 1998 Defective LPS signaling in C3H/HeJ and C57BL/10ScCr mice: mutations in tlr4 gene. Science 282:2085

Su GL 2002 Lipopolysaccharides in liver injury: molecular mechanisms of Kupffer cell activation. Am J Physiol (Gastroint & Liver Physiol) 283:G256–265

Suliman HB, Carraway MS, Piantadosi CA 2003a Postlipopolysaccharide oxidative damage of mitochondrial DNA. Am J Respir Crit Care Med 167:570–579

Suliman HB, Carraway MS, Welty-Wolf KE, Whorton AR, Piantadosi CA 2003b Lipolysaccharide stimulates mitochondrial biogenesis via activation of nuclear respiratory factor-1. J Biol Chem 278:41510–41518

Suliman HB, Welty-Wolf KE, Carraway MS, Tatro L, Piantadosi CA 2004 Lipopolysaccharide induces oxidative cardiac mitochondrial damage and biogenesis. Cardiovasc Res 64: 279–288

Suliman HB, Welty-Wolf KE, Carraway MS, Schwartz DA, Hollingsworth JW, Piantadosi CA 2005 Toll-like receptor 4 mediates mitochondrial DNA damage and biogenic responses to heat-killed E. coli. FASEB J 19:1531–1533

Takeda K, Kaisho T, Akira S 2003 Toll-like receptors. Ann Rev Immunol 21:335–376

Takeuchi O, Hoshino K, Kawai T et al 1999 Differential roles of TLR2 and TLR4 in recognition of Gram-negative and Gram-positive bacterial cell wall components. Immunity 11: 443–451

Taylor DE, Ghio AJ, Piantadosi CA 1995 Reactive oxygen species produced by liver mitochondria of septic rats. Arch Biochem Biophys 316:70–76

Tracey KJ, Beutler B, Lowry SF et al 1986 Shock and tissue injury induced by recombinant human cachectin. Science 234: 470–474

Tsan MF, Clark RN, Goyert SM, White JE 2001 Induction of TNF-α and MnSOD by endotoxin: role of membrane CD14 and Toll-like receptor-4. Am J Physiol (Cell Physiol) 280: C1422–1430

Welty-Wolf KE, Simonson SG, Huang Y-CT, Fracica PJ, Patterson JW, Piantadosi CA 1996 Ultrastructural changes in skeletal muscle mitochondria in Gram-negative sepsis. Shock 5:378–384

Wesche-Soldato DE, Lomas-Neira JL, Perl M, Jones L, Chung CS, Ayala A 2005 The role and regulation of apoptosis in sepsis. J Endotoxin Res 11:375–382

Yang H, Young DW, Gusovsky F, Chow JC 2000 Cellular events mediated by lipopolysaccharide-stimulated Toll-like receptor 4. MD-2 is required for activation of mitogen-activated protein kinase and Elk-1. J Biol Chem 275:20861

DISCUSSION

Griffiths: Clearly, with that considerable biogenesis going on, there will be a substrate requirement for nutrition containing the precursors for purines and pyrimidines. Are they limited?

Piantadosi: We haven't looked.

Griffiths: There isn't evidence for good salvage in humans for purines and pyrimidines.

Piantadosi: Not purines. At some point you have to recycle mitochondria, then of course, other processes will be limiting, and these may be mechanisms of biogenesis failure. We haven't tried to figure out what causes biogenic failure because we are first trying to understand the processes that regulate it.

Griffiths: This gets to the issue of calling it hibernation, which is the down-tuning of a synthetic process and turnover rather than the increased biogenesis you describe.

Piantadosi: These are non-lethal models. When we go to lethal models these processes do fail. It is a question of timing.

Singer: We touched on the issue of PARP earlier. You are suggesting that the mitochondrial DNA damage triggers biogenesis. Therefore, if you block PARP too early, would you potentially be delaying the process? Or do you think there is a timing issue?

Piantadosi: Timing is everything, in terms of interfering with repair processes. When you block PARP you are still left with DNA strand breaks.

Szabó: The story of DNA breaks and PARP is a complex one. The short answer is that if the cell survives, then the DNA breaks will eventually be repaired somehow. By blocking PARP you don't generally make the DNA breaks even more pronounced. It isn't PARP that is inducing the DNA breaks but it is the actual oxidative damage. As far as mitochondria and PARP are concerned, it is a mess. There are only a handful of papers suggesting even the presence of PARP in the mitochondria. We have seen poly ADP ribosylation of certain proteins in the mitochondria. It is well known that PARP is not part of the mitochondrial genome, so if it is there, it is coming from the nucleus. No one has a clue whether eukaryotic PARP is attached to the mitochondrial DNA, and if it is, what it is doing there. But we and others have certainly seen poly ADP ribosylation in isolated mitochondrial systems.

Piantadosi: There is endonuclease activity in mitochondria. The way mitochondria repair is different from nuclear repair. MtDNA is a small genome and the mitochondrion doesn't waste a lot of time trying to fix things. It destroys the badly damaged copies and replicates the good copies.

Singer: A question to you and Greet Van den Berghe: do you think the insulin story could also be regenerating through AKT?

Piantodosi: I think both things are true. If you stress the mitochondrion with glucose when it is damaged, there will be more reactive oxygen species (ROS) production. Hydrogen peroxide directly from the mitochondrion will activate AKT. What Greet says about glucose toxicity is right, but AKT is also an important pro-survival factor.

Van den Berghe: Both things could explain what we have seen, namely the difference between the muscle and the liver. The muscle is responsive to insulin and we have found AKT signals in the muscle biopsies. Perhaps that is the reason why the muscle is able to repair. The mitochondria don't look normal but they may be regenerated, and the liver can't regenerate because it is insulin resistant and there is no AKT signal there.

Piantadosi: Something is turning off the AKT in the liver. It may be related to insulin. You would think oxidant production would become high enough at some point to re-activate AKT in the liver. It does in the mouse. But humans may be different. There may be better ROS scavenging in the human liver. There are many reasons why that pathway might not be fully activated.

Ayala: I was interested in the Toll-like receptor 4 (TLR4) story and the nitric oxide (NO) story. These are two examples where if you really set down a true infection they don't work so well (TLR4$^{-/-}$ and iNOS$^{-/-}$ mice survive endotoxin challenge quite well, but do much poorer in models of polymicrobial sepsis/infection). This is also supported indirectly by the work with IRAK4-deficient humans. It is the NF-κB/TLR4 story. While these patients are very young they are highly susceptible to infection. Could you propose other mechanisms other than simply TLR4, that might drive this injury system?

Piantadosi: This is just one. You could look for stimulation of other Toll pathways. We chose TLR4 knockout mice because although they were reported to be endotoxin resistant, if you put them in sepsis and look long term, they get organ damage. They are endotoxin shock resistant but they are not damage resistant. We have found that NF-κB is needed for full expression of the mitochondrial recovery. Moreover, you have the possibility for several transcriptional activators to interact in order to get the full expression of biogenesis gene expression. When stress is high, multiple activators may be needed for full expression of genes for mitochondrial repair.

Cavaillon: I would be interested to know more about the status of mitochondria within the circulating leukocytes of septic patients. Depending on the answer, I would like to comment on the concept of sick cells.

Singer: Didier Payen has looked at monocytes. Essentially, the oxygen consumption is higher in the septic monocyte compared to a resting one. This seems to be related to the respiratory burst. When you stimulate them extrinsically with PMA, they cannot respond like a normal cell. The burst goes up a bit and the mitochondrial respiration changes only a tiny amount. In contrast, a normal healthy monocyte can double or treble the amount. It seems that they are working to capacity, but you can't push them to do anything more.

Piantadosi: The lymphocytes are susceptible to glutathione depletion, which has a big effect on the mitochondrial genome. Loss of mtDNA depresses oxidative phosphorylation and shortens the life of the lymphocyte. And if you give FAS ligand they are also more sensitive to receptor-mediated apoptosis.

Singer: Again, Didier has shown that if you give an IL10 antagonist you can restore the septic monocyte to normal.

Cavaillon: The lymphocyte experiments you mentioned were performed *in vitro*. This was not lymphocytes from patients. My comment about the sick cell is the following: the leukocytes are not sick, they are reprogrammed (Cavaillon et al 2005). They stop making some proteins, like tumour necrosis factor (TNF), but they continue to make other proteins such as IL1 and IL1Rα, of which the productions are never depressed.

Piantadosi: The lymphocytes stay well only as long as they have energy.

Fink: What is the stimulus for mitochondrial biogenesis in trained athletes?

Piantadosi: It depends on who you read. Oxidative stress might be involved.

Fink: Exercising muscle releases a lot of IL6, and I wondered whether this is involved in that signalling.

Griffiths: There is mechanical transduction in muscle.

Fink: If you want to confuse yourself hopelessly, read the IL6 literature for about two hours. There are data to suggest that exogenous IL6 is quite protective in sepsis models.

Piantadosi: I haven't looked: that is a great idea.

Griffiths: Are all mitochondria created equal?

Piantadosi: No.

Griffiths: Does this have implications for how they might be sacrificed?

Piantadosi: I think we are in the infancy of understanding mitochondrial adaptation. If you look at things that go up and down after cell stress, mitochondrial responses differ depending on the stimulus. But you have to give the cell a chance to make new mitochondria and pull them out at the right time to find the differences. These are regulated processes, for example, succinate is a signal for HIF-1 even when there is plenty of oxygen around.

Singer: Just as we were talking about the effects of animals or cells at different ages, mitochondria have different ages. The turnover is thought to be days, but no one knows for sure. The older mitochondria act differently in terms of ROS production. The heterogeneity of what you and we have shown means that not all mitochondria are equally affected.

Radermacher: When you do your experiments at different PO_2s, does this make a difference in terms of biogenesis?

Piantadosi: That's a good question. We have looked across a PO_2 continuum, and both extremes lead to new mitochondria. I think they are different mitochondria in each case: in hyperoxia there is a lot of MnSOD, and in hypoxia there is little change.

Griffiths: The complexity of the whole organ system is striking. I have always been puzzled by why different cells choose different options as to how they survive. I remember experiments years ago when we were looking at apoptosis in muscle. It was pretty easy to use ROS to make them go apoptotic as myocytes, but once they are in a big structure this isn't a signal they want to bother with.

Fink: This raises a point: there is an area of cell biology in our field that is untapped. Almost all of us doing this kind of work are looking at cells as isolated entities, yet in an organ such as the liver they work together. There is a lot of cell–cell communication. The organ only functions properly when all the guys are pulling their oars simultaneously.

Piantadosi: There is an example of this which we are working on. If you feed respiration deficient cells pyruvate and uridine, they survive. They up-regulate membrane oxidases and ROS production. Those ROS activate AKT and the pro-survival pathway in these and neighbouring cells.

Reference

Cavaillon JM, Adrie C, Fitting C, Adib-Conquy M 2005 Reprogramming of circulatory cells in sepsis and SIRS. J Endotoxin Res 11:311–320

Contributor index

Non-participating co-authors are indicated by asterisks. Entries in bold indicate papers; other entries refer to discussion contributions.

Subject index